CARDIAC DEVELOPMENT

PROGRESS IN EXPERIMENTAL CARDIOLOGY

Edited by Naranjan S. Dhalla, Ph.D., M.D. (Hon.), D.Sc. (Hon.)

1. S. Mochizuki, N. Takeda, M. Nagano, N.S. Dhalla (eds.): *The Ischemic Heart*. 1998.
   ISBN 0-7923-8105-X

2. N.S. Dhalla, P. Zahradka, I. Dixon, R. Beamish (eds.): *Angiotension II Receptor Blockade: Physiological and Clinical Implications*. 1998.
   ISBN 0-7923-8147-5

3. N. Takeda, M. Nagano, N.S. Dhalla (eds.): *The Hypertrophied Heart*. 2000.
   ISBN 0-7923-7714-9

4. B. Ostadal, M. Nagano, N.S. Dhalla (eds.): *Cardiac Development*. 2002.
   ISBN 1-4020-7052-7

CARDIAC DEVELOPMENT

Editors
BOHUSLAV OSTADAL, M.D., D.Sc.
Professor
Institute of Physiology
Academy of Sciences of the Czech Republic
Prague, Czech Republic

MAKOTO NAGANO, M.D., Ph.D.
Professor Emeritus
Jikei University School of Medicine
Tokyo, Japan

NARANJAN S. DHALLA, Ph.D., M.D. (Hon.), D.Sc. (Hon.)
Distinguished Professor and Director
Institute of Cardiovascular Sciences
St. Boniface General Hospital Research Centre
Faculty of Medicine, University of Manitoba
Winnipeg, Canada

KLUWER ACADEMIC PUBLISHERS
BOSTON

Distributors for North, Central and South America:
Kluwer Academic Publishers
101 Philip Drive
Assinippi Park
Norwell, Massachusetts 02061 USA
Telephone (781) 871-6600
Fax (781) 681-9045
E-Mail: kluwer@wkap.com

Distributors for all other countries:
Kluwer Academic Publishers Group
Post Office Box 322
3300 AH Dordrecht, THE NETHERLANDS
Telephone 31 786 576 000
Fax 31 786 576 474
E-Mail: services@wkap.nl

 Electronic Services <http://www.wkap.nl>

Library of Congress Cataloging-in-Publication Data

Cardiac development / editors, Bohuslav Ostadal, Makoto Nagano, Naranjan S. Dhalla.
    p. cm.— (Progress in experimental cardiology; 4)
    Includes bibliographical references and index.
    ISBN 1-40207-052-7 (alk. paper)
    1. Heart—Growth. I. Ostádal, Bohuslav. II. Nagano, Makoto, 1928– III. Dhalla, Naranjan S.
IV. Series.
QP111.4.C367 2002

612.1'7—dc21   2002016267

CONTENTS

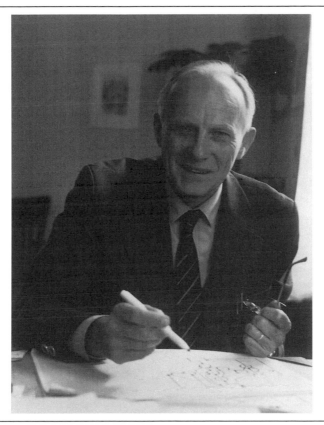

Dr. Pavel Braveny

This book is dedicated to Pavel Braveny to mark his distinguished achievements in the field of cardiovascular research and education.

PREFACE: A TRIBUTE TO PAVEL BRAVENY ON HIS 70th BIRTHDAY

The career of professor Pavel Bravený, M.D., PhD. is typically for the Central European space bound to a single location. Brno (celebrated through J.G. Mendel) was his birthplace in 1931, here he studied, rooted at the Masaryk University, raised his family and lived to see his grandchildren. Nevertheless, it has not been an idle, boring career without any satisfaction on one hand and baffling defeats on the other.

In 1951, at the very onset of his university studies, P. Bravený happened to appear in the Department of Physiology, where professor Vladislav Kruta, experimenttal cardiologist, just became the head. He chose P. Bravený his assistant two years later. However, P. Bravený due to unconcealed criticism was in an almost permanent conflict with the communist regime which did not tolerate anything except devotion. Thus, after graduation (1956) he was sent to a district hospital and his scientific career seemed to be over. But Kruta did not give up and managed to bring him back to his Department after a year as his closest coworker. The following period (1957–1970) was the most prolific era of the Kruta—Braveny tandem. In 1958 they introduced the concept of restitution of cardiac contractility into the analysis of interval-strength relationship and explained its diverse and seemingly incompatible manifestations by a single principle (later identified with the calcium handling of the heart muscle cell). P. Bravený showed already in 1962 that pulsus alternans is generated at the cellular level. He studied the mechanisms of aftercontractions, the inotropic effects of low temperature, strontium ions and arrived at the electro-mechanical relations. The political climate partly eased and thus, P. Bravený was allowed to work with professor F.L. Meijler in Amsterdam and with J.R. Blinks in Boston for a few months.

These thriving research activity of P. Bravený was halted by the political consequences of 1968 invasion of Czechoslovakia. Kruta was dismissed and so was his nearest ally. Their electrophysiological lab was gradually dismantled. PB was forced to accept a subordinate position of a clinical physiologist at the local Faculty Hospital. Although he profited in broadening his scope, the former productive work with his coworkers Sumbera and Simurda oriented to basic problems quantitatively dwindled. Even under these difficult conditions they were able—among others—to describe and later to explain the Na^+/Ca^{++} exchange current. However, the international contacts were almost completely interrupted and the future was all but promising. To compensate for this precarious situation, P. Bravený together with B. Ostadal founded the Czechoslovak Experimental Cardiology Study Group in 1972 which he presided for the next 25 years. It proved to be a wonderful satisfaction.

In 1982, as chance would have it again, an opportunity appeared to join the Department of Physiology at Kuwait University. P. Braveny spend four years there, teaching, doing some research, recovering former international contacts. Coming back home, he faced the same gloomy, motionless disfavor as before.

November 1989 turned P. Braveny's career upside down. Immediately after the fall of the communist regime, he was elected vice-dean and later dean of the Faculty of Medicine, promoted full professor in physiology and appointed the head of the Department of Physiology. From 1992 to 1998 P. Braveny served as the vice-rector of Masaryk University. His professional career culminated in his presidency of the XIV World Congress of ISHR in Prague. Understandably, in the following years, he become interested (in his tutor's footsteps) in history of physiology and published two monoghaphs (E. Babak and V. Kruta). This CV would be an incomplete one without mentioning his broad interests in natural sciences and in art, particularly music and painting. As a tutored amateur he has acquired certain success in the latter.

When reviewing P. Braveny's whole-life work, largely done under adverse circumstances with minimum financial support, his almost two hundred papers, innumerable essays and four monographs are a commensurate result. In appreciation, he was awarded honorary membership of the Czech Medical Society, Physiological Society and Cardiological Society, Gold Medal of Masaryk University, Ministry of Education Award etc.

Bohuslav Ostadal	Makoto Nagano	Naranjan S. Dhalla
Prague, Czech Republic	Tokyo, Japan	Winnipeg, Canada

CARDIAC DEVELOPMENT

B. Ostadal, M. Nagano and N.S. Dhalla (eds.).
CARDIAC DEVELOPMENT. Copyright © 2002.
Kluwer Academic Publishers. Boston.
All rights reserved.

COMPARATIVE GENETICS OF HEART DEVELOPMENT: CONSERVED CARDIOGENIC FACTORS IN *DROSOPHILA* AND VERTEBRATES

KATHLEEN GAJEWSKI* and ROBERT A. SCHULZ

Department of Biochemistry and Molecular Biology, Graduate Program in Genes & Development, The University of Texas M.D. Anderson Cancer Center, 1515 Holcombe Boulevard, Houston TX 77030, USA

Summary. Despite differences in structure and complexity, the hearts of *Drosophila* and vertebrates share important developmental characteristics. Five different transcription factors that play vital roles in the formation of the fly heart have also been shown to be necessary for the early steps in vertebrate cardiogenesis. Despite the divergence between the two groups, there is a high degree of functional conservation of these factors, which has made information gained in *Drosophila* relevant to the investigation of heart cell specification and tube formation in vertebrates. Additionally, the mechanisms that generate the diversity of cell types in the *Drosophila* heart may also be conserved in the later steps of vertebrate heart development.

Key words: Tinman/NKx2.5, Pannier/GATA, U-shaped/FOG, Mef2, Seven-up/COUP TF

INTRODUCTION

At first glance, the hearts of *Drosophila* and vertebrates could not look more dissimilar. The fly heart, or dorsal vessel, is a simple structure comprising a few different cell types. The actual heart tube is formed of a monolayer of cardial cells with both endothelial and myocardial characteristics. Flanking the cardial cells are several rows of nonmuscle pericardial cells. Their function is less clear, although membrane structures that resemble those of nephrocytes suggest that they have a role in the

* Correspondence to: Kathleen Gajewski, Department of Biochemistry and Molecular Biology-Box 117, The University of Texas M.D. Anderson Cancer Center, 1515 Holcombe Boulevard, Houston TX 77030, USA (Tel: 713-792-3729; Fax: 713-792-0329; e-mail: *kgajewski@odin.mdacc.tmc.edu*)

filtration of the hemolymph [1]. The heart is attached to the dorsal epidermis by segmentally repeated alary muscles. The *Drosophila* hemolymph is not contained within blood vessels; it circulates freely throughout the body, propelled by the peristaltic motions of the dorsal vessel. The lumen of the dorsal vessel is wider in the portion that spans the three posterior-most segments; this section is referred to as "the heart", while the anterior region encompassing four segments with the narrower lumen is termed "the aorta". In the heart portion of the dorsal vessel, there are three segmentally spaced pairs of specialized valves, called "ostia", that allow flow of the hemolymph into the sides of the dorsal vessel [2,3].

In contrast, a vertebrate heart is much more complex. The cardiac precursors separate into endothelial and myocardial populations. The endothelial cells will form a plexus of preendothelial tubes, which will combine to form a single endocardial heart tube. The heart tube is subsequently surrounded by myocardial and connective tissue layers [4]. A vertebrate heart is divided into multiple chambers separated by more complex valves and linked to an elaborate closed circulatory system.

Despite these differences, there are a number of similarities in the development of fly and vertebrate hearts. For example, fly heart cells arise from two regions of dorsal-most mesoderm; vertebrate heart precursors are formed from two regions of anterolateral plate mesoderm. In both cases, the two groups of heart cells migrate together to form a heart tube. The migration is to the dorsal surface in flies and in a ventral direction in vertebrates. Inductive signals from other tissues are vital for proper development of the heart; these signals originate from the overlying dorsal ectoderm in *Drosophila* embryos, while in developing vertebrate hearts they are received from the endoderm. Once the two rows of cardiac cells have aligned at the dorsal region of the fly embryo, the leading edges of the cardioblasts on each side come into contact. The cardioblasts then change shape, with the trailing edges curling forward to form a lumen [5]. This process resembles the formation of the preendothelial tubes of vertebrates, as well as that of the vertebrate capillary [6,7].

However, the similarities in the development of fly and vertebrate hearts are more striking in the conservation of genes involved in development. For example, transcription factors and signaling molecules that play a role in the specification of heart cells in the fly have been found in several vertebrate systems. However, often there are multiple versions of a given type of gene acting in vertebrate heart formation; such redundancy can complicate genetic analysis. In contrast, fruit flies often have a single version of a related gene playing a similar role.

Many important developmental genes have been discovered and characterized in *Drosophila*, and the information gained has then been applied to the study of analogous processes in more complex organisms. This review concentrates on five transcription factors- Tinman/Nkx, Pannier/GATA, U-shaped/FOG2, Mef2, and Seven-up/COUP TF- that play important roles in heart development and have been extensively studied in *Drosophila* and several species of vertebrates. The effects of perturbation of these factors on heart development are summarized in Tables 1 and 2.

Table 1. Effects of perturbation of early heart-expressed transcription factors

Gene	Alteration/mutation	Heart phenotype	Refereneces
Drosophila tinman	Null mutation	Heart cells absent	10, 11
Mouse Nkx2.5	Ectopic expression (whole embryo)	Temporary increase in *eve*-PCs	12
	Knockout	No looping of heart tube	39
Xenopus Nkx2.3, 2.5	Co-injection of dominant negative transcripts	Absence of heart	44, 45
	Ectopic expression	Enlarged heart	42, 43
Drosophila pannier	Null mutation	Loss of cardial cells, increase in *eve*-PCs	18
	Ectopic expression-mesoderm	Gain of cardial cells, loss of *eve*-PCs	18
Mouse GATA4	Knockout	Cardia bifida	75, 76
Mouse GATA5	Knockout	None, viable	76
Mouse GATA6	Knockout	Early death before heart development	78, 79
Chick GATA4, 5, 6	Antisense inhibition of all three transcripts	Heart tube fusion defects, cardia bifida	74
Xenopus GATA4	Dominant negative	Expansion of Nkx2.5 expression pattern	82
Drosophila u-shaped	Hypomorphic mutation, deletion	Gain of cardial cells, gain of *eve*-PCs, mesodermal migration defect-sporadic loss of heart cells	51
Mouse FOG2	Ectopic expression (mesoderm)	Loss of cardial cells	61
	Knockout	Thinning of the ventricular myocardium, valve defects, septal defects	94, 95

(*eve*-PCs = *eve*-expressing pericardial cells).

Table 2. Effects of perturbation of late heart-expressed transcription factors

Gene	Alteration/mutation	Heart phenotype	Refereneces
D-mef2	Hypomorphic mutation	Heart tube forms, but does not express myosin	99, 100 104
Mouse mef2B	Knockout	None, viable	109
Mouse mef2C	Knockout	No heart looping, absence of right ventricle, disruptions of vascular system	113, 114
Drosophila svp	Null mutation	Tinman expression expanded from 4 to 6 cardial cell pairs per segment	106
	Ectopic expression in tin -cardial cells	Severe reduction/loss of tin protein	106
Mouse COUP TFII	Knockout	Hemorrhaging around heart, underdevelopment of atrial chamber and sinus venosus, defective angiogenesis	151

Tinman

The first four members of the NK family of homeobox genes were identified during a screen of a *Drosophila* genomic library for homeotic genes with degenerate homeodomain probes [8]. Subsequent screens in other species have uncovered numerous other homologous genes. The proteins encoded by these genes act as transcriptional activators and are required for the proper development of many different tissues. All members of this family share a common protein motif of a homeodomain with an invariant tyrosine at position 54 of the homeodomain sequence. The majority of the genes in this group also have a 12-amino acid TN domain at the N-terminus and an NK2-SD domain just C-terminal to the homeodomain. One of the founding members of this family, the *Drosophila* gene *tinman* (*tin*), plays a major role in the development of the heart and other dorsal mesodermal derivatives. It is unique among genes that encode NK proteins in that it possesses a TN domain but lacks an NK2-SD domain [9].

Mutations of *tin* cause the absence of tissues derived from dorsal mesoderm. For example, embryos homozygous for *tin* null mutations lack heart, visceral muscle, and a number of dorsal somatic muscles [10,11]. In addition, the ectopic expression of *tin* causes a temporary increase in the numbers of *even-skipped* (*eve*)-expressing pericardial cells in the germ band-extended stages of from three to four cells to eight to ten cells per cluster, but the numbers of these cells return to normal in the later stages. No abnormalities are observed in the late-stage hearts of these embryos. Therefore, although *tin* is required for the formation of the *Drosophila* heart, it alone cannot specify a cardiac fate [12].

There are three distinct phases of *tin* expression in the *Drosophila* embryo. In the early stages, *tin* is found throughout the mesoderm. The enhancer element controlling early expression is located within the first intron of the *tin* gene, and Twist protein is required for this phase of expression [13]. Around stage 10, *tin* expression becomes restricted to the dorsal mesoderm. This changeover in the expression pattern is dependent on the Dpp signaling supplied by the overlying dorsal ectoderm. A Dpp-response region, located 3′ to the gene, has been characterized. It contains four important sequence elements; these include two identical *tin* binding sites, a site recognized by both *Mothers against Dpp* (*Mad*) and *Medea*, which are essential components of the Dpp signaling pathway, and a site that also binds *Mad*. Mutation of the *tin* sites in the region results in reporter gene expression in the dorsal ectoderm, suggesting the presence of a repressor in the ectoderm and *tin* autoregulation in the mesoderm [14]. It is during this restriction of *tin* to the dorsal mesoderm that the heart precursors are specified. Wingless signaling is also required for specification of these cells at this time, although its exact role remains to be determined [15]. During dorsal closure, the *tin* pattern is again reduced to expression in the pericardial cells and to four pairs of cardial cells per segment. The heart-specific element required for this phase also lies 3′ to the *tin* gene [13]. Dissection of this region has defined separate cardial and pericardial control elements. A pair of CREB consensus binding sites is needed for the late myocardial expression of tin [16].

So far, three downstream targets of *tin* in the *Drosophila* heart are known: *D-mef2*, the GATA factor *pannier* (*pnr*), and *β3-tubulin* [17–19]. A *tin*-dependent enhancer has been discovered upstream of *D-mef2*. The region contains two consensus *tin* binding sites (CTCAAGTGG) that are essential for enhancer function. Embryos carrying a 237-bp reporter construct that contains both sites initially express β-galactosidase at stage 11 in the newly formed heart precursors. In the later stages, expression in the cardial cells occurs in the four-pairs-per-segment pattern identical to that of *tin*. Unlike *tin*, however, there is no enhancer expression in the pericardial cells. Ectopic expression of *tin* via an *hs-tin* construct [11] causes expansion of β-galactosidase expression driven by this enhancer element, but not uniformly throughout the embryo [17]. The pattern is expanded into the dorsal mesoderm and procephalic regions but is significantly absent in the ventral region of the embryo. While the two *tin* sites are necessary for *D-mef2* enhancer expression in the cardial cells, they are not sufficient to cause its expression. A GATA consensus sequence near the second *tin* site is also required. Mutation of that site abolishes reporter expression in the cardial cells and causes *de novo* expression in the pericardial cells [20].

A pair of *tin* binding sites has also been found within a 457-bp region immediately upstream of the *pnr* gene. The protein encoded by *pnr* is a zinc finger protein of the GATA family of transcription factors and is described in more detail below. Reporter constructs carrying this *pnr* enhancer region show expression in the dorsal mesoderm and the amnioserosa [18]. Mutation of either *tin* site abolishes mesodermal expression, as does crossing the construct into a *tin* mutant background. When a *UAS-tin* construct is ectopically expressed via a *twi-GAL4* driver [21], the reporter gene is expressed throughout the mesoderm and along the ventral midline [22].

β3-tubulin is the first structural gene to be confirmed as a direct target of *tin*. *β3-tubulin* transcripts and protein are expressed in the cardial cells in a four pairs on/two pairs off-per-segment pattern in the late embryonic heart, reminiscent of the *tin* cardial cell pattern [19]. Three *tin* binding sites have been found in a 320-bp region upstream of the *β3-tubulin* gene. DNA footprinting and gel retardation assays have shown that the 5′-most site has a strong affinity for Tin protein and the middle site a weaker but significant affinity; however, interaction with the 3′-most site is barely detectable. A 333-bp reporter construct, which includes the strong-and moderate-affinity *tin* sites, is sufficient to drive reporter expression in four of six cardial cell pairs in the abdominal regions, but staining is absent in the thoracic region of the heart. Mutation of the strong-affinity *tin* site abolishes expression, but when the moderate-affinity site is altered, a weak heart expression pattern is observed. Therefore, unlike the *tin* sites in the *D-mef2* and *pnr* enhancers, the two *β3-tubulin* sites are not equivalent [19].

Vertebrate *tin* homologs

Searches for *tin* homologs in vertebrates have revealed related genes in zebrafish, *Xenopus*, chicken, mouse, and human. The first heart-expressed vertebrate NK genes identified, Nkx2.5 and 2.6, were isolated in a screen of an adult mouse heart cDNA library with oligonucleotides from the *tin* homeobox [23]. Seven different vertebrate *tin* homologs, Nkx 2.3, 2.5, 2.6, 2.7, 2.8, 2.9, and 2.10, are currently known [24–36]. The majority of these genes are expressed in the mesodermal region that will form heart and visceral muscle and in the endodermal tissues of the pharynx. Many members of this family are also expressed in a wider variety of embryonic tissues, such as the muscle of the tongue, the ectodermal and mesenchymal tissues of the pharynx, and the gut endoderm. All species so far examined express Nkx 2.5 in the cardiogenic lineage [9], and this gene shows the greatest conservation across different species. Expression of Nkx2.5 can first be detected at stage 5 in chick and 7.5 days postcoitum (dpc) in mouse, making it one of the earliest markers of heart commitment identified so far [23,27]. Mutations in the human homolog of Nkx2.5, Csx, have been linked to congenital heart defects [37].

Although vertebrate Nkx2.5 has the greatest functional and sequence similarity with *Drosophila tin*, the two proteins do not show a complete conservation of developmental function. For example, a chimeric construct of *tin* that has its homeodomain replaced with that of mouse Nkx2.5 can rescue heart development in *tin* mutant *Drosophila* embryos. However, although the entire Nkx2.5 protein inhibits fly cardiogenesis, it can only partially rescue formation of the visceral mesoderm. As the two proteins are considerably divergent outside the conserved TN and homeodomains, mouse Nkx2.5 can recognize *Drosophila tin* binding sites but lacks the ability to properly interact with *tin* cofactors [38].

Unlike mutations in *tin*, loss of Nkx2.5 function in mice does not eliminate the formation of heart. For example, in Nkx2.5 knockout mice, which die around 9.5 dpc, the heart tube forms but does not initiate looping. Except for a ventricle-specific myosin light chain (MLC2V), contractile proteins are produced [39]. Later in development, there is no production of eHAND (a bHLH protein) or CARP (an ankyrin repeat protein) in the Nkx2.5 null heart [40,41]. It is possible that the expression of multiple members of the Nkx family genes in the heart results in a redundancy of function. Recent experiments in *Xenopus* embryos support this theory. For example, two *tin* homologs, XNkx2.3 and 2.5 were found to be expressed in the developing *Xenopus* heart. Ectopic expression of either gene in the embryo resulted in an enlarged heart phenotype [42,43]. When dominant negative constructs for both genes were injected into *Xenopus* embryos, a synergistic effect was observed, and in the most extremely affected embryos, the heart failed to form. Conversely, the coinjection of either wildtype gene substantially reduced the severity of the mutant phenotypes [44,45].

Cardiac enhancer elements have been found upstream of the mouse *Nkx2.5* gene. A 505-bp region contains multiple GATA, NKE, bHLH, HMG, and HOX consensus binding sites. Transgenic mice carrying a reporter construct that includes this region showed early expression in anterior portions of the early heart, the spleen primordium, and pharyngeal region [46]. Gel shift assays showed that paired GATA sites in this element were recognized by GATA4. This protein is a transcription factor with two zinc finger regions and is encoded by a member of another family of genes that play an important role in the heart development of multiple species (see below). Mutation of the GATA sites abolished reporter activity in the heart, pharynx, and spleen [46].

Nkx2.5 is a direct activator of several cardiac genes. The first *Nkx2.5* responsive enhancer element identified was found in the proximal region of the cardiac atrial natriuretic factor (ANF) promoter [47]. In a co-transfection assay, the Nkx2.5 and GATA4 proteins synergistically activated the ANF promoter [48,49]. This interaction was specific for GATA4 and 5; the related genes *GATA1* and *GATA6* cannot act synergistically with *Nkx2.5* [48]. Combinatorial interactions between *Nkx2.5* and *GATA4* or *Nkx2.5* and serum response factor can activate transcription of the cardiac alpha–actin (α-CA) promoter [50]. The C-terminal zinc finger of GATA4 is critical for this interaction with *Nkx2.5*. It has been proposed that *GATA4* binds a repressor domain located in the C-terminal region of *Nkx2.5*, causing a conformational change that uncovers activation domains [48,50]. An upstream enhancer element for mouse *GATA6* has recently been characterized and a binding site for *Nkx2.5* is essential for heart expression of the gene [51]. In *Nkx2.5* mutant hearts, there are alterations in the heart expression patterns of genes such as brain natriuretic peptide (*BNP*), *CARP*, *eHAND*, *Irx4*, *MEF2C*, *Msx2*, *MLC2V*, and *N-myc* [39–41,52]. It remains to be determined whether these genes are affected directly or indirectly by *Nkx2.5*.

Pannier

Members of the GATA family of transcription factors play important roles in many developmental processes. These zinc finger proteins recognize a WGATAR consensus sequence, although there is considerable deviation in the sequences these factors will bind [53]. There are three GATA genes that have been uncovered in *Drosophila*: *pannier* (*pnr*), *serpent* (*srp*), and *dGATAc* or *grain* (*grn*). Mutations in these genes were isolated on the third chromosome by an Ethyl Methanesulfonate (EMS) mutagenesis screen [54]. The functions of *pnr* in the formation of dorsal ectoderm in the embryo and sensory bristles in the adult fruit fly have been well characterized [55–57]. The *srp* locus plays a role in hematopoicsis, gut formation, and fat body development

[58]. *grn* is required for development of the terminal structure of the embryo. It is also expressed in the gut and central nervous system in the midembryonic stages [59]. All three proteins have two conserved zinc-finger motifs but are highly divergent from one another outside this region. Additionally, *pnr* has a feature unique among the GATA family of proteins: two putative amphipathic alpha helices at the C-terminal end. This region of the protein has been postulated to act as a transcriptional activation domain [60].

Cross-sections of embryos stained with a *pnr* cRNA probe revealed a previously unknown domain of *pnr* expression in the dorsal-most mesoderm. This mesodermal expression of *pnr* is first detected at stage 11, the time when heart precursors are specified. In *pnr* mutants, cardiac cells are absent, and there is an expansion in the numbers of *eve*-expressing pericardial cells [18]. Ectopic expression of *pnr* using the *twistGAL4* driver resulted in the formation of many additional heart cells in the embryo. Since there are simultaneous reductions in cells from the visceral muscle and pericardial cell populations, it is most likely that these groups of cells, which also express *tin* in the mid stages, are recruited to form the ectopic cardial cells. Against this background of ectopic *pnr*, expression of the 237 bp *D-mef2* heart enhancer is expanded, but only in the dorsal mesoderm. When *tin* and *pnr* are both ectopically expressed via the *twistGAL4* driver, they can activate expression of the cardial specific enhancer throughout the mesoderm, as well as in the mesectodermal cells, which are normally fated to form the ventral midline. Therefore the actions of these two genes are sufficient to specify a cardiac fate. Since ectopically expressed *srp* cannot induce the formation of additional heart cells, the cardiogenic activity is specific to *pnr*, not a general function of GATA factors in flies [18].

Similar to results seen in vertebrates, *pnr* and *tin* physically interact and can act together to activate *D-mef2* in the cardiac cells. When co-transfected into mammalian CV-1 cells, both localize to the nucleus and can be co-immunoprecipitated [22]. In an *in vitro* assay with a *CAT* reporter gene linked to the *D-mef2* heart enhancer, *tin* and *pnr* act synergistically to activate reporter gene expression [61]. Since the combined action of *tin* and *pnr* is sufficient to specify cardiac cells, it is likely that they act together to activate other important heart genes.

At least two regions of the Pnr protein are required for its cardiogenic function. Mutations that disrupt the C-terminal zinc finger fail to act synergistically with *tin* in activating the *D-mef2* heart enhancer element; however, mutations in the N-terminal zinc finger have no effect. Deletion of the last 83 amino acids, which removes the helical regions, also abolishes cardiogenic activity. The homeodomain region of *tin* is required for its interaction with *pnr* and the resultant cardiogenic activity. A second domain, spanning amino acids 111–152, is also needed to specify heart cells [22].

Vertebrate GATA factors

GATA1, the first vertebrate GATA protein to be described, was isolated as an activator of globin genes [62]. Along with the related genes *GATA2* and *GATA3*, it plays a role in hematopoiesis [63–67]. A second subfamily of GATA factors, 4, 5, and 6, are expressed in unique but overlapping patterns in developing heart, gut, and gonad. GATA4 is expressed in the cardiogenic crescents of early mouse, chick, and frog embryos in a pattern reminiscent of that of Nkx2.5 [68–70]. In the later stages, GATA4 transcripts can be found in both the myocardial and endocardial layers of the heart [68]. Early expression of GATA5 and GATA6 is broader than that of GATA4, and occurs in a ventral area that encompasses the heart-forming region [69,70]. While these two factors are initially produced in both myocardial and endocardial cells, GATA5 is eventually limited to the endocardium and GATA6 to the myocardium of the late embryonic and postnatal heart [70–73]. While the GATA4, 5, and 6 proteins are divergent outside the zinc-finger domains, there is a high degree of conservation seen for each type of GATA factor between species. This conservation and the differences seen in their expression patterns suggest unique roles for each factor, but functional overlap has been observed. In studies of chick embryos, in which antisense oligonucleotides were used to selectively deplete GATA factors in the heart, interference with the transcripts of one or two of the three factors had no effect on development. Only when all three GATAs were targeted were heart phenotypes manifested. In the least severe cases, the embryos formed a single large heart tube that failed to loop. An intermediate phenotype was also observed, in which two heart tubes fused in the ventral midline. In the most severe cases, two bilateral beating and looping heart tubes (cardia bifida) were observed [74]. The cardia bifida phenotype is also seen in mouse GATA4 null embryos. The mutation causes death of the embryos between stages E9.5 and E10.5. Levels of GATA6 are up-regulated in these mutants, which could indicate that GATA6 can partially compensate for the loss of GATA4, but expression of other cardiac genes such as MLC2A, MLC2V, Nkx2.5, eHAND, and dHAND were unaffected [75,76]. However, GATA4-/- stem cells can form myocytes in the hearts of chimeric embryos [77]. GATA5 knockout mice are viable and exhibit no heart defects [76]. GATA6 null mice die early in development, due to defects in extra-embryonic tissues, before a heart phenotype can be observed [78,79]. Zebrafish GATA5 mutants exhibit a range of heart tube defects, including cardia bifida, and expression of Nkx2.5 is diminished [80]. These results suggest that GATA factors in vertebrates are necessary for proper heart tube formation, but are not needed for the differentiation of cardiac cells.

GATA factors are involved in the transcriptional activation of many important cardiac genes. As described in other sections of this review, GATA factors can synergize with Nkx2.5 and MEF2. NFAT3 also can associate with the C-terminal zinc finger of GATA4 to cooperatively activate the BNP promoter. This interaction may have an important bearing on the development of cardiac hypertrophy [81]. GATA factors can also exhibit inhibitory effects. Overexpression of GATA6 in Xenopus embryos prevents the expression of late genes that encode such proteins as cardiac actin and heart-specific myosin light chain. In wildtype embryos, the levels of GATA6 in the heart decrease prior to terminal differentiation, suggesting that GATA6 plays a role in maintaining a proliferative state [73]. A dominant negative form of GATA4, which inhibits transcription of GATA target genes when injected into Xenopus embryos, also causes an expansion of the Nkx2.5 transcript pattern, suggesting that one or more GATA targets negatively regulate Nkx2.5 [82]. Therefore, GATA factors can either activate or repress expression of Nkx2.5, depending on the cellular context. The GATA4 cofactor FOG2 (described below) is known to modulate GATA4 activity and may play a crucial role in defining the boundaries of Nkx2.5 expression.

Mouse GATA4 is 85% identical to the Drosophila factor pnr within the zinc-finger region, and the two proteins show a degree of functional conservation. Ectopic expression of a GATA4 construct in the mesoderm of the Drosophila embryo can induce the formation of additional cardial cells, although not to the same extent as pnr. This effect is specific for GATA4; similar expression of a GATA1 gene does not result in the production of ectopic cardial cells, despite the fact that the two proteins encoded share a 76% identity in the zinc finger region [18]. On the basis of amino acid and functional similarities, mouse GATA4 and pnr should be considered homologs, as should srp and mouse GATA1.

U-shaped

The first alleles of u-shaped (ush) were uncovered in a mutagenesis screen of the second chromosome [82]. Mutations in ush enhance the gain of bristle phenotype seen in flies heterozygous for dominant pnr alleles (pnr^D) [84]. All mutants of the pnr^D class have lesions in the N-terminal zinc finger [54,56]. The addition of Ush protein can inhibit transcriptional activation by both Pnr and chicken GATA1, but it has only a minimal effect on activation by Pnr^D mutant proteins. In two-hybrid binding assays, Ush interacts with wildtype Pnr, as well as with Pnr proteins with mutations in the far C-terminal region, but it cannot bind to Pnr^D mutants [60]. Therefore, Ush antagonizes Pnr transcriptional activation, and the N-terminal zinc finger of Pnr is required for Ush-mediated repression.

The ush locus encodes a protein with nine zinc-finger domains. Its overall structure is similar to that of the vertebrate Friend of GATA (FOG) proteins, FOG1 and FOG2, although the overall amino acid identity is low. The greatest degree of homology is seen between zinc fingers 6 and 8 of Ush and FOG2 [85]. The ush gene is expressed in a very dynamic pattern during embryogenesis. In addition to its expression in the dorsal ectoderm, it can be found in the precursors of hemocytes and the fat body, and in the cardiogenic mesoderm, at the time (stage 11) when heart precursors are specified [61]. An increased number of cardial cells is observed in embryos homozygous for hypomorphic ush alleles, or a deficiency that removes ush, the direct opposite of the phenotype observed in embryos with pnr loss of function mutations. The number of eve-expressing pericardial cells is also increased in ush mutants. This phenotype is seen in pnr mutants as well, suggesting that the combined action of ush and pnr is required to prevent overproduction of this type of pericardial cell [61]. Ectopic expression of ush throughout the mesoderm causes a decrease of up to 50% in the numbers of cardial cells in the heart tube, again opposite to the phenotype observed with the forced expression of pnr.

Ush can also abolish the synergistic activation of the *D-mef2* heart enhancer by *tin* and *pnr* [61]. It is likely that *pnr* and *ush* act as developmental switches that cause an alternation between the cardial and pericardial cell fates. In dorsal mesodermal cells in which *ush* and *pnr* are expressed together, the two proteins encoded by the genes form a repressor complex that inhibits cardial cell formation. When *pnr* is expressed alone in dorsal mesodermal cells, it acts synergistically with *tin* to promote a cardial cell fate and turn on cardial cell-specific genes. Mutations in the N-terminal zinc finger of *pnr* do not affect its cardiogenic activity, consistent with its proposed function of binding to Ush protein [22]. Ectopic mesodermal expression of the *ush* vertebrate homologs FOG1 or FOG2 causes a phenotype similar to that of ectopic Ush, which is a reduction in the number of cardial cells [86]. Therefore, despite the convergence in sequence, there is a degree of functional conservation between the proteins.

Embryos mutant for *ush* also exhibit defects in mesodermal cell migration. After formation of the ventral furrow, the mesodermal cells migrate dorsally until they form a monolayer, which is in close contact with the overlying ectoderm. This process is required to move the dorsal mesodermal cells into position to receive *dpp*-mediated signaling from the dorsal ectoderm [87]. Mutation in the *heartless* (*htl*) gene, which encodes a fibroblast growth factor receptor, causes severe defects in mesodermal migration, which results in the loss of dorsal mesodermal derivatives, with the heart showing the most severe effects [88,89]. In 50% of mutant *ush* embryos examined, disparities in cardial cell populations were seen, with some hemisegments having 8–12 cardial cells, while others had none. In some of the embryo cross-sections of *ush* mutants at stage 10, when the mesoderm should have formed a monolayer, showed regions in which cells had remained clustered, similar to an *htl* phenotype. Embryos transheterozygous for *ush* and *htl* have also shown this phenotype, which suggests that these two genes function in a common pathway to facilitate migration of the mesodermal cells [61].

Vertebrate FOG factors

There are two known FOG factors in vertebrates. FOG-1, which interacts with GATA1 and is essential for erythroid and megakaryocytic differentiation, was found in a yeast two-hybrid screen for GATA1-interacting proteins [90]. FOG-2, which was isolated during a search of expressed sequence tag databases, is co-expressed with GATA4 in the heart, starting at E8.5, and is also found in the brain and testis [85,90,91]. Similar to the interaction seen for Ush and Pnr proteins, FOG proteins interact with the N-terminal zinc finger of GATA proteins [85,91–93]. Transient transfection assays with FOG2 and GATA4 demonstrated variable effects of FOG2 on transcription. In Cos cells, FOG2 and GATA4 caused a 20-fold activation of the α-HMC promoter, but in primary neonatal rat cardiomyocytes, FOG2 prevented GATA4 upregulation of the same promoter [85]. In addition, FOG2 blocks GATA4-mediated activation of the ANF promoter in both 10T1/2 cell and cardiomyocyte backgrounds. GATA4-mediated activation of the BNP, cardiac troponin I, and cardiac troponin C promoters was also inhibited by FOG2 [85,91]. A mutant form of GATA with an E215K amino acid substitution in the N-terminal zinc finger could activate the BNP promoter to the same extent as wild-type GATA4, but FOG2 could not inhibit its transcriptional activity [91]. Therefore, FOG2 can act as a repressor or an activator of GATA4-mediated transcription, depending on the promoter and its cellular context.

Eliminating FOG2 function in the mouse embryo causes death between E12.5 to E13.5 and a multitude of heart defects. For example, there are changes in the gross morphology of the heart due to dilation of the atria and an absence of the ventricular apices. Pulsation of the mutant hearts is slower and weak. Additional defects include thinning of the ventricular myocardium and defects analogous to the human congenital malformation tetralogy of Fallot [94]. Affected mice also exhibit defects resembling tricuspid atresia [95]. However, no effects on ANF and BNP production have been observed despite transfection studies that suggested FOG2 plays a role in their regulation. Expression of the genes that encode Nkx2.5, IRX-4, MLC2A, MLC2V, cardiac troponin I, N-myc, phospholamban, GATA4, and GATA6 was also not changed. Tevosian et al. [94] reported a down-regulation of *eHAND* and *dHAND* transcripts and an up-regulation of *CARP*, although Svensson et al. [95] reported no effects on *dHAND*. Mutant hearts also failed to express the endothelial markers intercellular adhesion molecule-2 and FLK-1 (signal-transducing VEGF receptor-2), which suggests defects in the formation of the coronary vasculature. Expression of *FOG2* in the myocardium could rescue the formation of these vessels. Therefore, *FOG2* is needed for signaling by the myocardium to initiate coronary vessel formation, but these signals remain to be identified [94].

D-Mef2

Myocyte enhancer factor 2 (MEF2) was initially detected as a nuclear factor from differentiated C2 myotubes that bound an A/T- rich enhancer element in the muscle creatine kinase promoter [96]. MEF2 is a member of the MADS box of transcription factors. These proteins share a common 56-amino acid N-terminal domain (the MADS box), which is essential for DNA-binding activity and dimerization. MEF2 proteins also exhibit a unique feature, the MEF2 domain, which is just C-terminal to the MADS box. Genetic screens in *Drosophila* revealed a single *mef2* gene [97,98]. It is first expressed during invagination of the mesoderm and can be observed in all three muscle types later in development [99–101]. The early expression of *D-mef2* is dependent on activation by the bHLH factor *twist* [102]. It is also found in the Kenyon cells of the brain, which form the mushroom bodies [103]. Mutations of *D-mef2* do not prevent formation of the heart but do eliminate expression of late heart genes such as the myosin subunit genes [99,100,104]. *D-mef2* is expressed in all of the cardial cells but not in the pericardial cells. A *tin*-dependent enhancer (see above) drives expression in four of the six pairs of cardial cells per segment. A second later-acting heart enhancer drives expression in an identical pattern starting at stage 14 [105]. A third heart enhancer has been uncovered that drives *D-mef2* in the two pairs of cardial cells that do not express *tin* [106]. It is interesting to note that this enhancer also controls pharyngeal muscle expression [106]. Currently there are no characterized direct-target genes of D-mef2 in the heart, although on the basis of mutant phenotypes myosin is a candidate. It remains to be determined whether D-mef2 acts directly or indirectly to control expression of this late structural gene.

Vertebrate MEF2

Vertebrates have four separate mef2 genes: mef2A-D. They have a high degree of amino acid identity in the MADS-box and MEF2 domains, but are highly divergent in their C-terminal regions. Several alternative exons are present in the non-conserved regions of mef2A, C, and D, which results in multiple isoforms of the proteins [107]. The MEF2 proteins are produced in unique but overlapping patterns and can homodimerize and heterodimerize. D-mef2 shares an 85% amino acid identity with vertebrate mef2s in the MADS-box and MEF2 domains and can activate transcription through its binding site in mammalian cells [97,98]. mef2B and C are the first of these genes to be expressed in the heart, appearing in the precardiac mesoderm at E7.75 around the same time Nkx2.5 is seen. The other two mef2 genes are detected in myocardial cells about 12 hours later [108,109]. mef2 genes are also expressed in skeletal and visceral muscle and in the brain. Later in development, mef2A, B, and D transcripts become ubiquitous, but active protein is found almost exclusively in muscle and nerve cells [110–112].

mef2B knockout mice are viable, with no significant muscle defects [109]. The absence of mef2C, however, is lethal by E10.5 and causes severe cardiac abnormalities. Mutant embryos form a beating heart tube, but the contractions are slower and less rhythmic than those in a comparable wild-type heart. The mutant heart tube fails to loop and shows no morphological evidence of the future right ventricle. Transcripts of cardiac genes such as ANF, α-CA, α-myosin heavy chain (αHMC), and (MLC) are absent or severely reduced [113]. The absence of mef2C also causes severe disruptions of the vascular system, as a result of the defective differentiation of smooth muscle cells and failure of the endothelial cells to properly organize [114,115].

Mef2 is required for the optimal production of MLC2V, cardiac troponin T, cardiac troponin I, αHMC, and desmin. The promoters for the genes that encode these proteins contain Mef2 consensus sequences, and promoter activity decreases when these sites are mutated [116,121]. Although ANF and α-CA are not detectable in Mef2C null embryos, the ANF promoter has only one very low affinity mef2 site, and ectopic expression of Mef2 failed to activate endogenous α-CA or αMHC in explanted Xenopus ectoderm [42,122]. Mef2 can activate downstream genes with weak or absent Mef2 binding sites by interacting with GATA4. The physical interaction of the two proteins encoded has been confirmed through immunoprecipitation studies and in vitro pull downs. Mutation or deletion of the C-terminal zinc finger of GATA4 abolished this interaction with MEF2, but deletion of the N-terminal zinc finger merely reduced it. The MADS-box and MEF2 domains are required for the interaction, but Mef2 DNA binding is not; as shown by the fact that two different Mef2 mutants that lacked the ability to bind DNA could still associate with *GATA4* and synergistically activate an *ANF* reporter gene. *GATA6* could also synergize with *mef2*, but *GATA5* could not [122]. This mechanism of gene activation is reminiscent of interactions between Mef2 and MyoD/E12 in developing skeletal muscle. DNA binding by Mef2 is not required for a synergistic activation of transcription if the MyOD/E12 complex is bound to its consensus site [123].

Seven-up

The *Drosophila seven-up* (*svp*) gene encodes a protein with homology to chick oval-bumin upstream promoter (COUP) transcription factors and was identified in an enhancer trap screen for neurogenic genes. Two isoforms of the protein have been described [124]. Svp I is a 543-amino acid protein that contains a DNA-binding domain and a ligand-binding domain. The Svp I protein shares a 75% identity (over the entire protein) with human COUP transcription factor. Within the DNA binding domains, 94% of the identity is shared, and the putative ligand domains share a 93% identity. The Svp II isoform is a larger protein (746 amino acids) that results from a splicing variation. Svp II is identical to Svp I through the first 452 amino acids; after that point, which is in the middle of the ligand-binding domain, the sequences diverge greatly. This isoform shows no significant homology to any known proteins [124]. *svp* function in the *Drosophila* eye is well characterized, where it prevents outer photoreceptors from assuming the fate of an R7 inner photore-ceptor [124,125]. It also functions in the development of the fat body, controlling expression of the fat cell differentiation markers *Adh* and *DCg1* [125] and the pro-liferation of cells in the malpighian tubules [126].

In the heart, Svp is expressed in a segmentally repeating pattern of two pairs of cardial cells. Its expression is first detected at stage 11 [127]. These cells originate through asymmetric divisions of precursor cells and do not express Tin in the late stages of heart development [106,128,129]. The asymmetric divisions produce a car-dioblast and a pericardial cell [128]. In *svp* mutants, the expression pattern of Tin in the heart is expanded from four cell pairs per segment to six, suggesting a role for Svp in the repression of late *tin* expression in a subpopulation of heart cells. Expression of the 333-bp β3-*tubulin* reporter gene, which is under the direct control of *tin*, is expanded in an identical manner [106]. Ectopic expression of the two Svp isoforms in the four pairs of *tin*-expressing cardial cells produces two opposite results, in contrast to the findings from ectopic expression experiments in the malpighian tubules [127]. Misexpression of the Svp I construct results in a dramatic decrease in Tin protein in the cardial cells of the heart, but the Tin levels in the pericardial cells are unaffected. In contrast, the Svp II construct has no effect on late tin pro-duction in the four pairs of cardial cells [106]. Therefore the Svp I isoform acts late in heart development to inhibit the production of Tin in a subset of cardial cells. Although the mechanism of repression remains to be elucidated, a 100-bp region 3' to the *tin* gene has been uncovered that is necessary to block *tin* expression in the Svp-expressing cardial cells [16]. It is interesting that a comparable result occurs if *hedgehog* (*hh*) signaling is disrupted in mid-embryogenesis. When *hh*[ts] mutants are shifted to a nonpermissive temperature, ectopic Tin expression in the two pairs of cardioblasts is observed [130].

The functional consequences of these separate expression patterns in the two types of heart cells are not known, but the structure of the larval heart may provide some direction for investigation. For example, the cells that express Svp assume a different shape, remaining round and compact, in contrast to the cardial cells that express Tin, which become large and flattened. The Svp cells are also the first cardioblasts to be contacted by the alary muscles. The spacing of these pairs of cells also suggests that they could be instrumental in the formation of the ostia, which are spaced in a similar manner in the heart region of the dorsal vessel [1]. The possible role for *svp* in any of these events remains to be established.

Vertebrate COUP factors

COUP TF genes are members of the steroid hormone receptor superfamily. As their ligand is unknown, they are classified as orphan nuclear receptors. The first identified member of this group was chick ovalbumin upstream promoter-transcription factor (COUP-TF), which was detected through its binding of a repeat element in the chicken albumin promoter [131–133]. COUP TF proteins share several highly conserved domains. The DNA-binding domain contains two zinc fingers and recognizes an imperfect direct repeat of the AGGTCA sequence [131,132,134]. There are also two regions C-terminal to the binding domain that are homologous to regions of other steroid receptors that are crucial for the formation of a ligand-binding pocket [135]. COUP TF factors have been shown to inhibit transcriptional activation of the retinoid acid receptor, vitamin D receptor, and thyroid receptor [136–138]. The *Drosophila* homolog Svp acts as a repressor of *Ultraspiracle* (the *Drosophila* retinoid X receptor homolog) based hormonal signaling [139]. Several mechanisms of this repression have been proposed, including competition for binding sites by *COUP TF*, disruption of the binding complexes by *COUP TF*, competition for retinoid X receptors, active repression, and transrepression [136,137,139–146]. Since it was initially isolated as an activator of the chicken albumin gene, *COUP TF* can probably also act as a transactivator [147]. Although, regulation of *COUP TF* expression is not as well characterized, treatment of zebrafish embryos with retinoic acid alters the expression of *COUP TFII/svp[40]* in the hindbrain, suggesting that *COUP TF* and retinoids modulate each other's functions in development [148]. Sonic hedgehog has also been demonstrated to induce *COUP TFII* mRNA synthesis in cell culture [147,149,150].

A heart phenotype has been observed for the mouse *COUP TFII* gene. *COUP TFII* is expressed in mesenchymal cells in a number of developing organs, including the heart [147,151]. It is first detected in the myocardium of the sinus venosus during looping of the heart tube. Later in development, *COUP TFII* is also expressed in the common atrium. A targeted disruption of *COUP TFII* produced a particular phenotype in heterozygous mice: those carrying one disrupted copy of *COUP TFII* were one third smaller than their wild-type littermates, and 66% died before weaning. In addition, homozygous mutant *COUP TFII* mice died before E11.5, and the hearts were often hemorrhagic. The atrial chamber and sinus venosus were also smaller and less developed than those in the wild-type animals, although staining for smooth muscle actin revealed that the myocardium had differentiated appropriately. The anterior and posterior cardial veins were collapsed or missing, and angiogenesis was defective. Transcription of the angiogenic factor angiopoietin I (ANG1) was severely reduced in the mutants [152]. ANG1 is a receptor for TIE2, a receptor tyrosine kinase; both play an important role in the development of the heart and vascular system via mesenchymal-endothelial signaling [153–155]. The expression pattern of ANG-1 overlaps that of *COUP TFII*, and mutations of either *Ang1* or *Tie2* result in defects in the atrial chamber and vascular development. However, *COUP TFII*-mediated defects are more severe, which implies that there are additional direct or indirect targets for *COUP TFII* in the heart [152].

CONCLUSIONS

The expression of common genes during heart development has made the information gained from studies of *Drosophila* cardiogenesis useful for those who seek to understand the mechanisms of heart cell specification and tube formation in vertebrates. Although the vertebrate circulatory system is much more elaborate than that of the fruit fly, there may be useful information about later stages of heart development to be gained from *Drosophila*. On the basis of patterns of gene expression, there are at least two types of cardiac cells, and four types of pericardial cells [128]. The functional relevance of these differences is yet undetermined, and the characterization of the genetic pathways that generate them is incomplete. The larval heart also shows differences in structure along its anteroposterior axis, which hint at a role for homeotic genes in their generation. The mechanisms that determine the different fates of these heart cells may also be conserved in more complex animals.

REFERENCES

1. Rugendorff A, Younossi-Hartenstein A, Hartenstein V. 1994. Embryonic origin and differentiation of the *Drosophila* heart. Roux's Arch Dev Biol 203:266–280.
2. Rizki TM. 1978. The circulatory system and associated cells and tissues. In: The Genetics and Biology of *Drosophila*. Ed. M Ashburner and TRF Wright, 397–452. London and New York: Academic Press.
3. Bate M. 1993. The mesoderm and its derivatives. In: The Development of *Drosophila melanogaster*. Ed. M Bate and AM Arias, 1013–1090. Plainview, NY: Cold Spring Harbor Laboratory Press.
4. Fishman MC, Chien KR. 1997. Fashioning the vertebrate heart: earliest embryonic decisions. Development 124:2099–2117. Review.
5. Haag TA, Haag NP, Lekven AC, Hartenstein V. 1999. The role of cell adhesion molecules in *Drosophila* heart morphogenesis: *faint sausage, shotgun/DE-cadherin*, and *laminin A* are required for discrete stages in heart development. Dev Biol 208:56–69.
6. Grant DS, Tashiro K, Segui-Real B, Yamada Y, Martin GR, Kleinman HK. 1989. Two different laminin domains mediate the differentiation of human endothelial cells into capillary-like structures in vitro. Cell 58:933–943.
7. Sugi Y, Markwald RR. 1996. Formation and early morphogenesis of endocardial endothelial precursor cells and the role of endoderm. Dev Biol 175:66–83.
8. Kim Y, Nirenberg M. 1989. *Drosophila* NK-homeobox genes. Proc Natl Acad Sci USA 86:7716–7720.
9. Harvey RP. 1996. NK-2 homeobox genes and heart development. Dev Biol 178:203–216.

10. Azpiazu N, Frasch M. 1993. *tinman* and *bagpipe*: two homeo box genes that determine cell fates in the dorsal mesoderm of *Drosophila*. Genes Dev 7:1325–1340.
11. Bodmer R. 1993. The gene *tinman* is required for specification of the heart and visceral muscles in *Drosophila*. Development 118:719–729.
12. Yin Z, Frasch M. 1998. Regulation and function of *tinman* during dorsal mesoderm induction and heart specification in *Drosophila*. Dev Genet 22:187–200.
13. Yin Z, Xu XL, Frasch M. 1997. Regulation of the *twist* target gene *tinman* by modular *cis*-regulatory elements during early mesoderm development. Development 124:4871–4982.
14. Xu X, Yin Z, Hudson JB, Ferguson EL, Frasch M. 1998. Smad proteins act in combination with synergistic and antagonistic regulators to target Dpp responses to the *Drosophila* ectoderm. Genes Dev 12:2354–2370.
15. Wu X, Golden K, Bodmer R. 1995. Heart development in *Drosophila* requires the segment polarity gene *wingless*. Dev Biol 169:619–628.
16. Venkatesh T, Park M, Ocorr K, Nemaceck J, Golden K, Wemple M, Bodmer R. 2000. Cardiac enhancer activity of the homeobox gene *tinman* depends on CREB consensus binding sites in *Drosophila*. Genesis 26:55–66.
17. Gajewski K, Kim Y, Lee YM, Olson EN, Schulz RA. 1997. D-mef2 is a target for Tinman activation during *Drosophila* heart development. EMBO J 16:515–522.
18. Gajewski K, Fossett N, Molkentin JD, Schulz RA. 1999. The zinc finger proteins Pannier and GATA4 function as cardiogenic factors in *Drosophila*. Development 126:5679–5688.
19. Kremser T, Gajewski K, Schulz RA, Renkawitz-Pohl R. 1999. Tinman regulates the transcription of the *beta3 tubulin* gene (*betaTub60D*) in the dorsal vessel of *Drosophila*. Dev Biol 216:327–339.
20. Gajewski K, Kim Y, Choi CY, Schulz RA. 1998. Combinatorial control of *Drosophila* mef2 gene expression in cardiac and somatic muscle cell lineages. Dev Genes Evol 208:382–392.
21. Baylies MK, Bate M. 1996. *twist*: A myogenic switch in *Drosophila*. Science 272:1481–1484.
22. Gajewski K, Zhang Q, Choi CY, Fossett N, Dang A, Kim YH, Kim Y, Schulz RA. 2001. Pannier is a transcriptional target and partner of Tinman during *Drosophila* cardiogenesis. Dev Biol 233:425–436.
23. Lints TJ, Parsons LM, Hartley L, Li R, Andrews JE, Robb L, Harvey RP. 1995. Myogenic and morphogenic defects in the heart tubes of murine embryos lacking the homeo box gene *Nkx-2.5*. Genes Dev 9:1654–1666.
24. Komuro I, Izumo S. 1993. *Csx*: a murine homeobox-containing gene specifically expressed in the developing heart. Proc Natl Acad Sci USA 90:8145–8149.
25. Tonissen KF, Drysdale TA, Lints TJ, Harvey RP, Krieg PA. 1994. *XNkx-2.5*, a *Xenopus* gene related to *Nkx-2.5* and *tinman*: evidence for a conserved role in cardiac development. Dev Biol 162:235–328.
26. Evans SM, Yan W, Murillo MP, Ponce J, Papalopulu N. 1995. *tinman*, a *Drosophila* homeobox gene required for heart and visceral mesoderm specification, may be represented by a family of genes in vertebrates: *XNkx-2.3*, a second vertebrate homologue of *tinman*. Development 121:3889–3899.
27. Schultheiss TM, Xydas S, Lassar AB. 1995. Induction of avian cardiac myogenesis by anterior endoderm. Development 121:4204–4214.
28. Buchberger A, Pabst O, Brand T, Seidl K, Arnold HH. 1996. Chick *NKx-2.3* represents a novel family member of vertebrate homologs to the *Drosophila* homeobox gene *tinman*: different expression of *cNKx-2.3* and *cNKx-2.5* during heart and gut development. Mech Dev 56:151–163.
29. Chen JN, Fishman MC. 1996. Zebrafish *tinman* homolog demarcates the heart field and initiates myocardial differentiation. Development 122:3809–3816.
30. Lee KH, Xu Q, Breitbart RE. 1996. A new *tinman*-related gene, nkx2.7, anticipates the expression of *nkx2.5* and *nkx2.3* in Zebrafish heart and pharyngeal endoderm. Dev Biol 180:722–731.
31. Nikolova M, Chen X, Lufkin T. 1997. Nkx2.6 expression is transiently and specifically restricted to the branchial region of pharyngeal-stage mouse embryos. Mech Dev 69:215–218.
32. Pabst O, Scheider A, Brand T, Arnold HH. 1997. The mouse Nkx2-3 homeobox gene is expressed in gut mesenchyme during pre- and postnatal mouse development. Dev Dynam 209:29–35.
33. Reecy JM, Yamada M, Cummings K, Sosic D, Chen CY, Eichele G, Olson EN, Schwartz RJ. 1997. Chicken Nkx-2.8: a novel homeobox gene expressed in early heart progenitor cells in pharyngeal pouch-3 and -3 endoderm. Dev Bio 188:295–311.
34. Biben C, Hatzistavrou T, Harvey RP. 1998. Expression of NK-2 class homeobox gene Nkx2-6 in foregut endoderm and heart. Mech Dev 73:125–127.

35. Newman CS, Krieg PA. 1998. Tinman-related genes expressed during heart development in *Xenopus*. Dev Genet 22:230–238.
36. Newman CS, Reecy J, Grow MW, Ni K, Boettger T, Kessel M, Schwartz RJ, Krieg PA. 2000. Transient cardiac expression of the tinman-family homeobox gene, XNkx2-10. Mech Dev 91:369–373.
37. Schott JJ, Benson DW, Basson CT, Pease W, Silberbach GM, Moak JP, Maron BJ, Seidman CE, Seidman JG. 1998. Congenital heart disease caused by mutations in the transcription factor NKX2-5. Science 281:108–111.
38. Ranganayakulu G, Elliot DA, Harvey RP, Olson EN. 1998. Divergent roles for NK-2 class homeobox genes in cardiogenesis in flies and mice. Development 125:3037–3048.
39. Lyons I, Parsons LM, Hartley L, Li R, Andrews JE, Robb L, Harvey RP. 1995. Myogenic and morphogenetic defects in the heart tubes of murine embryos lacking the homeo box gene Nkx2-5. Genes Dev 9:1654–1666.
40. Biben C, Harvey RP. 1997. Homeodomain factor *Nkx2-5* controls left-right asymmetric expression of bHLH eHand during murine heart development. Genes Dev 11:1357–1369.
41. Zou Y, Evans S, Chen J, Kuo HC, Harvey RP, Chien KR. 1997. CARP, a cardiac ankyrin repeat protein, is downstream in the Nkx2-5 homeobox gene pathway. Development 124:793–804.
42. Fu YC, Izumo S. 1995. Cardiac myogenesis-overexpression of xcsx2 or xmef2a in whole *Xenopus* embryos induces the precocious expression of xmhc-α gene. Roux Arch Dev Biol 205:198–202.
43. Cleaver OB, Patterson KD, Krieg PA. 1996. Overexpression of the tinman-related genes XNkx-2.5 and XNkx-2.3 in *Xenopus* embryos results in myocardial hyperplasia. Development 122:3549–3556.
44. Fu Y, Yan W, Mihun TJ, Evans SM. 1998. Vertebrate *tinman* homologues *XNKx2-3* and *XNKx2-5* are required for heart formation in a functionally redundant manner. Development 125:4439–4449.
45. Grow MW, Krieg PA. 1998. Tinman function is essential for vertebrate heart development: Elimination of cardiac differentiation by dominant inhibitory mutants of the tinman-related genes, XNkx2-3 and XNkx2-5. Dev Biol 204:187–196.
46. Searcy RD, Vincent EB, Liberatore CM, Yutzey KE. 1998. A GATA-dependent nkx-2.5 regulatory element activates early cardiac gene expression in transgenic mice. Development 125:4461–4470.
47. Durocher D, Chen CY, Ardati A, Schwartz RJ, Nemer M. 1996. The atrial natriuretic factor promoter is a downstream target for Nkx-2.5 in the myocardium. Mol Cell Biol 16:4648–4655.
48. Durocher D, Charron F, Warren R, Schwartz RJ, Nemer M. 1997. The cardiac transcription factors Nkx2-5 and GATA-4 are mutual cofactors. EMBO J 16:5687–5696.
49. Lee Y, Shioi T, Kasahara H, Jobe SM, Wiese RJ, Markham BE, Izumo S. 1998. The cardiac tissue-restricted homeobox protein Csx/Nkx2.5 physically associates with the zinc finger protein GATA4 and cooperatively activates atrial natriuretic factor gene expression. Mol Cell Biol 18:3120–3129.
50. Sepulveda JL, Belaguli N, Nigam V, Chen CY, Nemer M, Schwartz RJ. 1998. GATA-4 and Nkx-2.5 coactivate Nkx-2 DNA binding targets: role for regulating early cardiac gene expression. Mol Cell Biol 18:3405–3415.
51. Molkentin JD, Antos C, Mercer B, Taigen T, Miano JM, Olson EN. 2000. Direct activation of a GATA6 cardiac enhancer by Nkx2.5: evidence for a reinforcing regulatory network of Nkx2.5 and GATA transcription factors in the developing heart. Dev Biol 217:301–309.
52. Bruneau BG, Bao ZZ, Tanaka M, Schott JJ, Izumo S, Cepko CL, Seidman JG, Seidman CE. 2000. Cardiac expression of the ventricle-specific homeobox gene Irx4 is modulated by Nkx2-5 and dHand. Dev Biol 217:266–277.
53. Merika M, Orkin SH. 1993. DNA-binding specificity of GATA family transcription factors. Mol Cell Biol 13:3999–4010.
54. Jürgens G, Wiechaus E, Nüsslein-Volhard C, Kluding H. 1984. Mutations affecting the pattern of the larval cuticle in *Drosophila melanogaster*. II. Zygotic loci on the third chromosome. Roux's Arch Dev Biol 193:283–295.
55. Ramain P, Heitzler P, Haenlin M, Simpson P. 1993. *pannier*, a negative regulator of *achaete* and *scute* in *Drosophila*, encodes a zinc finger protein with homology to the vertebrate transcription factor GATA-1. Development 199:1277–1291.
56. Winick J, Abel T, Leonard MW, Michelson AM, Chardon-Loriaux I, Holmgren RA, Maniatis T, Engel JD. 1993. A GATA family transcription factor is expressed along the embryonic dorsoventral axis in *Drosophila melanogaster*. Development 119:1055–1065.
57. Heitzler P, Haenlin M, Ramain P, Calleja M, Simpson P. 1996. A genetic analysis of *pannier*, a gene necessary for viability of dorsal tissues and bristle positioning in *Drosophila*. Genetics 143:1271–1286.
58. Rehorn KP, Thelen H, Michelson AM, Reuter R. 1996. A molecular aspect of hematopoiesis and endoderm development common to vertebrates and *Drosophila*. Development 122:4023–4031.

59. Lin WH, Huang LH, Yeh JY, Hoheisel J, Lehrach H, Sun YH, Tsai SF. 1995. Expression of a *Drosophila* GATA transcription factor in multiple tissues in the developing embryos: identification of homozygous lethal mutants with P-element insertion at the promoter region. J Biol Chem 270: 25150–25158.
60. Haenlin M, Cubadda Y, Blondeau F, Heitzler P, Lutz Y, Simpson P, Ramain P. 1997. Transcriptional activity of pannier is regulated by heterodimerization of the GATA DNA-binding domain with a cofactor encoded by the *u-shaped* gene of *Drosophila*. Genes Dev 11:3096–3108.
61. Fossett N, Zhang Q, Gajewski K, Choi CY, Kim Y, Schulz RA. 2000. The multitype zinc-finger protein U-shaped functions in heart cell specification in the *Drosophila* embryo. Proc Natl Acad Sci USA 97:7348–7353.
62. Orkin SH. 1995. Hematopoiesis: how does it happen? Curr Opin Cell Biol 7:870–877. Review.
63. Pevny L, Simon MC, Robertson E, Klein WH, Tsai SF, D'Agati V, Orkin SH, Costantini F. 1991. Erythroid differentiation in chimeric mice blocked by a targeted mutation in the gene for transcription factor GATA-1. Nature 349:257–260.
64. Tsai FY, Keller G, Kuo FC, Weiss M, Chen J, Rosenblatt M, Alt FW, Orkin SH. 1994. An early haematopoietic defect in mice lacking the transcription factor GATA-2. Nature 371:221–226.
65. Pandolfi PP, Roth ME, Karis A, Leonard MW, Dzierzak E, Grosveld FG, Engel JD, Lindenbaum MH. 1995. Targeted disruption of the GATA3 gene causes severe abnormalities in the nervous system and in fetal liver haematopoiesis. Nat Genet 11:40–44.
66. Simon MC. 1995. Gotta have GATA. Nat Genet 11:9–11.
67. Zheng W, Flavell RA. 1997. The transcription factor GATA-3 is necessary and sufficient for Th2 cytokine gene expression in CD4 cells. Cell 89:587–596.
68. Heikinheimo M, Scandrett JM, Wilson DB. 1994. Localization of transcription factor to regions of the mouse embryo involved in cardiac development. Dev Biol 164:361–373.
69. Laverriere AC, MacNeill C, Mueller C, Poelmann RE, Burch JBE, Evans T. 1994. *GATA 4/5/6*, a subfamily of three transcription factors transcribed in developing heart and gut. J Biol Chem 269:23177–23184.
70. Jiang Y, Evans T. 1996. The Xenopus *GATA-4/5/6* genes are associated with cardiac specification and can regulate cardiac-specific transcription during embryogenesis. Dev Biol 174:257–270.
71. Kelley C, Blumberg H, Zon LI, Evans T. 1993. *GATA-4* is a novel transcription factor expressed in the endocardium of the developing heart. Development 118:817–827.
72. Morrisey EE, Ip HS, Lu MM, Parmacek MS. 1996. *GATA-6*: a zinc finger transcription factor that is expressed in multiple cell lineages derived from lateral mesoderm. Dev Biol 177:309–322.
73. Gove C, Walmsley M, Nijjar S, Bertwistle D, Guille M, Partington G, Bomford A, Patient R. 1997. Over-expression of GATA-6 in *Xenopus* embryos blocks differentiation of heart precursors. EMBO J 16:355–368.
74. Jiang Y, Tarzami S, Burch JBE, Evans T. 1998. Common role for each of the *GATA-4/5/6* genes in the regulation of cardiac morphogenesis. Dev Genet 22:263–277.
75. Kuo CT, Morrisey EE, Anandappa R, Sigrist K, Lu MM, Parmacek MS, Soudais C, Leiden JM. 1997. GATA-4 transcription factor is required for ventral morphogenesis and heart tube formation. Genes Dev 11:1048–1060.
76. Molkentin JD, Lin Q, Duncan SA, Olson EN. 1997. Requirement of the transcription factor GATA4 for heart tube formation and ventral morphogenesis. Genes Dev 11:1061–1072.
77. Narita N, Bielinska M, Wilson DB. 1996. Cardiomyocyte differentiation by GATA-4-deficient embryonic stem cells. Development 122:3755–3764.
78. Morrisey EE, Tang Z, Sigrist K, Lu MM, Jiang F, Ip HS, Parmacek MS. 1998. GATA6 regulates HNF4 and is required for differentiation of visceral endoderm in the mouse embryo. Genes Dev 12:3579–3590.
79. Koutsourakis M, Langeveld A, Patient R, Beddington R, Grosveld F. 1999. The transcription factor GATA6 is essential for early extraembryonic development. Development 126:723–732.
80. Reiter JF, Alexander J, Rodaway A, Yelon D, Patient R, Holder N, Stainier DYR. 1999. Gata5 is required for the development of the heart and endoderm in zebrafish. Genes Dev 13:2983–2995.
81. Molkentin JD, Lu JR, Antos CL, Markham B, Richardson J, Robbins J, Grant SR, Olson EN. 1998. A calcineurin-dependent transcriptional pathway for cardiac hypertrophy. Cell 93:215–228.
82. Jiang Y, Drysdale TA, Evans T. 1999. A role for GATA-4/5/6 in the regulation of Nkx2.5 expression with implications for patterning of the precardiac field. Dev Biol 16:57–71.

83. Nüsslein-Volhard C, Wiechaus E, Kluding H. 1984. Mutations affecting the pattern of the larval cuticle in *Drosophila melanogaster*. I. Zygotic loci on the second chromosome. Roux Arch Dev Biol 193:297–282.

84. Cubadda Y, Heitzler P, Ray RP, Bourouis M, Ramain P, Gelbart W, Simpson P, Haenlin M. 1997. *u-shaped* encodes a zinc finger protein that regulates the proneural genes *acheate* and *scute* during the formation of bristles in *Drosophila*. Genes Dev 11:3083–3095.

85. Lu JR, McKinsey TA, Xu H, Wang DZ, Richardson JA, Olson EN. 1999. FOG-2, a heart- and brain-enriched cofactor for GATA transcription factors. Mol Cell Biol 19:4495–4502.

86. Fossett N, Tevosian SG, Gajewski R, Zhang Q, Orkin SH, Schulz RA. 2001. The friend of GATA proteins U-shaped, FOG-1, and FOG-2 function as negative regulators of blood, heart, and eye development in *Drosophila*. Proc Natl Acad Sci USA 98:7342–7347.

87. Frasch M. 1995. Induction of visceral and cardiac mesoderm by ectodermal Dpp in the early *Drosophila* embryo. Nature 374:464–467.

88. Beiman M, Shilo B, Volk T. 1996. *Heartless*, a *Drosophila* FGF receptor homolog, is essential for cell migration and establishment of several mesodermal lineages. Genes Dev 10:2993–3002.

89. Gisselbrecht S, Skeath J, Doe C, Michelson A. 1996. *Heartless* encodes a fibroblast growth factor receptor (DFR1/DFGF-R2) involved in the directional migration of early mesodermal cells in the *Drosophila* embryo. Genes Dev 10:3003–3017.

90. Tsang AP, Visvader JE, Turner CA, Fujiwara Y, Yu C, Weiss MJ, Crossley M, Orkin SH. 1997. FOG, a multitype zinc finger protein, acts as a cofactor for transcription factor GATA-1 in erythroid and megakaryocytic differentiation. Cell 90:109–119.

91. Svensson EC, Tufts RL, Polk CE, Leiden JM. 1999. Molecular cloning of FOG-2: a modulator of transcription factor GATA-4 in cardiomyocytes. Proc Natl Acad Sci USA 96:956–961.

92. Tevosian SG, Deconinck AE, Cantor AB, Rieff HI, Fujiwara Y, Corfas G, Orkin SH. 1999. FOG-2: a novel GATA-family cofactor related to multitype zinc-finger proteins Friend of GATA-1 and U-shaped. Proc Natl Acad Sci USA 96:950–955.

93. Fox AH, Kowalski K, King GF, Mackay JP, Crossley M. 1998. Key residues characteristic of GATA N-fingers are recognized by FOG. J Biol Chem 273:33595–33603.

94. Tevosian SG, Deconinck AE, Tanaka M, Schinke M, Litovsky SH, Izumo S, Fujiwara Y, Orkin SH. 2000. FOG-2, a cofactor for GATA transcription factors, is essential for heart morphogenesis and development of coronary vessels from epicardium. Cell 101:729–739.

95. Svensson EC, Huggins GS, Lin H, Clendenin C, Jiang F, Tufts R, Dardik FB, Leiden JM. 2000. A syndrome of tricuspid atresia in mice with a targeted mutation of the gene encoding Fog-2. Nat Genet 25:353–356.

96. Gossett LA, Kelven DJ, Sternberg EA, Olson EN. 1989. A new myocyte-specific enhancer-binding factor that recognizes a conserved element associated with multiple muscle-specific genes. Mol Cell Biol 15:1870–1878.

97. Lilly B, Galewsky S, Firulli AB, Schulz RA, Olson EN. 1994. D-MEF2: a MADS box transcription factor expressed in differentiating mesoderm and muscle cell lineages during *Drosophila* embryogenesis. Proc Natl Acad Sci USA 91:5662–5666.

98. Nguyen HT, Bodmer R, Abmayr SM, McDermott JC, Spoerel NA. 1994. *D-mef2*: a *Drosophila* mesoderm-specific MADS box-containing gene with a biphasic expression profile during embryogenesis. Proc Natl Acad Sci USA 91:7520–7524.

99. Bour BA, O'Brien MA, Lockwood WL, Goldstein ES, Bodmer R, Taghert PH, Abmayr SM, Nguyen HT. 1995. Drosophila MEF2, a transcription factor that is essential for myogenesis. Genes Dev 9:730–741.

100. Lilly B, Zhao B, Ranganayakulu G, Paterson B, Schulz RA, Olson EN. 1995. Requirement of MADS domain transcription factor D-MEF2 for muscle formation in *Drosophila*. Science 267:688–693.

101. Taylor MV, Beatty KE, Hunter HK, Baylies MK. 1995. *Drosophila* MEF2 is regulated by *twist* and is expressed in both the primordia and differentiated cells of the embryonic somatic, visceral, and heart musculature. Mech Dev 50:26–41.

102. Cripps RM, Black BL, Zhao B, Lien CL, Schulz RA, Olson EN. 1998. The myogenic regulatory gene Mef2 is a direct target for transcriptional activation by Twist during *Drosophila* myogenesis. Genes Dev 12:422–434.

103. Schulz RA, Chromey C, Lu MF, Zhao B, Olson EN. 1996. Expression of the D-MEF2 transcription factor in the *Drosophila* brain suggests a role in neuronal cell differentiation. Oncogene 12:1827–1831.

104. Ranganayakulu G, Zhoa B, Dokidis A, Molentin JD, Olson EN, Schulz RA. 1995. A series of mutations in the D-MEF2 transcription factor reveal multiple functions in larval and adult myogenesis in *Drosophila*. Dev Biol 171:169–181.
105. Nguyen HT, Xu X. 1998. *Drosophila* mef2 expression during mesoderm development is controlled by a complex array of cis-acting regulatory modules. Dev Biol 204:550–566.
106. Gajewski K, Choi CY, Kim Y, Schulz RA. 2000. Genetically distinct cardial cells within the *Drosophila* heart. Genesis, in press.
107. Martin JF, Miano JM, Hustad CM, Copeland NG, Jenkins NA, Olson EN. 1994. A Mef2 gene that generates a muscle-specific isoform via alternative mRNA splicing. Mol Cell Biol 14:1647–1656.
108. Edmondson DG, Lyons GE, Martin JF, Olson EN. 1994. MEF2 gene expression marks the cardiac and skeletal muscle lineages during mouse embryogenesis. Development 120:1251–1263.
109. Molkentin JD, Firulli AB, Black BL, Martin JF, Hustad CM, Copeland N, Jenkins N, Lyons G, Olson EN. 1996. MEF2B is a potent transactivator expressed in early myogenic lineages. Mol Cell Biol 16:3814–3824.
110. Yu YT, Breitbart RE, Smoot LB, Lee Y, Mahdavi V, Nadal-Ginard B. 1992. Human myocyte-specific enhancer factor 2 comprises a group of tissue-restricted MADS box transcription factors. Genes Dev 6:1783–1798.
111. Leifer D, Golden J, Kowall NW. 1994. Myocyte-specific enhancer binding factor 2C expression in human brain development. Neuroscience 63:1067–1079.
112. Leifer D, Krainc D, Yu YT, McDermott J, Breitbart RE, Heng J, Neve RL, Kosofsky B, Nadal-Ginard B, Lipton SA. 1993. MEF2C, a MADS/MEF2-family transcription factor expressed in a laminar distribution in cerebral cortex. Proc Natl Acad Sci USA 90:1546–1550.
113. Lin Q, Schwarz J, Bucana C, Olson EN. 1997. Control of mouse cardiac morphogenesis and myogenesis by transcription factor MEF2C. Science 276:1404–1407.
114. Lin Q, Lu J, Yangisawa H, Webb R, Lyons GE, Richardson JA, Olson EN. 1998. Requirement of the MADS-box transcription factor MEF2C for vascular development. Development 125:4565–4574.
115. Bi W, Drake CJ, Schwarz JJ. 1999. The transcription factor MEF2C-null mouse exhibits complex vascular malformations and reduced cardiac expression of angiopoietin I and VEGF. Dev Biol 211:255–267.
116. Iannello RC, Mar JH, Ordahl CP. 1991. Characterization of a promoter element required for transcription in myocardial cells. J Biol Chem 266:3309–3316.
117. Zhu H, Garcia AV, Ross RS, Evans SM, Chien KR. 1991. A conserved 28-base-pair element (HF-1) in the rat cardiac myosin light-chain-2 gene confers cardiac-specific and α-adrenergic-inducible expression in cultured neonatal rat myocardial cells. Mol Cell Biol 11:2273–2281.
118. Yu YT, Breitbart RE, Smoot LB, Lee Y, Mahdavi V, Nadal-Ginard B. 1992. Human myocyte-specific enhancer factor 2 comprises a group of tissue-restricted MADS box transcription factors. Genes Dev 6:1783–1798.
119. Molkentin JD, Markham BE. 1993. Myocyte-specific enhancer-binding factor (MEF-2) regulates α-cardiac myosin heavy chain gene expression *in vitro* and *in vivo*. J Biol Chem 268:19512–19520.
120. Kuisk IR, Li H, Tran D, Capetanaki Y. 1996. A single MEF2 site governs desmin transcription in both heart and skeletal muscle during mouse embryogenesis. Dev Biol 174:1–13.
121. Di Lisi R, Millino C, Calabria E, Altruda F, Schiaffino S, Ausoni S. 1998. Combinatorial cis-acting elements control tissue-specific activation of the cardiac troponin I gene *in vitro* and *in vivo*. J Biol Chem 273:25371–25380.
122. Morin S, Charron F, Robitaille L, Nemer M. 2000. GATA-dependent recruitment of MEF2 protein to target promoters. EMBO J 19:2046–2055.
123. Black BL, Molkentin JD, Olson EN. 1998. Multiple roles for the MyoD basic region in transmission of transcriptional activation signals and interaction with MEF2. Mol Cell Biol 18:69–77.
124. Mlodzik M, Hiromi Y, Weber U, Goodman CS, Rubin GM. 1990. The *Drosophila* seven-up gene, a member of the steroid receptor gene superfamily, controls photoreceptor cell fates. Cell 60:211–224.
125. Hiromi Y, Mlodzik M, West SR, Rubin GM, Goodman CS. 1993. Ectopic expression of *seven-up* causes cell fate changes during ommatidial assembly. Development 118:1123–1135.
126. Hoshizaki DK, Blackburn T, Price C, Ghosh M, Miles K, Ragucci M, Sweis R. 1994. Embryonic fat-cell lineage in *Drosophila melanogaster*. Development 120:2489–2499.
127. Kerber B, Fellert S, Hoch M. 1998. *Seven-up*, the *Drosophila* homolog of the COUP-TF orphan receptors, controls cell proliferation in the insect kidney. Genes Dev 12:1781–1786.

128. Ward EJ, Skeath JB. 2000. Characterization of a novel subset of cardial cells and their progenitors in the *Drosophila* embryo. Development 127:4959–4969.
129. Bodmer R, Frasch M. 1999. Genetic determination of *Drosophila* heart development. In: Heart development. Ed. N Rosethal and R Harvey, 65–90. San Diego: Academic Press.
130. Frémion F, Astier M, Zaffran S, Guillen A, Homburger V, Sémériva M. 1999. The heterotrimeric protein G_0 is required for the formation of heart epithelium in *Drosophila*. J Cell Biol 145: 1063–1076.
131. Pastoric M, Wang H, Elbrecht A, Tsai SY, Tsai MJ, O'Malley BW. 1986. Control of transcription initiation *in vitro* requires binding of a transcription factor to the distal promoter of the ovalbumin gene. Mol Cell Biol 6:2784–2791.
132. Sagami I, Tsai SY, Wang H, Tsai MJ, O'Malley BW. 1986. Identification of two factors required for transcription of the ovalbumin gene. Mol Cell Biol 6:4259–4267.
133. Wang LH, Tsai SY, Cook RG, Beattie WG, Tsai MJ, O'Malley BW. 1989. COUP transcription factor is a member of the steroid receptor superfamily. Nature 340:163–166.
134. Tsai SY, Sagami I, Wang H, Tsai MJ, O'Malley BW. 1987. Interactions between a DNA-binding transcription factor (COUP) and a non-DNA binding factor (S300-II). Cell 50:701–709.
135. Renaud JP, Rochel N, Ruff M, Vivat V, Chambon P, Gronemyer H, Moras D. 1995. Crystal structure of the RAR-gamma ligand-binding domain bound to all-*trans* retinoic acid. Nature 378:681–689.
136. Cooney AJ, Tsai SY, O'Malley BW, Tsai MJ. 1992. Chicken ovalbumin upstream promoter transcription factor (COUP-TF) dimers bind to different GGTCA response elements, allowing COUP-TF to repress hormonal induction of the vitamin D3, thyroid hormone, and retinoic acid receptors. Mol Cell Biol 12:4153–4163.
137. Kliewer SA, Umesono K, Heyman RA, Mangelsdorf DJ, Dyck JA, Evans RM. 1992. Retinoid X receptor-COUP-TF interactions modulate retinoic acid signaling. Proc Natl Acad Sci USA 89:1448–1452.
138. Tran P, Zhang XK, Salbert G, Hermann T, Lehmann JM, Pfahl M. 1992. COUP orphan receptors are negative regulators of retinoic acid response pathways. Mol Cell Biol 12:4666–4676.
139. Cooney AJ, Leng X, Tsai SY, O'Malley BW, Tsai MJ. 1993. Multiple mechanisms of chicken ovalbumin upstream promoter transcription factor-dependent repression of transactivation by the vitamin D, thyroid hormone, and retinoic acid receptors. J Biol Chem 268:4152–4160.
140. Zelhof A, Yao TP, Chen JD, Evans R, McKeown M. 1995. *Seven-up* inhibits Ultraspiracle-based signaling pathways *in vitro* and *in vivo*. Molec Cell Biol 15:6736–6745.
141. Berrodin TJ, Marks MS, Ozato K, Linney E, Lazar MA. 1992. Heterodimerization among thyroid hormone receptor, retinoic acid receptor, retinoid X receptor, chicken ovalbumin upstream promoter transcription factor, and an endogenous liver protein. Mol Endocrinol 6:1468–1478.
142. Widom RL, Rhee M, Karathanasis SK. 1992. Repression by ARP-1 sensitizes apolipoprotein AI gene responsiveness to RXR alpha and retinoic acid. Mol Cell Biol 12:3380–3389.
143. Casanova J, Helmer E, Selmi-Ruby S, Qi JS, Au-Fliegner M, Desai-Yajnik V, Koudinova N, Yarm F, Raaka BM, Samuels HH. 1994. Functional evidence for ligand-dependent dissociation of thyroid hormone and retinoic acid receptors from an inhibitory cellular factor. Mol Cell Biol 14:5756–5765.
144. Chen JD, Evans RM. 1995. A transcriptional co-repressor that interacts with nuclear hormone receptors. Nature 377:454–457.
145. Horlein AJ, Naar AM, Heinzel T, Torchia J, Gloss B, Kurokawa R, Ryan A, Kamei Y, Soderstrom M, Glass CK, Rosenfeld MG. 1995. Ligand-independent repression by the thyroid hormone receptor mediated by a nuclear receptor co-repressor. Nature 377:397–404.
146. Leng X, Cooney AJ, Tsai SY, Tsai MJ. 1996. Molecular mechanisms of COUP-TF-mediated transcriptional repression: evidence for transrepression and active repression. Mol Cell Biol 16:2332–2340.
147. Tsai SY, Tsai MJ. 1997. Chick ovalbumin upstream promoter-transcription factors (COUP TFs): coming of age. Endocr Rev 18:229–240.
148. Fjose A, Weber U, Mlodzik M. 1995. A novel vertebrate svp-related nuclear receptor is expressed as a step gradient in developing rhombomeres and is affected by retinoic acid. Mech Dev 52: 233–246.
149. Krishnan V, Elberg G, Tsai MJ, Tsai SY. 1997. Identification of a novel sonic hedgehog response element in the chicken ovalbumin upstream promoter-transcription factor II promoter. Mol Endocrinol 11:1458–1466.

150. Krishnan V, Pereira FA, Qiu Y, Chen CH, Beachy PA, Tsai SY, Tsai MJ. 1997. Mediation of sonic hedgehog-induced expression of COUP-TFII by a protein phosphatase. Science 278:1947–1950.
151. Pereira FA, Qiu Y, Tsai MJ, Tsai SY. 1995. Chicken ovalbumin upstream promoter transcription factor (COUP-TF): expression during embryogenesis. J Steroid Biochem Mol Biol 53:503–508. Review.
152. Pereira FA, Qiu Y, Zhou G, Tsai MJ, Tsai SY. 1999. The orphan nuclear receptor COUP-TFII is required for angiogenesis and heart development. Genes Dev 13:1037–1049.
153. Sato TN, Tozawa Y, Deutsch U, Wolburg-Buchholz K, Fujiwara Y, Gendron-Maguire M, Gridley T, Wolburg H, Risau W, Qin Y. 1995. Distinct roles of the receptor tyrosine kinases Tie-1 and Tie-2 in blood vessel formation. Nature 376:70–74.
154. Suri C, Jones PF, Patan S, Bartunkova S, Maisonpierre PC, Davis S, Sato TN, Yancopoulos GD. 1996. Requisite role of angiopoietin-1, a ligand for the TIE2 receptor, during embryonic angiogenesis. Cell 87:1171–1180.
155. Maisonpierre PC, Suri C, Jones PF, Bartunkova S, Wiegand SJ, Radziejewski C, Compton D, McClain J, Aldrich TH, Papadopoulos N, Daly TJ, Davis S, Sato TN, Yancopoulos GD. 1997. Angiopoietin-2, a natural antagonist for Tie2 that disrupts *in vivo* angiogenesis. Science 277:55–60.

B. Ostadal, M. Nagano and N.S. Dhalla (eds.).
CARDIAC DEVELOPMENT. Copyright © 2002.
Kluwer Academic Publishers. Boston.

MICROVASCULAR BED IN MAMMALIAN HEARTS FROM BIRTH TO DEATH OF THE ORGANISM

KAREL RAKUSAN and NICHOLAS CICUTTI

Department of Cellular and Molecular Medicine, Faculty of Medicine, University of Ottawa, Ottawa, Ontario, Canada

Summary. Morphometric data on postnatal cardiac vascularization are reviewed in conjunction with concurrent events which may influence coronary angiogenesis. The postnatal development may be divided into three distinct stages: 1) early postnatal stage, characterized by marked proliferation of coronary capillaries and arterioles, maturation of the vascular walls and establishment of the adult type architecture of the microvascular bed, 2) adult stage of stable growth, which, nevertheless lags behind the growth of the myocyte mass and, 3) senescent stage—with a disappearance of capillaries and arterioles as well as increased heterogeneity of capillary spacing.

Key words: microcirculation, capillaries, arterioles, heart growth, cardiac development

INTRODUCTION

The microvascular bed is that portion of the total vascular bed which is not visible to the naked eye, i.e. smaller than about $300\,\mu m$. It is the second largest volume component of myocardial tissue (after the volume of myocytes) and the cells of the microvascular walls (endothelial cells, pericytes and smooth muscle cells) are the second largest group of myocardial cells (not much less than cardiac fibroblasts). In the present review we will concentrate only on the postnatal development of arterioles and capillaries, because little information is available on capillary venules and

Correspondence: Dr. K. Rakusan, Dept. of Cell. Mol. Medicine, University of Ottawa, 451 Smyth Rd. K1H 8M5, Ottawa, Ontario Canada. Tel: (613) 562-5800 ext. 8384; Fax: (613) 562-5464; e mail: krakusan@uottawa.ca

lymphatic capillaries. The postnatal changes in the coronary microvascular bed may be divided into three distinct stages: 1) early postnatal development stage, 2) "adult" stage of stable growth, and 3) senescent stage.

EARLY POSTNATAL STAGE

The early postnatal stage is characterized by marked proliferation of arterioles and capillaries. This occurs following a wave of cardiac myocyte proliferation which takes place mainly during the late fetal stages and wanes shortly after birth. On the other hand, the peak of vascular formation occurs during the early postnatal period. According to our estimate, close to half of the capillaries present in the adult rat heart are formed during the relatively short period of 3–4 postnatal weeks [1]. This may be illustrated by a 5–6 fold increase in capillary density during this period, which occurs in spite of rapidly increasing cardiac mass and myocyte size. Thus, the number of myocytes supplied by a single capillary decreases exponentially [2]. Such results are also supported by evidence of a higher percentage of endothelial cells entering the cell cycle found in the early postnatal period than in adult rat heart [3]. In addition, the study of Groningen and coworkers [4] described that the surface density of the capillaries in the rat heart increases during the first two postnatal weeks in spite of decreasing capillary volume density, resulting in a larger number of capillaries with smaller capillary diameter. The formation of new capillaries probably takes place on the distal (venular) part of the capillary bed [5]. This is associated with decreasing heterogeneity of capillary spacing, i. e. more regular orientation of capillaries [2,4].

Maturation of the capillary walls also takes place during the early postnatal period. Basal laminae of developing coronary capillaries are morphologically and biochemically mature by the end of the first postnatal week. Also during this period, the number of plasmalemmal vesicles increases and they are becoming more uniformly distributed [6].

The growth rate of arterioles during the early postnatal period in human hearts is even higher than that of capillaries: the number of capillaries per arteriole on a myocardial tissue cross-section decreases from 500 in infant hearts to 397 in children and 347 in adult hearts [7]. Arteriolar density in the rat heart also increases during the early postnatal period [8]. Most of the postnatal arteriolar formation in the rat heart occurs during the first four weeks after birth: the proportion of immature arterioles in the sample of arterioles from 1-day old rat heart is about 22%, which decreases to 12% on day 5, 8% day 12 and decreases to close to zero by postnatal day 28 [9]. Proliferation of arterioles is confined mainly to the smallest vessels as illustrated by changes in the frequency distribution of arteriolar size in rat hearts of various ages, depicted in Fig. 1. Newborn hearts are characterized by a higher incidence of larger arterioles while the arterioles of smaller caliber are predominant in older hearts as a reflection of their postnatal formation (Rakusan and Kolar, unpublished data). A similar phenomenon was also described during the postnatal development of human hearts [7].

ARTERIOLAR SIZE IN THE RAT HEART:

CHANGES IN FREQUENCY DISTRIBUTION WITH AGE

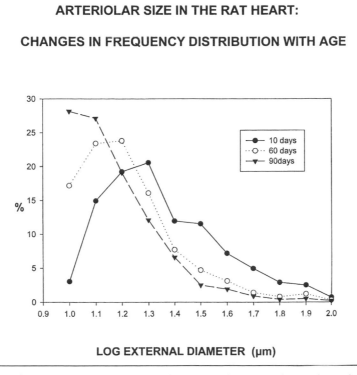

Figure 1. Relative frequency of arteriolar size (log external diameter) in hearts of rats of various ages. Rakusan and Kolar, unpublished data.

The early postnatal period is not only characterized by a rapid formation of the coronary microvascular bed but the tissue growth response to various internal and external stimuli is also enhanced. For instance, exercise normalizes capillarization in hearts from rats with spontaneous hypertension when initiated before puberty, but not in adult hearts [10]. Capillary density in thyroxine-treated rats is more elevated when the treatment begins before puberty [10]. This applies also to clearly pathological stimuli: in our own studies we have found almost normal capillarization in cardiac hypertrophy induced by pressure overload in both young human and rabbit hearts, while the same stimulus in adult hearts resulted in cardiac hypertrophy characterized by a decreased capillary supply [11,12]. It is also possible to stimulate capillary growth in the rat heart during the early postnatal period by chemical sympathectomy [13], while injections of protamine during this period has an inhibitory effect on capillary growth in both rat and sheep hearts [1,14]. The effect of protamine may be at least partially related to its inhibitory effect on FGF (see below). Finally, Godecke [15] described in a model of myoglobin knockout mice a significant increase in the coronary capillary density which was likely partially responsible for their normal physical performance and resistance to hypoxia.

All these changes, are, of course, possible only due to preceding and simultaneous changes at the molecular level. The most important angiogenic growth factors are probably peptides belonging to the VEGF family, which is endothelial cell specific and the FGF family, which regulates the whole tissue growth response. Immunoreactivity for VEGF remains high during the early postnatal period (VEGF mRNA and VEGF protein levels). According to Gerber and coworkers [16], VEGF is required for growth and survival in neonatal mice. They found increased mortality, stunted body growth and impaired organ development after inactivation of VEGF protein or after administration of VEGF receptor chimeric protein which inactivates the VEGF receptor. Interestingly, this dependence is lost after the fourth postnatal week. Engelmann and coworkers [17] described a decrease in FGF-1 immunoreactivity in the rat heart after birth which disappeared after the 3rd–4th postnatal weeks. FGF receptor flg is abundant in the fetal hearts, decreases around the birth with an additional peak in the 5th–7th postnatal week followed by a decrease to minimal values an the adult hearts. Tomanek and coworkers [18] report rather pronounced expression of FGF-2 mRNA during the early prenatal phases of vascularization in the rat heart (E14 and E15), which decreases afterwards but develops a second peak during the first postnatal week of postnatal life. By the end of the first postnatal month, the expression is once again reduced to the low levels encountered in adult hearts. Also the ventricular expression of types I, II and IV collagen transcripts reach their maximum during the first 2–3 postnatal weeks [19].

Normal cardiac and somatic growth is known to be also modulated by angiotensin II. Everett and coworkers described the upregulation of the AT_1 and AT_2 genes at the early postnatal stage of developing rat hearts [20]. For instance, AT_1 mRNA levels are highest in 19 day fetal hearts, are still high by postnatal day 10 and decrease afterwards. Also Shanmugam and Samberg [21] reported increased AT_1 and AT_2 expressions in rat heart following the birth, reaching a maximum at day 2 and decreasing afterwards.

"ADULT" STAGE OF STABLE GROWTH

The adult stage starts around the weaning period and covers most of the life span of the organism. Much of the available information originates from studies of rat hearts. During the postnatal development of the rat heart, microvascular architecture is firmly established by postnatal weeks 3–4 and the subsequent stages are mainly quantitative. Like many biological phenomena, it might be characterized by the allometric formula $y = ax^b$. For instance, the increase in cardiac mass in rats following the early postnatal period is almost entirely due to an increase in the size of cardiac myocytes. Because the total number of myocytes in this period is more or less constant and their shape (length-to-width ratio) remains the same, the allometric exponent b is equal to 1 [22,23]. The increase in myocyte size is in three dimensions, i.e. due to increases in both myocyte cross-section and myocyte length. Exponent b for an increase in total myocyte length would be therefore close to 0.3. The increase in aggregate length of capillaries exceeds that of total

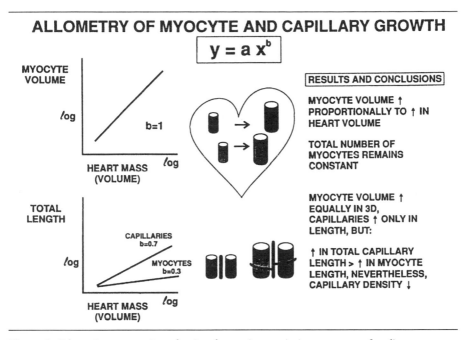

Figure 2. Schematic representation of major changes in quantitative parameters of cardiac myocytes and capillaries during the stable adult stage of postnatal development. The rate of growth of capillary and arteriolar length exceeds the increase in myocyte length, nevertheless, it does not match the increase in myocyte volume, leading to a relative dilution of these vessels. Reprinted from K. Rakusan/Coronary Angiogenesis, 1999, p.135, with permission from Elsevier Science.

myocyte length with b being 0.7–0.8 [23,24]. Nevertheless, coronary capillary numerical and length densities decrease, due to increases in myocyte cross-sectional area (see Fig. 2). The rate of growth of small arteries and arterioles in the rat heart during this period is similar to that of capillaries, i.e. $b = 0.7$ [25]. Thus, coronary angiogenesis during the adult stage decreases considerably but does not disappear completely.

The developmental stage would also predispose the vascular growth response to pathological stimuli. For instance, human cardiac hypertrophy due to pressure overload, when induced in the perinatal period is characterized by a normal or near normal vascularization, indicating proportional growth of myocyte and vascular components. In contrast, the same stimulus in the adult stage results in decreasing capillary density as a reflexion of an inadequate vascular growth response [11].

SENESCENT STAGE

After a long and stable adult stage in which the growth characteristics are reasonably described by the allometric formula, the final, senescent stage is more labile. It

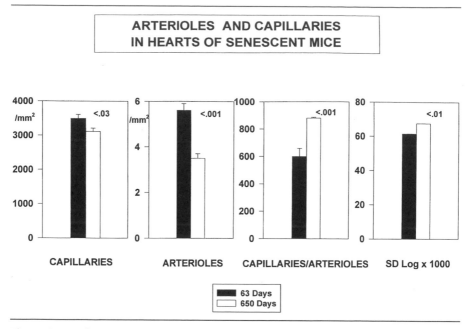

Figure 3. Morphometric data on vascularization of young and senescent mice hearts. SD log is an index of heterogeneity of capillary spacing. Based on data from Rakusan and Nagai [28].

is sometimes difficult to distinguish between signs of "normal aging" and those that reflect pathological events in senescence. The onset of this stage is poorly defined, depending on the species and its strain. In the case of most rat and mice strains, it starts around two years of age.

Senescent hearts are characterized by decreasing numerical densities of capillaries and arterioles. The decrease in coronary arteriolar density with aging is even more pronounced than the decrease in capillary density in murine, rat and canine hearts [26–28]. This is the result of the anatomical arrangement of the microvascular bed. The vast capillary network receives blood from several terminal arterioles and even when one arteriole becomes obliterated, perfusion of its respective capillaries can, to a large extent, be maintained by the remaining vessels of the network. The average size of arterioles in the senescent murine heart is therefore larger when compared to adult values. This is due to prevalence of larger vessels in the total population of arterioles, which is the result of disappearance of the smallest arterioles.

Typical results of morphometric analysis of senescent hearts are depicted in Fig. 3. This is based on our own analysis of the hearts from 63 and 650 days old mice [28]. The decrease in arteriolar numerical density exceeds the decrease in capillary density. Therefore, the number of capillaries per arteriole on a tissue cross-section increases significantly with age. The capillary bed becomes once again less regularly oriented in the senescent hearts, as reflected by a significant increase in heterogeneity of capillary spacing. Thus, changes in the coronary microvascular bed during aging seem to resemble a reverse picture to changes in neonatal hearts.

REFERENCES

1. Rakusan K, Turek Z. 1985. Protamine inhibits capillary formation in growing rat hearts. Circ Res 57:393–398.
2. Rakusan K. 1999. Vascularization of the heart during normal and pathological growth. In: Coronary Angiogenesis. Ed. K. Rakusan, 129–153. Stanford: JAI Press.
3. Heron MI, Rakusan K. 1995. Proliferating cell nuclear antigen (PCNA) detection of cellular proliferation in hypothyroid and hyperthyroid rat hearts. J Mol Cell Cardiol 27:1393–1403.812
4. Van Groningen JP, Wenink ACG, Testers LHM. 1991. Myocardial capillaries: increase in number by splitting of existing vessels. Anat Embryol 184:65–70.
5. Tomanek RJ, Doty MK, Snadra A. 1998. Early coronary angiogenesis in response to thyroxine. Growth characteristics and upregulation of basic fibroblast growth factor. Circ Res 82:587–593.
6. Porter GA, Bankston PW. 1987. Maturation of myocardial capillaries in the fetal and neonatal rat: An ultrastructural study with a morphometric analysis of the vesicle population. Am J Anat 178: 116–125.
7. Rakusan K, Cicutti N, Flanagan MF. 1994. Changes in the microvascular network during cardiac growth, development and aging. Cel Mol Biol Res 40:117–122.
8. Heron MI, Rakusan K. 1996. Short- and long-term effects of neonatal hypo- and hyperthyroidism on coronary arterioles in rat. Am J Physiol 271:H1746–H1754.
9. Heron MI, Kuo C, Rakusan K. 1999. Arteriolar growth in the postnatal rat heart. Microvasc Res 58:183–186.
10. Tomanek RJ. 1992. Age as a modulator of capillary angiogenesis. Circulation 86:183–186.
11. Rakusan K, Flanagan MF, Geva T, Southern J, Van Praag R. 1992. Morphometry of human coronary capillaries during normal growth and the effect of age in left ventricular pressure-overload hypertrophy. Circulation 86:38–46.
12. Rakusan K, Rochemont W, Braasch W, Tschopp H, Bing RJ. 1967. Capacity of the terminal vascular bed during normal growth, in cardiomegaly and in cardiac atrophy. Circ Res 21:209–215.
13. Tomanek RJ. 1989. Sympathetic nerves modify mitochondrial and capillary growth in normotensive and hypertensive rats. J Mol Cell Cardiol 21:755–764.
14. Flanagan MF, Fujii AM, Colan SD, Flanagan RG, Lock JE. 1991. Myocardial angiogenesis and coronary perfusion in left ventricular pressure overload hypertrophy in the young lamb. Circ Res 68: 1458–1470.
15. Godecke A, Flogel U, Zanger K, Ding K, Ding Z, Hirchenhain J, Decking U, Schrader J. 1999. Disruption of myoglobin in mice induces multiple compensatory mechanisms. Proc Nat Acad Sci USA 96:10495–10500.
16. Gerber HP, Hillian KJ, Ryan AM, Wright BD, Radtke F, Agnet M, Ferrara N. 1999. VEGF is required for growth and survival in neonatal mice. Development 126:1149–1159.
17. Engelmann GL, Dionne CA, Jaye MC. 1993. Acidic fibroblast growth factor and heart development. A role in myocyte proliferation and capillary angiogenesis. Circ Res 72:1285–1292.
18. Tomanek RJ, Haung L, Suvarna PR, O'Brien LS, Ratajska A, Sandra A. 1996. Coronary vascularization during development in the rat and its relationship to basic fibroblast growth factor. Cardiovasc Res 31:116–126.
19. Engelmann GL. 1993. Coordinate gene expression during neonatal rat heart development. A possible role for the myocyte in extracellular matrix biogenesis and capillary angiogenesis. Cardiovasc Res 27:1598–1605.
20. Everett AD, Fisher A, Tufro-Mc Reddie A, Harris M. 1997. Developmental regulation of angiotensin type 1 and 2 receptor gene expression and heart growth. J Mol Cell Cardiol 29:141–148.
21. Shanmugam S, Samberg K. 1996. Ontogeny of angiotensin II receptors. Cell Biol Int 20:169–176.
22. Korecky B, Rakusan K. 1978. Normal and hypertrophic growth of the rat heart: changes in cell dimensions and number. Am J Physiol 234:H123–H128.
23. Mattfeldt T, Mall G. 1987. Growth of capillaries and myocardial cells in the normal rat heart. J Mol Cell Cardiol 19:1237–1246.
24. Rakusan K, Jelinek J, Korecky B, Soukupova M, Poupa O. 1965. Postnatal development of muscle fibres and capillaries in the rat heart. Physiol Bohemoslov 14:32–37.

25. Wiest G, Gharehbaghi H, Amann K, Simon T, Masttfeldt T, Mall G. 1992. Physiological growth of arteries in the rat heart parallels the growth of capillaries, but not of myocytes. J Mol Cell Cardiol 24:1423–1431.
26. Anversa P, Capasso JM. 1991. Loss of intermediate-sized coronary arteries and capillary proliferation after left ventricular failure in rats. Am J Physiol 260:H1552–H1560.
27. Anversa P, Li P, Sonnenblick EH, Olivetti G. 1994. Effects of aging on quantitative structural properties of coronary vasculature in rats. Am J Physiol 267:H1062–H1073.
28. Rakusan K, Nagai J. 1994. Morphometry of arterioles and capillaries in hearts of senescent mice. Cardiovasc Res 28:969–972.

B. Ostadal, M. Nagano and N.S. Dhalla (eds.).
CARDIAC DEVELOPMENT. Copyright © 2002.
Kluwer Academic Publishers. Boston.

EXPRESSION OF ANGIOPOIETINS (-1 AND -2) IN EMBRYONIC RAT HEARTS DURING CORONARY VESSEL DEVELOPMENT

ANNA RATAJSKA,[1] MAŁGORZATA MYKA,[1] ELŻBIETA FIEJKA,[1] ALICJA JÓZKOWICZ, and JÓZEF DULAK

[1] Department of Pathological Anatomy, Medical University of Warsaw, Poland
[2] Department of Clinical Biochemistry, Collegium Medicum of Jagiellonian University in Krakow, Poland
[3] Institute of Molecular Biology, Jagiellonian University of Kraków, Poland and Department of Cardiology, University of Innsbruck, Austria

Summary. In order to characterize the temporal expression and localization of Ang-1 and Ang-2 during prenatal coronary neovascularization we studied rat hearts from the avascular stage (embryonic day ED12) until the end of the prenatal life (ED21). During the earliest stages of vascularization (ED13) angiopoietins (Angs) were distributed within the cells of atria and ventricles, subsequently (ED14–16) the prominent reaction was additionally found between cardiac myocytes (mostly around and/or within the capillary walls) and in the trabecular system of the heart. This immunostaining pattern persisted through the end of the prenatal life (ED17–21). Ang-1 and -2 immunoreactivity was absent within the cushion tissue and the heart valves, where vessels are not formed; the proteins were found neither within the walls of vessels with already developed media nor within the walls of the epicardial sinusoidal vessels devoid of pericytes/smooth muscle cells. Immunogold staining in transmission electron microscope indicate that Ang-1 and Ang-2 were localized within the wall of forming vessels: in the space between the endothelial cells and the mural cells. Western blot resulted in identification of the Ang-1 and Ang-2 proteins in the early, middle and late vascular hearts. RT-PCR with the primers for rat Ang-1 gene identified transcript of 160 bp length in hearts during the all neovascularization steps. Similarly, RT-PCR with Ang-2 designed primers identified a 330 bp fragment, which was expressed in the rat hearts during the stages of ED12–ED21. Our data indicate that both Angs are expressed during coronary vessel embryogenesis. Their spatial distribution and time course expression implicates their role in the maturation of the coronary vessel wall.

Corresponding author: Anna Ratajska, Department of Pathological Anatomy, Medical University of Warsaw, 02-004 Chałubińskiego 5, Warsaw, Poland. Tel: +48-22-628-10-41 ext. 73; Fax: +48-22-629-98-92; e-mail: arataj@ib.amwaw.edu.pl

Key words: Angiopoietin-1, Angiopoietin-2, Coronary vessel development, Rat, Embryonic heart

INTRODUCTION

Angiopoietin's (Ang) family of growth factors have been recently described to be involved in neovascularization during embryonic vessel development [1–4] and post-natal angiogenesis [5–9]. Ang-1 and Ang-2 are ligands for Tie-2 tyrosine kinase receptor on vascular endothelial cells and their precursors. Ang-1 stimulates angiogenic response by stabilizing the vessel wall and sustaining its survival [2]. Transgenic mice (ang-1$^{-/-}$) die on embryonic day (ED) 12.5 with the lack of the periendothelial cells and collagen fibers within the early vasculature in the head region of the embryo [2]. This indicates that Ang-1 plays a role in mediating reciprocal interaction between endothelium and the surrounding mesenchyme. Ang-1 deficient mouse exibit a lack of the heart trabecule compared with the wild type of animals. Ang-2, on the other hand acts as a natural antagonist of Ang-1 interaction with Tie-2 receptor [3]. While acting together with VEGF Ang-2 stimulates vessel growth and enhances an angiogenic response whereas in the absence of VEGF it hampers vascular growth and causes vessel regression [3,9]. VEGF has been already shown to play a role in coronary tube formation in vitro [10], and is spatially and temporally related with coronary vasculo- and angiogenesis [11].

Data on Angs expression and localization during distinct steps of coronary vessel development are lacking. Here we describe the Ang-1 and Ang-2 protein and gene expression and protein localization during embryonic heart development in rats compared with coronary vessels formation. We propose that Ang-1 and Ang-2 are temporally and spatially related to certain steps of the angiogenic cascade in the fetal heart.

MATERIALS AND METHODS

Animals and tissue harvesting

Rat pregnant dams at different gestational day were used for the experiments. The day 0 of pregnancy was established by the presence of spermatozoa in the early morning vaginal smear. The fetuses were removed from the uteri at different stages of heart development beginning from ED12 till the end of the fetal life (ED21). Ether and chloral hydrate anesthesia was used at the time of sacrifice. Hearts were dissected in Tris-Tyrode (pH 7.4) solution and collected and treated in four different ways:

1. formalin-fixed, dehydrated and routinely processed for paraffin embedding,
2. fixed in 4% paraformaldehyde for immuno-electron microscopy,
3. frozen, for Western blot,
4. immersed in denaturing solution (containing GTC—guanidinium thiocyanate, β-mercaptoethanol and N-laurosarcosyl) solution and kept frozen until RNA extraction.

Immunohistochemistry

Paraffin sections were deparaffinized in xylene, ethanol, washed in TBS (Tris buffered saline: 0.05 M Tris, 0.15 M NaCl, pH 7.8), microwaved 2 times in 10 mM citric acid buffer (pH 6.0), cooled and washed in TBS again. The sections were incubated overnight at 4°C with anti-angiopoietin-1 or -2 antibody (dilution 1:300 in TBS containing 1%BSA (bovine serum albumin) (Santa Cruz Biotechnology, Inc.). We utilized an affinity-purified goat polyclonal antibody to Ang-1 reacting with the epitope corresponding to amino acid sequence mapping at the carboxy terminus of the Ang-1, and anti-Ang-2 antibodies reacting with the epitope localized at the amino terminus of Ang-2. Then the sections were washed several times in TBS, and incubated for 30 min. with biotinylated anti-goat IgG (Sigma), (appropriate dilution in TBS with 1%BSA). After washing with TBS the sections were incubated with streptavidin-alkaline phosphatase complex (Sigma) in TBS, pH 7.8 containing 1%BSA, incubated for 30 min, and thoroughly washed in TBS. Subsequently substrate NBT/BCIP (Nitro Blue Tetrazolium Chloride and 3-Bromo-4-Chloro-3-Indoxyl Phosphate) (DAKO) was overlaid on sections and immunoreaction was assessed under the light microscope. Enzymatic reaction was stopped by immersing the slides in distilled water. Sections were mounted in glycerogel. For each set of staining the control slide was treated the same way except for the first step in which the primary antibody was omitted.

To mark the growing coronary vasculature an immunohistochemical staining was performed with *Griffonia simplicifolia I* lectin, a marker of endothelial cells in rodents [12,13].

Immunogold transmission electron microscopy

After fixation for 3 hours in 4% paraformaldehyde the hearts were rinsed in PBS, dehydrated in series of increasing ethanol concentrations and embedded in LRWhite resin (Polysciences). Polymerization was performed at 50°C for 24 hours. Ultrathin sections mounted on nickel grids were stained with anti-Ang-1 or anti-Ang-2 antibodies (1:300 dilution in PBS + 1%BSA), rinsed in PBS and then stained with anti-goat IgG gold (10 nm) conjugate (1:100 in PBS + 1%BSA). Subsequently grids were rinsed in PBS as above, air dried and contrasted with uranyl acetate. Negative control grids were always stained as above except for the omission of the primary antibody (anti-Ang-1 or Ang-2). Grids were viewed in JEOL S100 transmission electron microscope.

Western blot

Hearts were homogenized on ice in the presence of (lytic buffer) extracting 10 mM Tris-Cl buffer containing 1%Triton X-100, 1%deoxycholate and 0.1% SDS (sodium dodecyl sulphate) with protease inhibitor (1 µM PMSF = phenylmethylsulfonyl fluoride). Then the samples were centrifuged and electrophoresed on a 12% polyacrylamide gel, with protein content of 20 µg per lane; subsequently transferred to PVDF membranes (BioRad), and probed with anti-angiopoietin 1 or -Ang-2 antibodies raised in goat (Santa Cruz Biotechnology, Inc). An alkaline phosphatase anti-goat antibody (Santa Cruz Biotechnology, Inc) and BCIP/NBT (BioRad) reagent were used to visualize Ang-1 or Ang-2 specific bands. Control membranes were treated the same way except for the incubation with the primary antibody (which was omitted). To control the specificity of antibodies additional gels were run with the control peptides (Ang-1, and Ang-2, respectively at concentration of 50–100 ng per lane), transferred, and further the PVDF membranes incubated with the respective anti-Ang-1 and anti-Ang-2 antibodies. The specific bands were only observed with Ang-1 peptide and anti-Ang-1 antibody and Ang-2 peptide with anti-Ang-2 antibody. The cross-reactivity between Ang-1 peptide and Ang-2 antibody and Ang-2 peptide and anti-Ang-1 was never observed.

RT-PCR

Expression of Ang-1 and Ang-2 genes was tested by RT-PCR performed on 400 ng of total RNA. Total RNA was isolated from the embryonic hearts by guanidinium thiocyanate extraction according to Chomczyński and Sacchi [14]. The RNA concentration and purity were controlled spetrofotometrically by measuring its optical density at 260/280 nm. RNA was diluted in RNA-se free water and kept deep frozen. Reverse transcription PCR (RT-PCR) was performed using Access RT-PCR kit (Promega, Madison, USA). RT step (45 min) was performed at 48°C followed by 3 minute denaturation at 94°C. Subsequently 40 PCR cycles were performed at the temperature profile 94°C–30 sec, 57°C–30 sec and 68°C–30 sec for Ang-1 amplification and 94°C–30 sec, 65°C–30 sec, and 68°C for Ang-2 amplification. Final elongation was done at 68°C for 10 min.

The primers for rat Ang-1 and Ang-2 genes were designed on the basis of partial rat sequences deposited in the Gene Bank (accession No. AF030376 and AF030378, respectively). The sequence of the primers for Ang-1 were 5′-GAGATGGCCCA GATACAACAG for sense and 5′-GCAGTTGGATTTCAAGACGGG for antisense primer. The product length was 160 bp. The sequence for Ang-2 primers were 5′-TACAAAGAGGGCTTCGGGAGCCC and 5′-AGGACCACATGCGTCGAAC CACC for sense and antisense, respectively. The product length was 330 bp. Detection of rat GAPDH mRNA (PCR product 573 bp) was used as a control for RNA isolation. The PCR products stained with ethidium bromide were separated by the standard 3% agarose gel electrophoresis performed at 75 V. The detection of RNA was confirmed by negative results of PCR reaction when RT step was omitted and AMV reverse transcriptase was not included.

RESULTS

Immunohistochemistry

During the earliest stages of heart vascularization (ED13) both Ang-1 and Ang-2 antigens were distributed within the atria and the ventricles with a strong immunoreaction within the heart trabecule. Subsequently (ED14–16) a prominent staining was additionally found in the form of a punctate (patchy) pattern overlaid over the positively stained ventricular and atrial walls (Fig. 1). The immunoreactivity was

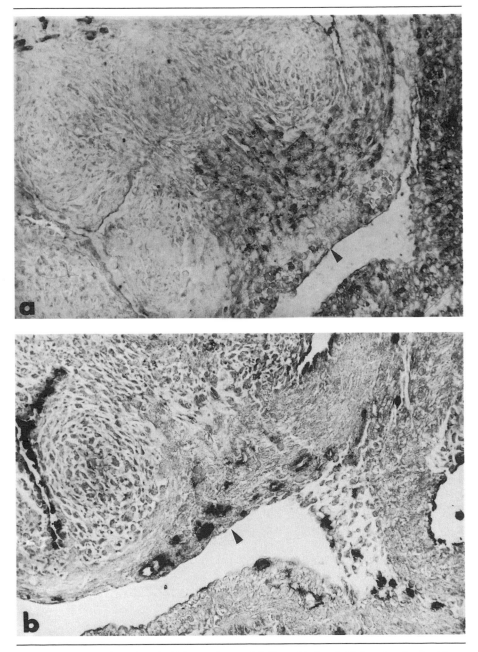

Figure 1. ED15 (a–b) and ED16 (c) hearts. Immunolabeling with Ang-1 (a), Ang-2 antibodies (c) and Griffonia simplicifolia I lectin (b). The latter specifically marks vessels. (a) and (b) are adjacent (consecutive) sections taken from the area of the outflow tract. Patchy character of staining with an intense immunolabeling in some areas prevails. Sinusoidal vessels (arrowheads in a and b) within the outflow tract and the cushion tissue are negative.

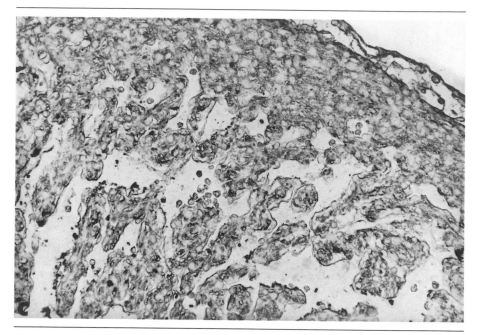

Figure 1. *Continued*

absent within the early vascular structures of the subepicardium (Fig. 1a) and in the media of the multilayered vascular walls. Similarly, the staining was absent within the cushion tissue and the heart valves, devoid of vasculature. During the late stages of embryonic life (ED17–21) Angs distribution was located within the myocardium of the ventricles and atria with a conspicuous, patchy character of staining. Epicardium was also positively stained with anti-angs antibodies.

Immunogold-TEM

In ED13 hearts immunolabeling with Ang-1 antibodies was only found within undifferentiated cardiac myocytes and mesenchymal cells. Similar distribution was observed with anti-Ang-2 antibodies.

In ED15 hearts immunogold particles of Ang-1 and Ang-2 specificity were found within cardiac myocytes and mesenchymal (endothelial-like cells, pericyte-like/smooth muscle-like). In addition, immunolabeling was found between cells of forming vessels within the immature connective tissue. In cardiac myocytes gold deposits were distributed between myofibrils and within the rough endoplasmic reticulum. The most intensive immunogold deposits were found in mesenchymal cells—endothelial-like cells of both Ang-1 and Ang-2 specificity (Fig. 2). They were localized mostly within the vesicles (Golgi and/or endoplasmic reticulum vesicles) indicating that both proteins were heavily expressed in synthetizing cells and/or in

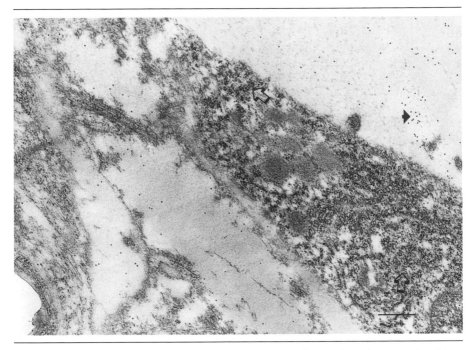

Figure 2. Mesenchymal cell of ED15 heart. Ang-1 is present in the cytoplasm (open arrow) and in the intercellular space (black arrow). Gold particles are distributed within the vesicles and the rough endoplasmic reticulum. Bar = 1 μm.

metabolically active cells. In the later stages of development (ED17 and ED19) distribution of angiopoietins was observed in cardiac myocytes, in adjacent endothelial cells of newly formed vessels and particularly in the space between the cells. After the contact between cells has been established the immunogold particles of Ang-1 and Ang-2 specificity were not found in the intercellular space. Within the forming vessel wall at the stage of mural cell attachment to the primitive endothelial cell the distribution of Angs was found in the space between interacting cells (Fig. 3). Such deposits were not found in areas outside of the lumen within the adventitia with mature collagen fibers.

Western blot

Angiopoietin—corresponding bands were consistently found in hearts beginning from the onset of vascularization (ED13) through the middle (ED14–16) till the late (ED17–21) stages of coronary vessel formation. Ang-1 was detected as two bands: of 70 kDa and weaker about 50 kDa; similarly, Ang-2 was detected as two bands: one with a strong staining intensity corresponding to 70 kDa and a weaker band migrating at 50 kDa (Fig. 4). In avascular hearts (ED12) both proteins were also detected.

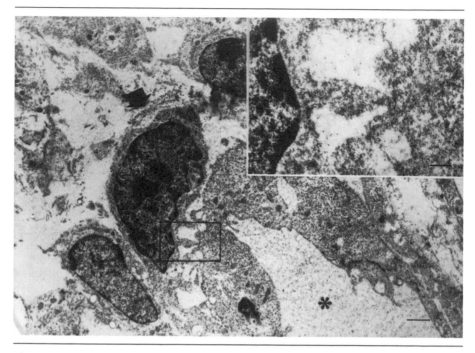

Figure 3. ED17 heart. The wall of a forming arteriole (asterisk) with the endothelial cell and the mural cell attaching to it; the latter cell marked by arrow. The boxed area is represented in insert. An intensive immunogold labeling with anti-Ang-1 antibodies in the space between these cells (between the cellular processes). Bar (picture) = 1 μm, (insert) = 0.6 μm.

RT-PCR

With the primers designed on the basis of rat sequences of Ang-1 gene the transcript of 160 bp was identified in the heart homogenates at all stages examined (ED12 till ED21). RT-PCR with Ang-2 gene primers identified fragment about 330 bp during the same studied stages (Fig. 5a,b).

DISCUSSION

This study is the first to demonstrate the Ang-1 and Ang-2 expression and distribution in the rat hearts compared to coronary vessel formation and differentiation.

Our immunohistochemical findings indicate that both angiopoietins (-1 and -2) are present in developing myocardium at the onset and during subsequent stages of the heart vascularization and their localization corresponds to the angiogenic areas within the heart. A detailed TEM immunogold labeling reveal that Ang-1 and Ang-2 are present in the sites of certain angiogenic activities, like intercellular interactions within the walls of the newly formed vessel: between endothelial cells and mural cells (of pericyte/smooth muscle cell) and between endothelial cells and the adjacent cardiac myocytes. The proteins were also found within the cytoplasm of

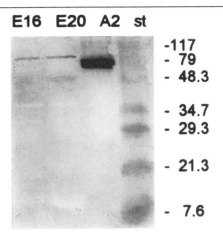

Ang-2

Figure 4. Western blot analysis demonstrating Ang-2 presence within the embryonic hearts at different stages of development (ED16 & ED20) compared with the carboxyterminal fragment of the purified Angiopoietin 2 (A2); st—molecular weight standards. The immunospecific bands occur as two isoforms: strong at about 70 kDa and weak at about 50 kDa. They correspond to glycosylated and unglycosylated form of angiopoietins.

developing cardiac myocytes and within the endothelial cells and mural cells themselves. The mRNA for Ang-1 and for Ang-2 are expressed before the onset of the heart vascularization and during all steps of the prenatal vascularization. Western blot exibits the expression of the immunoreactive proteins with both Ang-1 or Ang-2 antibodies in heart homogenates during all stages of heart vascularization.

Angiopoietins have been shown to activate differently the Tie-2 receptor: while Ang-1 appears to stimulate endothelial cell sprouting in vitro and in vivo [15,16] and to influence the vessel stability by recruitment of the periendothelial cells and interaction with the extracellular matrix [2], Ang-2 seems to inhibit the Ang-1-Tie-2 activation by receptor-dependent interaction [3,17]. Our detailed immunogold TEM staining indicates that at the onset of vascularization Angs are expressed only within cells while during the stage of an intense vasculogenic process (ED15) and late stages (ED17,19) both Angs are mostly found in the space between interacting cells (within the vessel wall and within the space between cardiac myocytes and the endothelial cells of capillaries). Since ED15 coronary vessels have been shown to acquire the second layer of cells (the primitive media) [18]. This would be consistent with the notion that Angs play a role in maturation and stabilization of the vessel wall when mural cells are attaching to the endothelial cell. Our immunogold studies confirm this hypothesis. In other reports Ang-1 has been found to influence the "sealing" of the vascular wall [19]. On the contrary Ang-2, in addition to being the Tie-2 receptor antagonist, when acting in the presence of VEGF Ang-2 stimulates angiogenesis, whereas in the absence

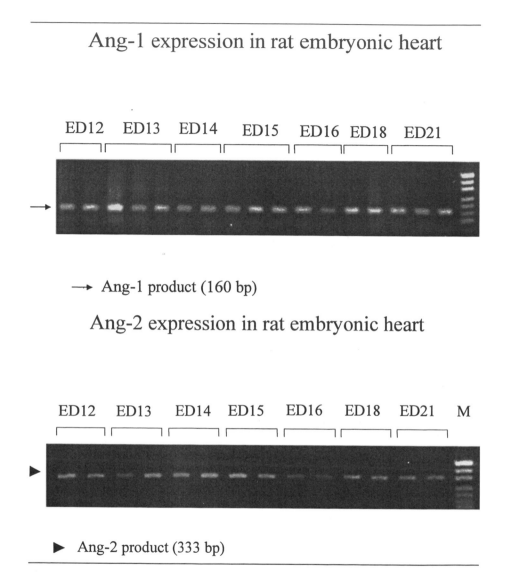

Ang-1 expression in rat embryonic heart

ED12 ED13 ED14 ED15 ED16 ED18 ED21

⟶ Ang-1 product (160 bp)

Ang-2 expression in rat embryonic heart

ED12 ED13 ED14 ED15 ED16 ED18 ED21 M

▶ Ang-2 product (333 bp)

Figure 5. RTPCR with Ang-1 (a) and Ang-2 (b) specific primers. The presence of mRNA is observed in all stages of heart vascularization and in avascular stage (ED12).

of VEGF Ang-2 may cause the vessel regression [5,17,20–22]. In our previous paper [11] we have already demonstrated that VEGF gene expression and protein distribution coincides with vasculogenic and angiogenic process of the fetal rat heart. In this study we have shown that angiopoietins are also expressed during the stages of coronary vessel development. These studies are consistent with the earlier suggestion that angiogenesis/vasculogenesis involves many growth factors which may interact in the specific time course [23,24]. According to our results they may interact in a specific spatial manner within the developing heart. The precise role of a particular molecule (Ang-1 or Ang-2) can not be exactly predicted within local environment since many other factors like presence of activators and inhibitors and local concentration of each [25] may differently influence the angiogenic cascade. RT-PCR study indicates that Ang-1 gene and Ang-2 gene expression are permanently found before the onset and during the vascularization steps of the embryonic hearts, which suggests that mRNAs are constantly synthetized in hearts or/and are very stable during second half of the prenatal life. Although an existence of Ang-1 splice variants has been reported in different cell cultures [26], the primers for the Ang-1 gene designed by us detected only a single band.

Ang-1 is considered to stimulate angiogenesis by modulating an interaction of endothelial cells with the other cellular components of the primitive vessel (mesenchymal, pericyte-like, smooth muscle-like) as well as with the extracellular matrix [26]. Our study demonstrates, that within the later stages of heart development the pattern of immunoreactive Ang-1 and Ang-2 is similar and corresponds to the pattern of VEGF distribution and coronary vessel formation. Similar pattern of Ang-1 and Ang-2 codistribution in highly vascularization sites has been reported to occur in pathologic postnatal angiogenesis [27].

Their presence within the particular time point and the spatial distribution of forming vascular wall (in the endothelial cells and their precursors as well as between endothelial cells and attaching mural cells) suggests that both factors are playing an important role in certain steps of neovascularization. For example, we have never observed in our study the Ang-1 and Ang–2 presence in sinusoidal vessels devoid of pericytes and in multilayered vessels with attached and differentiated smooth muscle cells of the media. These observations might support the above statement.

ACKNOWLEDGMENTS

The technical assistance of Anna Podbielska, Maria Michniewska and Jadwiga Powałko is greatly appreciated. The paper was supported by KBN grant (401/P05/97/13) and funds of the Medical University of Warsaw.

REFERENCES

1. Davis S, Aldrich TH, Jones PF, Acheson A, Compton DL, Jain V, Ryan TE, Bruno J, Radziejewski C, Maisonpierre PC, Yancopoulos GD. 1996. Isolation of angiopoietin-1, a ligand for the TIE2 receptor, by secretion-trap expression cloning. Cell 87:1161–1169.
2. Suri C, Jones PF, Patan S, Bartunkova S, Maisonpierre PC, Davis S, Sato TN, Yancopoulos GD. 1996. Requisite role of angiopoietin-1, a ligand for the TIE2 receptor, during embryonic angiogenesis. Cell 87:1171–1180.
3. Maisonpierre PC, Suri C, Jones PF, Bartunkova S, Wiegand SJ, Radziejewski C, Compton D, McClain J, Aldrich TH, Papadopoulos N, Daly TJ, Davis S, Sato TN, Yancopoulos GD. 1997. Angiopoietin-2, a natural antagonist for Tie2 that disrupts in vivo angiogenesis. Science 277:55–60.
4. Valenzuela DM, Griffiths JA, Rojas J, Aldrich TH, Jones PF, Zhou H, McClain J, Copeland NG, Gilbert DJ, Jenkins NA, Huang T, Papadopoulos N, Maissonpierre PC, Davis S, Yancopoulos GD. 1999. Angiopoietins 3 and 4: diverging gene counterparts in mice and humans. Proc Natl Acad Sci USA 96:1904–1909.

5. Asahara T, Chen D, Takahashi T, Fujikawa K, Kearney M, Magner M, Yancopoulos GD, Isner JM. 1998. Tie2 receptor ligands, angiopoietin-1 and angiopoietin-2 modulate VEGF-induced postnatal neovascularization. Circ Res 83:233–240.

6. Laurén J, Gunji Y, Alitalo K. 1998. Is angiopoietin-2 necessary for the initiation of tumor angiogenesis? Am J Pathol 153:1333–1339.

7. Mandriota SJ, Pepper MS. 1998. Regulation of angiopoietin-2 mRNA levels in bovine microvascular endothelial cells by cytokines and hypoxia. Circ Res 83:852–859.

8. Shyu K-G, Manor O, Magner M, Yancopoulos GD, Isner JM. 1998. Direct intramuscular injection of plasmid DNA encoding angiopoietin-1 but not angiopoietin-2 augments revascularization in the rabbit ischemic hindlimb. Circulation 98:2081–2087.

9. Holash J, Maisonpierre PC, Compton D, Boland P, Alexander CR, Zagzag D, Yancopoulos GD, Wiegand SJ. 1999. Vessel cooption, regression, and growth in tumors mediated by angiopoietins and VEGF. Science 284:1994–1998.

10. Ratajska A, Torry RJ, Kitten GT, Kolker SJ, Tomanek RJ. 1995. Modulation of cell migration and vessel formation by vascular endothelial growth factor and basic fibroblast growth factor in cultured embryonic heart. Dev Dyn 203:399–407.

11. Tomanek RJ, Ratajska A, Kitten GT, Yue X, Sandra A. 1999. Vascular endothelial growth factor expression coincides with coronary vasculogenesis and angiogenesis. Dev Dyn 215:54–61.

12. Alroy J, Goyal V, Skutelsky E. 1987. Lectin histochemistry of mammalian endothelium. Histochemistry 86:603–607.

13. Tomanek RJ, Haung L, Suvarna PR, O'Brien LC, Ratajska A, Sandra A. 1996. Coronary vascularization during development in the rat and its relationship to basic fibroblast growth factor. Cardiovasc Res 31:E116–E126.

14. Chomczyński P, Sacchi N. 1987. Single-step method of RNA isolation by acid guanidinium thiocyanate-phenol-chloroform extraction. Anal Biochem 162:156–159.

15. Koblizek TI, Weiss C, Yancopoulos GD, Deutsch U, Risau W. 1998. Angiopoietin-1 induces sprouting angiogenesis in vitro. Current Biol 8:529–532.

16. Suri C, McClain J, Thurston G, McDonald DM, Zhou H, Oldmixon EH, Sato TN, Yancopoulos GD. 1998. Increased vascularization in mice overexpressing angiopoietin-1. Science 282:468–471.

17. Davis S, Yancopoulos GD. 1999. The angiopoietins: yin and yang in angiogenesis. Curr Topisc Microbiol Immunol 237:173–185.

18. Ratajska A, Fiejka E. 1999. Prenatal development of coronary arteries in the rat: morphologic patterns. Anat & Embryol 200:533–540.

19. Thurston G, Suri C, Smith K, McClain J, Sato TN, Yancopoulos GD, McDonald DM. 1999. Leakage-resistant blood vessels in mice transgenically overexpressing angiopoietin-1. Science 286:2511–2514.

20. Goede V, Schmidt T, Kimmina S, Kozian D, Augustin HG. 1998. Analysis of blood vessel maturation processes during cyclic ovarian angiogenesis. Lab Invest 78:1385–1394.

21. Peters KG. 1998. Vascular endothelial growth factor and the angiopoietins. Working together to build a better blood vessel. Circ Res 83:342–343.

22. Holash J, Wiegand SJ, Yancopoulos GD. 1999. New model of tumor angiogenesis: dynamic balance between vessel regression and growth mediated by angiopoietins and VEGF. Oncogene 18:5356–5362.

23. Folkman J, D'Amore PA. 1996. Blood vessel formation: what is its molecular basis? Cell 87: 1153–1156.

24. Yancopoulos GD, Klagsbrun M, Folkman J. 1998. Vasculogenesis, angiogenesis, and growth factors: ephrins enter the fray at the border. Cell 93:661–664.

25. Drake CJ, Little CD. 1999. VEGF and vascular fusion: implications for normal and pathological vessels J Histochem Cytochem 47:1351–1355.

26. Huang YQ, Li JJ, Karpatkin S. 2000. Identification of a family of alternatively spliced mRNA species of angiopoietin-1. Blood 95:1993–1999.

27. Otani A, Takagi H, Oh H, Koyama S, Matsumura M, Honda Y. 1999 Expressions of angiopoietins and Tie-2 in human choroidal neovascular membranes. Invest Ophtalmol & Visual Science 40: 1912–1920.

B. Ostadal, M. Nagano and N.S. Dhalla (eds.
CARDIAC DEVELOPMENT. Copyright ©
Kluwer Academic Publishers. Boston.
All rights reserved.

THE DEVELOPMENT OF THE VENTRICULAR CONDUCTION SYSTEM: TRANSGENIC INSIGHTS

DIEGO FRANCO* and ANTOON F.M. MOORMAN

Experimental Molecular and Cardiology Group, Academic Medical Centre, University of Amsterdam, Amsterdam, The Netherlands

Summary. Over the last century, extensive literature has been devoted to the understanding of the origin of the cardiac conduction system. First descriptions suggested that the ventricular conduction has a myocardial origin, although more recently this common wisdom was challenged by the fact that several neural markers are specifically expressed in the developing conduction system, leading to the hypothesis of an extracardiac origin. Cell tracing experiments in chicken embryos have recently demonstrated a myocardial origin for several components of the ventricular conduction system, i.e. peripheral Purkinje network, although the origin of the bundle branches and the atrioventricular node remain controversial.

During the last years, the analysis of the transcriptional potential of truncated *cis*-acting elements of several gene loci have provided transgenic lines with restricted (compartment-specific) expression during cardiac development that can shed light into the developmental origin of distinct regions of the heart. A truncated human desmin promoter and a *KCNE1* knock-in transgene show that β-galactosidase expression is confined to the ventricular conduction system in the fetal/adult stage. In this study we have investigated the early expression profile of these two transgenic lines and compared them with the endogenous gene expression. Analyses of desmin transgenics reveal that myocardial cells from the early straight tube contribute to the atrioventricular node and the bundle branches, whereas *KCNE1*-transgenics reveal a substantial contribution of the interventricular ring to those structures. These

* Current address (author for correspondence): Diego Franco, Department of Experimental Biology, Faculty of Experimental and Health Sciences, Building B-3, University of Jaén, Paraje Las Lagunillas s/n, 23071 JAÉN, SPAIN. Phone: 34-953-002604; Fax: 34-953-012141; e-mail: dfranco@ujaen.es

data reinforce the notion that the atrioventricular node and bundle of His have a myocardial origin.

Key words: conduction system, KCNE1, desmin, transgenics

INTRODUCTION

Within the cardiac muscle two types of myocardial components are distinguished: the conduction system and the working atrial and ventricular myocardium. The adult conduction system is formed from separate morphological components which exert distinct functions. The sinoatrial (SAN) and atrioventricular (AVN) nodes are slow-conducting myocardial regions, whereas the atrioventricular bundle (bundle of His), the right and left bundle branches and the peripheral Purkinje fiber network (PPN), are fast-conducting pathways (see for a review 1).

In the early tubular heart ("primary myocardium"), no morphological components of the CS can be traced although there is already a leading pacemaker activity at the venous pole of the heart [2,3]. Soon after the atrial and ventricular chamber balloon out at the outer curvature of the heart [4] a sequential activation of the atria and ventricles can be recorded as an ECG [3]. The origin of the cardiac conduction system is still controversial. We have previously advocated that the atrioventricular node and the His bundle are derived from the "primary myocardium" (see e.g. 1,5). More recently, Gourdie et al. [6] have elegantly demonstrated by retroviral targetting that subendocardial Purkinje fiber cells share a common lineage origin with the working ventricular myocardial cells in chicken. Based on several studies in the rabbit heart, it was suggested that the atrioventricular node and the bundle of His have a neural crest origin [7–9].

In line with their distinct functional properties, the different components of the ventricular conduction system display specific patterns of gene expression (see for a review 1). Detailed analyses of the expression profile of sarcomeric genes have revealed that the conduction system myocytes share similar expression profile as the remnants of the "primary myocardium". However, the ventricular conduction system is more advanced with respect to the expression of connexins, suggesting that the 'electrical phenotype' is more developed. Recently, two transgenic mice models, a truncated human desmin promoter driving *nlacZ* reporter gene and a knock-in of the *KCNE1* gene, have been described to be specifically confined to the ventricular conduction system in mice [10,11]. However, detailed analyses of the embryonic expression profile have not been performed.

In the present study we have analysed the expression profile of the desmin–*nlacZ* and the *KCNE1-nlacZ* knock-in transgenics during embryonic cardiac development and compared with the endogenous gene. First expression of desmin–*lacZ* transgenes is observed within the cardiac crescent. Subsequently it becomes confined mostly to the outflow tract and interventricular ring. With further development, transgene expression is observed in scattered cells within the ventricular conduction system. A similar expression is observed for KCNE-*nlacZ*, although first expression of the transgene is only observed at E10.5, in line with the onset of the endogenous gene. These data indicate that precursors of the atrioventricular node and bundle of His are present as early as at the straight tubular stage, supporting the notion that these structures have a myocardial origin.

MATERIAL AND METHODS

Transgenic mice

The generation of desmin-*nlacZ* and minK-*lacZ* transgenic mice and their transgene expression pattern in adult heart have been previously described [10,11].

Embryos

Heterozygous and homozygous adult specimens, and embryos ranging from embryonic day (E) 7 to E18.5 for each transgenic line (CS7BL6/J background) were analysed. The day of plug was taken as E0.5. Embryos were excised from the uterus and the thoracic wall was removed (E12 to E16) exposing the heart to allow maximal penetrance of fixatives and reagents. Adult hearts were dissected at the arterial and venous pole of the heart, keeping intact the caval and pulmonary veins. Specimens were briefly fixed in 4% freshly prepared formaldehyde and rinsed twice in phosphate-buffered saline (PBS). Some specimens were rinsed in increasing sucrose gradients (10%, 20% and 30% in PBS) for 2 hours at each step, embedded in OCT (Miles Inc., USA) and frozen. Freeze cryotome serial sections of 7–10 µm were cut, mounted onto gelatin-coated slides, and stored at −20°C until use.

In toto X-gal histochemical staining

Specimens were briefly fixed in freshly prepared in 4% formaldehyde (30 min–1 hour) before histochemical detection of β-galactosidase. Incubation in X-gal solution at 37°C was performed for periods of 30 min to overnight as detailed elsewhere [12]. Subsequently, whole-mount embryos and adult hearts were postfixed in 4% freshly made formaldehyde for 4 hours to overnight and conserved in 70% ethanol until analysed.

β-galactosidase in cryosections

Sections were rinsed briefly in PBS and incubated at 37°C (1 hr–overnight) in X-gal reagent. After a brief rinse in PBS for 5 min, alternative sections were washed in bidistilled water for 5 min, counterstained with azofloxine or eosin (1%) for 5 min, dehydrated and mounted in Entellan (Merck).

Inmmunohistochemistry

Specific primary monoclonal antibody against desmin, human α-myosin heavy chain and β-myosin heavy chain [13] were used. The visualization of the primary antibody bindings was performed using a secondary antibody coupled to alkaline phosphatase as previously described [12].

Whole-mount in situ hybridization

Complementary RNA probes against mouse MLC2a [14] and MLC2v [15] and *KCNE1* (1–512 nt; 16,171) mRNAs were labeled with digoxigenin–UTP by *in vitro* transcription according to standard protocols [18]. Hybridisation conditions were as described by Moorman et al. [19].

RESULTS

Transgene expression in desmin-nlacZ mice

The first expression of the *nlacZ* reporter gene is observed at the cardiac crescent stage (E7.5) in desmin-*nlacZ* embryos. Scattered β-galactosidase positive cells are present in the left and right crescents (Fig. 1a). At the straight tubular stage, expression of β-galactosidase remains scattered along the entire cardiac tube (Fig. 1b). First signs of regionalized expression of the desmin-*nlacZ* transgenics is observed as the cardiac tube loops rightwards (E8.5–9.0). At this stage, β-galactosidase positive cells become confined to the most distal part of the outflow region and to the myocardium forming the interventricular groove (Fig. 1c). No positive cells can be observed in the atrial or ventricular chamber myocardium. With further development, as the heart acquires distinct right and left chambers (E12.5), the expression of the β-galactosidase reporter remains mainly confined to the distal outflow tract and the myocardium surrounding the interventricular junction (Fig. 1d,e). Analyses of cross sections demonstrate that most of the β-galactosidase positive cells are located in the subendocardial portion of the interventricular septum (Fig. 1f). In late embryonic (E14.5) and fetal (E16.5) stages, the expression of scattered positive cells can be observed in different components of the conduction system, i.e. atrioventricular node, bundle of His and bundle branches (Fig. 1g).

Endogenous desmin expression

The expression of desmin has been evaluated using immunohistochemistry in tissue sections. First expression of endogenous desmin is observed at the cardiac crescent stage [20]. At the embryonic stage (E10.5), expression of desmin is similar in distinct cardiac compartment. Within the ventricles the trabeculated component displays higher expression levels as compared with the compact myocardial component. With further development (E14.5 onwards), differential expression of desmin is observed between the right and left ventricles during embryonic and fetal stages (Fig. 1h). Interestingly, endogenous desmin expression is enhanced in the bundle branches (Fig. 1i) whereas the expression levels in the atrioventricular node and bundle of His are similar to those observed in the atrial and ventricular working myocardium.

→

Figure 1. Ventral views of whole-mount β-galactosidase staining of desmin-*nlacZ* transgenic embryos at E7.5 (A), E8.5 (B), E9.5 (C) and E12.5 (D). Transversal sections of desmin-*nlacZ* mouse embryos stained for β-galactosidase corresponding to E12.5 (E) and E16.5 (F) stages. Transversal sections of E16.5 mouse hearts stained immunohistochemically against desmin (G,H).

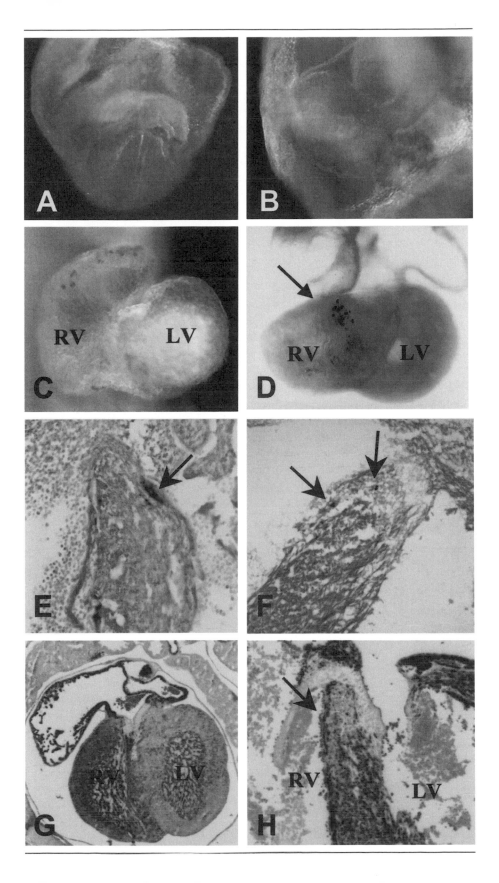

Transgene expression in KCNE1-nlacZ mice

First expression of the β-galactosidase reporter gene is observed at the embryonic heart stage (E10.5) in the *KCNE1-nlacZ* mice. β-galactosidase positive cells are mainly confined to the outflow tract, the myocardium of the interventricular junction and the atrioventricular canal (Fig. 2a,b). With further development (E12.5), the expression of the β-galactosidase reporter gene becomes confined to the outflow tract myocardium, the top of the interventricular septum extending to some degree into the septal trabeculations of both left and right cardiac chambers, and to the right atrioventricular junction (Fig. 2c,d). The expression pattern of the β-galactosidase reporter gene remains similar at later embryonic stages (E14.5). At fetal stages (E16.5), β-galactosidase positive cells are mainly restricted to distinct components of the conduction system; atrioventricular node, bundle of His and bundle branches, similar to the situation observed in adult stages (Fig. 2e,f). Some scattered positive cells can still be observed at this stage in the myocardium of the aortic and pulmonary outlets, reminiscent of the early expression in the developing outflow tract (data not shown).

Endogenous KCNE1 expression

The expression profile of *KCNE1* has been evaluated using whole-mount *in situ* hybridisation. First expression of *KCNE1* transcripts is observed in all myocardial compartments at the embryonic stage (E10.5). *KCNE1* transcripts display higher expression levels in the outflow tract myocardium as compared to the ventricular and atrial chambers [27]. With development (E12.5), expression of *KCNE1* becomes confined to the ventricular myocardium. Within the ventricular myocardium, *KCNE1* mRNA is highly expressed in the ventricular septum as compared to the right and left ventricular free walls. At E14.5, *KCNE1* transcripts become preferentially expressed in distinct components of the ventricular conduction system, i.e. atrioventricular node and bundle of His, although *KCNE1* remains to be expressed in the ventricular working myocardium (Fig. 2g,h). At fetal stages (E16.5), *KCNE1* is preferentially expressed in the compact myocardial layers of the ventricular chambers. Interestingly, similar levels of expression of *KCNE1* are observed in the ventricular conduction system at this stage, as compared with the surrounding ventricular working myocardium.

DISCUSSION

In the present study we show the distribution profile of two independent transgenic mice that are relevant for the understanding of the embryonic development of the

Figure 2. Ventral (A) and dorsal (B) views of whole mount β-galactosidase staining of KCNE1-*nlacZ* transgenic embryos at E10.5. Tranversal sections of KNCE1-*nlacZ* mouse embryos stained for β-galactosidase corresponding to E12.5 (C,D) and adult (E,F) stages. Distribution of KCNE1 transcripts in transverse sections corresponding to E12.5 mouse hearts (G,H).

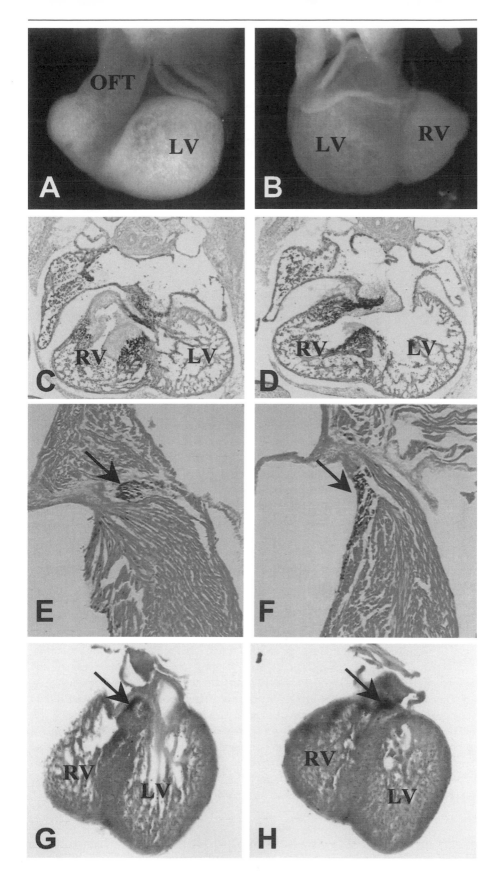

ventricular conduction system. The expression profile of desmin-*nlacZ* transgenics suggest that myocardial cells already present in the straight cardiac tube contribute to specific regions of the embryonic heart tube characterized by a slow conduction. During late embryonic stages, desmin-*nlacZ* transgenics display an expression profile of the β-galactosidase mainly restricted to the atrioventricular node and bundle of His. Secondly, the expression profile of KCNE1-*nlacZ* transgenic mice is also restricted to the slow conducting components of the embryonic heart and with further development, becomes confined preferentially to the conduction system. These data support the notion that distinct components of the conduction system are derived from myocardial precursors.

Recently, Gourdie et al. [6] have convincingly demonstrated that peripheral Purkinje fibers share their developmental origin with normal working ventricular myocardial cells by retroviral labelling. However, discrepancies still emerge regarding the developmental origin of the atrioventricular node, bundle of His and bundle branches [21]. In an attempt to discern their developmental origin, Cheng et al. [22] have performed retroviral labelling experiments in early developing chicken embryos. Injections with retroviruses at embryonic stages (HH14) led to few positive cells in the atrioventricular ring and bundle of His of fetal chicken hearts (HH39). Based on these results, these authors suggested that the atrioventricular node and bundle of His are formed by local recruitment of myocytes that do not originate from the slow components of the embryonic heart. Our results with the desmin-*nlacZ* and KCNE1-*nlacZ* can be compared to those originated with the retroviral experiments, keeping in mind the caveat of using transgenic mice as molecular markers. Expression of desmin-*nlacZ* transgene in the early tubular heart comprises the entire myocardial component but, with further development, the transgene expression in the embryonic heart is confined to the outflow tract and interventricular ring. Furthermore, only scattered cells can be discerned in the fetal conduction system in desmin-*nlacZ* embryos (similar to the retroviral experiments). An alternative explanation to that of Cheng et al. [22] is derived from the fact that slow conducting regions such as the outflow tract, inner curvature and atrioventricular canal [23–25] display lower rates of division than the surrounding fast-conducting atrial and ventricular chamber myocardium [26]. Therefore, the relative contribution of the slow conducting regions to the formed heart is, of necessity, smaller to that of the fast conducting regions. In this line of thinking, it is therefore not surprising that the primordial contribution of the straight myocardial tube and the slow conducting components of the embryonic heart to distinct components of the formed ventricular conduction system is limited. They can be therefore missed by targeting experiments, although this fact does not exclude a direct contribution of the straight tube to the atrioventricular canal and bundle of His.

The profile of transgene expression in desmin-*nlacZ* and the KCNE1-*nlacZ* embryos is comparable at similar developmental stages, reinforcing the notion that the same myocardial regions of the embryonic heart (i.e. interventricular ring) contribute to specific components of the ventricular conduction system. The differences on the onset of transgene expression between desmin-*nlacZ* and KCNE1-*nlacZ* might be related to distinct temporal expression of their respective endogenous genes. Desmin is expressed already at the cardiac crescent stage [20] whereas KCNE1 is first observed at the embryonic stage (27; this study). Secondly, the confinement of desmin-*nlacZ* driven transgene expression to distinct areas of the embryonic heart and fetal conduction system might related to the fact that a truncated promoter of the human desmin gene is used in these transgenics [10], which might only be able to active expression in those regions in which the endogenous gene is highly expressed. On the other hand, the restricted expression profile of β-galactosidase to the developing ventricular conduction system in KCNE1-*nlacZ* transgenics is more difficult to reconcile with the endogenous expression profile [11]. In fact, the generation of a knock-in strategy would imply that the expression profile of the reporter gene should be similar to the endogenous gene. We observed several discrepancies between endogenous KCNE1 and KCNE1-*nlacZ* driven β-galactosidase expression, which leads to the hypothesis that sequences located in the KCNE1 coding sequence might play a role on its own regulation.

ACKNOWELEDGMENTS

We are indebted with S. Kupershmidt and D. Roden for kindly providing the KCNE1-*nlacZ* transgenics, and with Z. Li and D. Paulin for kindly providing the desmin-*nlacZ* transgenics. We will to thank C. de Gier-de Vries for excellent technical assistance and C. Hersbach for excellent photographic help. D. Franco is supported by NWO (902-16-219) and the Dutch Heart Foundation (97206).

REFERENCES

1. Moorman AFM, de Jong F, Denyn MMFJ, Lamers WH. 1998. Development of the conduction system. Circ Res 82:629–644.
2. Kamino K, Hirota A, Fujii S. 1981. Localization of pacemaking activity in early embryonic heart monitored using voltage-sensitive dye. Nature 290:595–597.
3. Van Mierop LHS. 1967. Localization of pacemaker in chick embryo heart at the time of initiation of heartbeat. Am J Physiol 212:407–415.
4. Christoffels VM, Habets PEMH, Franco D, Campione M, de Jong F, Lamers WH, Bao Z-Z, Palmer S, Biben C, Harvey RP, Moorman AFM. 2000. Chamber formation and morphogenesis in the developing mammalian heart. Dev Biol 223:266–278.
5. Moorman AFM, Lamers WH. 1994. Molecular anatomy of the developing heart. Trends Cardiovasc Med 4:257–264.
6. Gourdie RG, Mima T, Thompson RP, Mikawa T. 1995. Terminal diversification of the myocyte lineage generates Purkinje fibers of the cardiac conduction system. Development 121:1423–1431.
7. Gorza L, Saggin L, Sartore S, Ausoni S. 1988. An embryonic-like myosin heavy chain is transiently expressed in nodal conduction tissue of the rat heart. J Mol Cell Cardiol 20:931–941.
8. Gorza L, Vitadello M. 1989. Distribution of conduction system fibers in the developing and adult rabbit heart revealed by an antineurofilament antibody. Circ Res 65:360–369.
9. Gorza L, Vettore S, Vitadello M. 1994. Molecular and cellular diversity of heart system myocytes. Trends Cardiovasc Res 4:153–159.
10. Li Z, Marchard P, Humbert J, Babinet C, Paulin D. 1993. Desmin sequence elements regulating skeletal muscle-specific expression in transgenic mice. Development 117:947–959.
11. Kupershmidt S, Yang T, Anderson ME, Wessels A, Niswender KD, Magnuson MA, Roden DM. 1999. Replacement by homologous recombination of the minK gene with lacZ reveals restriction of minK expression to the mouse cardiac conduction system. Circ Res 84:146–152.

12. Franco D, de Boer PAJ, de Gier-de Vries C, Lamers WH, Moorman AFM. 2001. Methods on in situ hybridization, immunohistochemistry and β-galactosidase reporter gene detection. Eur J Morphol 39:3–25.

13. Wessels A, Vermeulen JLM, Virágh S, Kálmán F, Lamers WH, Moorman AFM. 1991. Spatial distribution of "tissue specific" antigens in the developing human heart and skeletal muscle: II. An immunohistochemical analysis of myosin heavy chain isoform expression patterns in the embryonic heart. Anat Rec 229:355–368.

14. Kubalak SW, Miller-Hance WC, O'Brien TX, Dyson E, Chien KR. 1994. (1994) Chamber specification of atrial myosin light chain-2 expression precedes septation during murine cardiogenesis. J Biol Chem 269:16961–16970.

15. O'Brien TX, Lee KJ, Chien KR. 1993. Positional specification of ventricular myosin light chain 2 expression in the primitive murine heart tube. Proc Natl Acad Sci USA 90:5157–5161.

16. Lesage F, Attali B, Lazdunski M, Barharin J. 1992. IsK, a slowly activating voltage-sensitive K+ channel. Characterization of multiple cDNAs and gene organization in the mouse. FEBS Lett 301:168–172.

17. Demolombe S, Franco D, de Boer P, Kupershmidt S, Roden D, Pereon Y, Jarry A, Moorman AFM, Escande D. 2001. Differential expression of KvLQT1 and its regulator IsK in mouse epithelia. Am J Physiol 280:C359–372.

18. Hogan B, Beddington R, Costantini F, Lacy E. 1994. In: *Manipulating the mouse embryo* Cold Spring Harbor Laboratory Press.

19. Moorman AFM, Houweling AC, de Boer PAJ, Christoffels VM. 2001. Sensitive Nonradioactive detection of mRNA in tissue sections: novel application of the whole-mount in situ hybridization protocol. J Histochem Cytochem 49:1–8.

20. Schaart G, Viebahn C, Langmann W, Ramaekers F. 1989. Desmin and titin expression in early postimplantation mouse embryos. Development 107:585–596.

21. Gourdie RG, Kubalak S, Mikawa T. 1999. Conducting the embryonic heart: orchestrating development of specialized cardiac tissues. Trends Cardiovasc Res 9:18–26.

22. Cheng G, Litchenberg WH, Cole GJ, Mikawa T, Thompson RP, Gourdie RG. 1999. Development of the cardiac conduction system involves recruitment within a multipotent cardiomyogenic lineage. Development 126:5041–5049.

23. De Jong F, Opthof T, Wilde AAM, Janse MJ, Charles R, Lamers WH, Moorman AFM. 1992. Persisting zones of slow impulse conduction in developing chicken hearts. Circ Res 71:240–250.

24. Moorman AFM, Vermeulen JML, Koban MU, Schwartz K, Lamers WH, Boheler KR. 1995. Patterns of expression of sarcoplasmic reticulum Ca^{2+}ATPase and phospholamban mRNAs during rat heart development. Circ Res 76:616–625.

25. Moorman AFM, Schumacher CA, de Boer PAJ, Hagoort J, Bezstarosti K, van den Hoff MJB, Wagenaar GTM, Lamers JMJ, Wuytack F, Christoffels VM, Fiolet JWT. 2000. Presence of functional sarcoplasmic reticulum in the developing heart and its confinement to chamber myocardium. Dev Biol 223:279–290.

26. Thompson RP, Soles-Rosenthal P, Cheng G. 2000. Origin and fate of cardiac conduction tissue. In: 5th International Symposium on Etiology and Morphogenesis of congenital Heart Disease. EB Clark, A Takao (Eds). 2000. Futura Publishing Co., Armonk, NY.

27. Franco D, Demolombe S, Kupershmidt S, Roden D, Escande D, Moorman AFM. 2001. Divergent expression domains of K+ channel (I_{Ks} and I_{Kr}) subunits during mouse heart development. Cardiovasc Res 52:65–75.

B. Ostadal, M. Nagano and N.S. Dhalla (eds.).
CARDIAC DEVELOPMENT. Copyright © 2002.
Kluwer Academic Publishers. Boston.
All rights reserved.

CELL INTERACTIONS WITH EXTRACELLULAR MATRIX DURING PERINATAL DEVELOPMENT OF MYOCARDIUM

JANE-LYSE SAMUEL, PHILIPPE RATAJCZAK, and LYDIE RAPPAPORT

Unité 127 INSERM, IFR Circulation, Université D Diderot, Hôpital Lariboisière, 41 bd de la Chapelle, Paris 75475 France

Summary. Cardiac morphogenesis is dependent on the coordinated and programmed expression of cell surface receptors that can mediate interactions of cells with extracellular matrix (ECM) components, which in turn promote either cell adhesion or migration and determine the phenotype. Besides, the role of the membrane receptors as anchoring proteins for cytoskeleton appears prominent, the complex being implicated in different intracellular signaling cascades. A broad range of cellular processes involved in ontogenesis including, cell proliferation, growth and differentiation depend on cytokines but also on the nature of ECM components, ECM-activated receptors, induced alterations in cytoskeleton elements and transducing signals.

During perinatal myocardial growth, cardiomyocytes rapidly loose their ability to multiply and they hypertrophy, fibroblasts proliferate; the composition of the interstitial tissue varies and accompanies the remodeling of the arterial wall. It is not clear yet at which extend the expression of adhesive proteins such as fibronectin, laminin, cell surface receptors, (integrins and dystroglycans), and cytoskeleton associated proteins (vinculin, FAK, dystrophin) is coordinated and programmed in myocardium during the perinatal period of growth. We'll review the present knowledge concerning the expression of some of these proteins during perinatal cardiac growth.

Key words: fibronectin, integrins, desmin, laminin, heart

Corresponding author: L Rappaport, Unité 127 INSERM, IFR Circulation, Université D. Diderot, Hôpital Lariboisière, 41 bd de la chapelle, Paris 75475 France. Tel: 33 (1) 44-63-17-40/21; Fax: 33 (1) 48-74-23-15; e-mail: lydie.rappaport@inserm.lrb.ap-hop-paris.fr

Cardiac morphogenesis is dependent on the coordinated and programmed expression of cell surface receptors that can mediate cell-cell associations and interactions of cells with extracellular matrix (ECM) components, which in turn promote either adhesion or migration and determine cell phenotype. Besides, the role of the membrane receptors as anchoring proteins for cytoskeleton being implicated in multiple interaction sites and different intracellular signalling cascades appears more and more prominent [1]. A broad range of cellular processes involved in development, including, proliferation, cell growth and differentiation, apoptosis depend on cytokines but also notably on the nature of ECM components, ECM-activated receptors, induced alterations in cytoskeleton elements and transducing signals.

During perinatal myocardial growth, cardiomyocytes rapidly loose their ability to multiply and they hypertrophy, fibroblasts proliferate; the composition of the interstitial tissue varies and accompanies the remodeling of the arterial wall. At which extend the expression of components of ECM adhesive proteins (fibronectin, laminin, proteoglycans, etc), cell surface receptors, (integrins and dystroglycans), and cytoskeleton associated proteins (vinculin, FAK, dystrophin) is coordinated and programmed during the fetal and postnatal development of the heart is not clear yet. We'll review the present knowledge concerning the expression of some of these components during perinatal cardiac growth.

EXTRACELLULAR MATRIX ADHESIVE PROTEINS

Adhesive proteins constitute with ECM proteins a network surrounding and supporting myocardial constitutive cells. Adhesive proteins such as laminin, fibronectin, type IV and VI collagens are closely related to proteoglycans and metalloproteinases [2,3] and their interactions with cell membrane receptors activate communication between the extracellular and intracellular environment and favor cell adhesion [4,5]. Proteoglycans contribute to the architecture of the extracellular matrix network, bind growth factors and promote tissular remodeling and cell migration [6].

The ability of the cells constitutive of the myocardium to synthesize adhesive matrix components strongly differs. Fibroblasts and smooth muscle cells (SMCs) produce and release type III collagen and fibronectin (FN); myocytes and endothelial cells produce types IV and VI collagens. Laminin is synthetized by SMC, cardiac myocytes and endothelial cells.

Both the expression and distribution of isoforms of major adhesive proteins vary during heart development in a specific manner [7]. In the rat, type 1 collagen predominates, whatever the phase of the development, while type III collagen progressively increases in the first months of life. In fetal rat hearts, the procollagen III mRNAs are mostly abundant in the epicardium and in aortic valves. Ultrastructural analysis from mutant mice reveals that type III collagen is essential for normal collagen I fibrillogenesis in the cardiovascular system [8].

Fibronectin is initially secreted from the cell as a soluble protein within extracellular matrix. Fibronectin protomers polymerize to form insoluble multimeric FN. Only this insoluble and fibrillar FN can act as an adhesive ligand and regulate cell function. In contrast with other ECM components, FN polymerization requires specific cellular interactions with cell surface receptors, involves actin and microtubule cytoskeleton and Rho family of small GTPases [9]. Three regions of alternative splicing, that are not expressed in adult, have been described in rodents and humans.

In embryo, in rat [10] as in human [11], mRNAs coding for FN are abundant in epicardial interstitial cells and in endocardial endothelial cells. Few days before birth, when vasculogenesis develops, FN mRNAs and protein increase in coronary arterie SMCs. Then their expression progressively decreases in postnatal life and in the adult [12]. Quantitative expression of total FN mRNAs in the rat myocardium is abundant in the embryo, decreases in the fetus and in postnatal life, and reaches a level which is 10 fold less in the adult compared with the fetus. The two alternately spliced isoforms EIIIA and EIIIB, which represent more than 40% of FN mRNAs in the early stages of fetal development, decrease progressively in a parallel manner during intra-uterine and postnatal life, to represent less than 10% of total FN mRNAs in the adult. In fact, FN isoforms EIIIA and EIIIB mRNAs appear as markers of a cardiac immature phenotype, whatever the cell type. However, the control of growth and differentiation in the rat heart seems to depend mostly on plasmatic FN (p-FN). Indeed, in FN knockout mice, p-FN of maternal origin is sufficient to allow the early stages of a normal differentiation in the embryonic heart [13].

Laminins are a large family of heterotrimeric extracellular matrix proteins that, in addition to having structural roles, take part in the regulation of processes such as cell migration, differentiation, and proliferation. The protein is composed of three associated chains (α, β and γ), encoded by different genes. Laminin includes functional domains that bind collagen IV, nidogen, proteoglycans and transmembrane receptors [2]. At the membrane level, depending on its isoforms, the laminin, can bind to integrins or other receptors, such as dystroglycans.

In the heart, laminin is a structural component of the basal membrane forming one of the links between extracellular domains and the cytoskeleton and/or myofibrils in the cardiomyocytes. Laminin 2, also called merosin ($\alpha 2$, $\beta 1, \gamma 1$), predominates and a deficiency in its expression is characterized by a loss of cytoskeleton-extracellular matrix linkage, that results in a muscular dystrophy and dilated cardiomyopathy [14,15]. The laminin $\alpha 4$ chain associates to chain β and γ to form laminins 8 and 9. In the developing rat heart, laminin 2 is poorly expressed in the fetus, but accumulates during post-natal growth and then decreases between 3 and 30 weeks of age. Similarly, in human, the level of $\alpha 2$ mRNA decreases progressively during post-natal life [16]. The protein binds to integrin alpha 6 beta 1 [17]. In human aorta, SMC maturation is marked by a transition in the expression of laminin isoforms from $\alpha 1 \beta 1 \gamma 1$ to $\alpha 1 \beta 2 \gamma 1$ [18].

Taken together, the expression of adhesive proteins varies in a specific manner, depending on the stage of ontogenic development. The abundance of FN mRNAs in the rat heart at the embryonic stage corresponds to the phase of cell proliferation and migration, while the increase and/or the decrease in laminin and collagen at the perinatal stage are associated with heart growth.

Several experimental evidences suggest that adhesive proteins, such as laminin and FN, whose synthesis and deposition are influenced by mechanical stretch and mediated by growth factors [19] may in turn have diverse effects on cell growth and

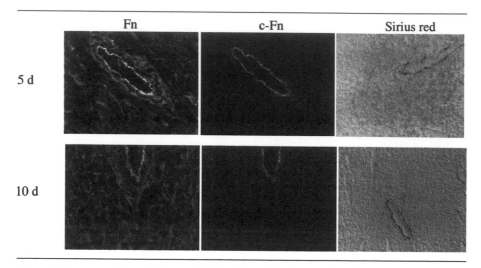

Figure 1. Immunostaining of fibronectin either plasmatic (Fn) or newly synthetized (cFn) in 5 day and 10 day old rat myocardium. Note the absence of collagen (Sirius red) and the distribution of c-Fn at the level of the only endothelial cells at these stages. (Objectives ×20)

modulate cells phenotype [20]. Antibodies directed against the FN arginine-glycine-aspartic acid fragment, the RGD peptide, block this property. The interaction of this fragment with extracellular matrix integrins results in the activation of the extracellular signal–regulated kinase ERK2 and c-Jun NH2-terminal kinase (JNK) in rat cardiac fibroblasts. This signaling pathway is initiated by mechanical stretch and is matrix-specific and integrin dependent [21,22]. Plating of SMCs on FN shifts their phenotype towards a less mature type, that is associated with changes in integrin activity and signaling pathways, modulating cell proliferation and migration [23]. Laminin mediates cell processes with opposite characterisitics and specificity than those depending on FN [20,24]. Rat fetal cardiac myocytes, that do not synthesize their own matrix, adhere to FN, collagen-I and -III, whereas isolated adult cardiac myocytes preferentially adhere to laminin and collagen IV [24]. Type IV collagen favors endothelial cells migration and this process is partially prevented by laminin and matrigel.

Tenascins are a family of large multimeric extracellular matrix proteins, including tenascin-C (TN-C), tenascin-R, and tenascin-X (TN-X), the later being predominantly expressed in heart and skeletal muscle [25]. TN-X protein, but not TN-C, binds to heparin, FN, laminin or collagens and is associated with the extracellular matrix of muscle tissues and blood vessels [26]. During development, TN-X expression begins in migrating cells of the epicardium in the E12 heart in rat. After epicardium is complete, TN-X is expressed in the sub-epicardial space in association with developing blood vessels and later by non-myocyte cells dispersed through the myocardial wall, thus suggesting a role in connective tissue cell migration and late muscle morphogenesis [27]. *In vitro*, TN-C mRNA and protein accu-

	5 days	10 days

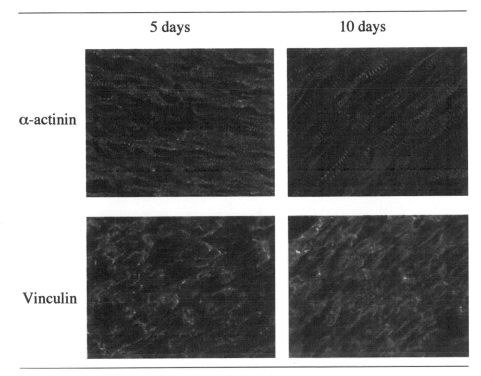

Figure 2. Distribution of α-actinin and vinculin throughout myocardium of 5 and 10 day old rats. Note the increase in size of the myocytes. (Objectives ×20)

mulations are induced by mechanical strain in neonatal rat cardiomyocytes, in an amplitude-dependent manner. Stimulation occurs through a nuclear factor-kappaB-dependent and an angiotensin II independent mechanism [28].

Thrombospondin is an adhesive glycoprotein that plays a role in tissue genesis and repair and angiogenesis. Cardiac myocytes show positive staining for thrombospondin at day 10 of gestation and this expression continues throughout development of the myocardium, together with that of one of its receptors syndecan [29].

Metalloproteinases (MMP) are a family of multigenic proteins that favor or inhibit matrix degradation and thus play an important role in cardiac remodeling [30]. Collagenases (MMP-1) cleave collagens in fragments that constitute the substrate of other, less specific proteases, such as gelatinases (MMP-2), responsible for the degradation of type IV collagen and FN [31]. The presence of collagenases and interleukin-1alpha has been detected on the surface of cardiomyocytes and mesenchymal cells at times when the heart is undergoing acute remodeling during septation and trabeculation [32]. However, transgenic mice with constitutive expression of human collagenase (MMP-1) appeared normal at birth until weaning, when compared with their wild-type littermates. However they had a 25% increase in mortality rate over 6 months and compensatory cardiomyocyte hypertrophy with an increased expres-

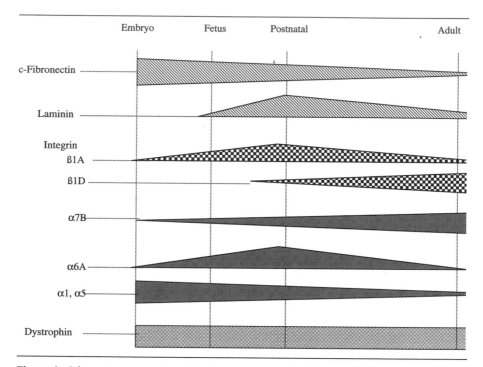

Figure 3. Schematic representation of the timing expression of two adhesive proteins (fibronectin and laminin), integrin chains, and a cytoskeletal protein (dystrophin) in developing heart. The schema is based on data of the litterature that are cited in the text.

sion of collagen type-III. At 12 months of age, the chronic expression of MMP-1 produced a loss of interstitial collagen associated with a disruption of the myocardial extracellular matrix that coincided with a deterioration of systolic and diastolic function and progressive heart failure [33].

ADHESIVE PROTEIN RECEPTORS

Integrins and dystroglycans are mechanoreceptors that transduce mechanical forces and changes in ECM and adhesive structures, through signals from the extracellular compartment to the cytoskeleton and viceversa, see for a review [22]. Binding of extracellular matrix proteins to their receptors induces the activation of kinases and ionic channels and the reorganization of cytoskeletal proteins in a focal adhesion region. Integrin activation also induces the synthesis of metalloproteinases, collagens, and gelatinases, which regulate the synthesis and type of extracellular matrix proteins. Thus, by connecting the cytoskeleton to the extracellular matrix and mediating cell-matrix interactions, integrins control cell ability to perceive its environment, to respond to changes in its environment, to alter its environment

[3] and to participate to cell motility, division, differentiation and programmed death [34].

Integrins are a family of transmembrane proteins composed of heterodimers of multiple isoforms of two covalently bound different chains, alpha (120–150 kDa) and beta (110–190 kDa) that are coded by different genes [5]. With their extracellular domain they bind extracellular and cell surface molecules and with their cytoplasmic domains they bind to cytoskeletal and signaling proteins, thus mediating transmembrane signaling from extracellular environment and vice versa. Integrins that are not bound to ECM ligands are generally distributed diffusely over the cell surface and appear not to be linked to the cytoskeleton [35]. The affinity of integrins to their ECM ligands is low (Kd 10^{-6} M), but ligands have a high density (10^5–10^6 molecules per cell). Alternative splicing leads to variations in the sequence of both extra and intra cellular domains and many integrin splice variants are specifically expressed in tissues and during development. Their expression is cell and ligand specific, several integrins being able to bind a same component of the ECM.

In heart muscle, cytoplasmic domain variants include members of the beta-1, beta-3, beta-4, alpha-3, alpha-6 and alpha-7 subtypes, but little information is available on the expression pattern of integrins during the transition from active cardiomyocyte proliferation to terminal differentiation. Cell-matrix interactions via beta-1 integrins appear necessary for differentiation and maintenance of a specialized phenotype of cardiac muscle cells [36] and for the maintenance of myofibrillar organization [37]. Beta-1 integrin blocking antibodies arrested the cell cycle at the fetal but not at the neonatal stage of development, thus suggesting that cell attachment via beta-1 integrins is involved in regulation of cell cycle [38]. Adenovirus-mediated overexpression of beta-1 integrin increases the hypertrophic response of neonatal rat ventricular myocytes to catecholamines, while suppression of integrin signaling by overexpression of free beta-1 integrin cytoplasmic domain inhibits this response [39]. Integrin beta-1A isoform is widely expressed in non muscle cell types and is present in fetal striated muscle cells including cardiomyocytes, whereas integrin beta-1D isoform is specifically expressed in cardiac and skeletal muscle cells of adult mammals. Integrin beta-1D isoform is localized near the Z lines [40] and mechanical forces stabilize its cellular level together with that of vinculin, possibly through the formation and maintenance of focal adhesion and costameres [41]. Thus, beta-1D isoform could increase ligand binding and FN matrix assembly and contribute to contraction by reinforcing the cytoskeleton-matrix linkage [42]. Beta-1D integrin subunit would be less efficient than beta-1A in mediating the signaling that regulates cell motility and responses of cells to mechanical stress [43]. *In vitro,* integrin beta-1A, and at a lesser extend beta-1D, are able to activate integrin-mediated signaling via FAK [40], but it remains to determine whether beta-1D isoform transmits in cardiac myocytes different signals from those transmitted by beta-1A in non muscle cells [44]. Inactivation of integrin beta-1D subunit, in knockout studies, induces a mild cardiomyopathy [42]. Changes in the expression of the beta-1A and beta-1D isoforms during cardiac development may be associated to the changes in cellular attachment and intracellular signaling, responsible for the diminished proliferative potential of cardiomyocytes.

Furthermore, beta-1 integrin subunits can dimerize with different alpha subunits. In fetal and neonatal cardiac myocytes, beta-1 integrin combines with alpha 1, 3, 5, 6, 7 subunits to mediate cell attachment to laminin, collagen and FN [44,45]. The increase in the amount of integrin beta-1 chain during development together with the absence of expression of both alpha-1 and alpha-5-chains is probably responsible for the poor attachment of adult cardiomyocytes on either collagen type I or FN [38]. Beta-1A-alpha-5 complex would play an essential role in the proliferation of fetal cells, that is eventually lost during early neonatal development when the laminin receptors beta-1D-alpha-6 and beta-1D-alpha-7 become increasingly expressed. However, alpha-6 and alpha-7 integrins and their variants appear to have different roles in laminin controlled cell adhesion and migration [46]. Alpha-6A expression would be favored under conditions that stimulate cardiac muscle differentiation [47], while at the adult stage, the only alpha-7 subunit persists [38,48]. The latter forms a complex with the beta-1D isoform, that is codistributed with vinculin, at both costamere and intercalated disc levels [43].

FORMATION OF FOCAL ADHESION REGIONS

Integrins modulate signals instigated by ionic channels, hormone growth factor receptors and their binding to extracellular matrix proteins induces their clustering, the activation of kinases and ionic channels and the reorganization of cytoskeletal proteins in a focal adhesion regions [49,50]. The clustering of integrins appears to be driven from within the cell by the Rho-family of Ras-related GTP binding proteins, that regulate the actin cytoskeleton [51]. Despite an apparent redundancy, many integrins have specific functions, see for a review [52]. Beta-1 and beta-3 containing integrins share the ability to promote the assembly of focal adhesions. Paxillin is tighly associated with the alpha-4 integrin and serves as a scaffold for the recruitment of signaling molecules. In vitro, binding of paxillin to alpha-4 integrin opposes cell spreading and focal adhesion plaque formation but facilitates cell migration [53].

At the level of the focal adhesion plaques, p125 FAK is activated after either binding of ECM matrix proteins to integrins or by growth factors, such as endothelin-1, Ang II, vasopressin and PDGF. Other intracellular signaling molecules, such as Ras, Raf, c-src, phosphatidylinositol 3 kinase, phospholipase C, are associated to focal adhesion contacts and activate different signaling pathways (MAPK, PEK, JNK) [50]. In vitro, in fibroblasts, MAP kinase activity is stimulated by Ang II but also in response to the activation of either alpha-v beta-3 or alpha-v beta-1 integrins by FN and collagen respectively. In cultured rat cardiac myocytes, Vascular Endothelial Growth Factor (VEGF) induces tyrosine phosphorylation and activation of p125 (FAK), which is translocated from perinuclear sites to the focal adhesion plaque, while paxillin is phosphorylated on tyrosine sites. In parallel, the adhesive interactions between cardiac myocytes and ECM are increased [54].

As an example, both in vivo and in vitro experiments lead Rabinovitch and coll to propose a functional paradigm for ECM-dependent cell survival whereby metalloproteinases (MMPs) upregulate TN-C by generating beta-3 integrin ligands in type I collagen. In turn, alpha-v beta-3 interactions with TN-C alter smooth muscle cell shape and increase EGF-R clustering and EGF-dependent growth. Conversely, suppression of MMPs downregulates TN-C and induces apoptosis [55,56]. Similarly, the proliferative response of human fetal ventricular myocytes to EGF requires the synthesis of collagen as well as attachement to specific alpha/beta-1 integrin heterodimers [57].

THE CYTOSKELETON

The interactions between cells and ECM components are essential in the morphogenesis of the developing heart. They are mediated in part by transmembrane proteins, such as integrins, dystro-glycans and by cytoskeletal proteins, such as α-actinin, vinculin, talin, dystrophin, and other proteins. Cytoskeletal proteins are associated to kinases, such as focal adhesion kinase (FAK), extracellular-signal-regulated kinase (ERK), Jun amino-terminal kinase (JNK), protein kinase C (PKC), integrin stimulated kinase (ISK) etc and participate to the transduction of signals from the cell to the matrix and vice versa. Phosphorylation of some of these proteins induces changes in structural conformations, which in turn can influence cell geometry and function [50].

Vinculin is a critical cytoskeletal compound that functions in the regulation of cell adhesion and mobility that are essential for normal embryonic morphogenesis. In the cardiomyocyte, vinculin appears as essential in the linkage of cytoskeletal actin filaments to the plasma membrane. The protein is colocalized at the level of costameres with integrins [45] and present at the level of fascia adherens junctions in the intercalated discs [58]. Vinculin determines cell shape and the arrangement and organization of developing myofibrils [59]. In vinculin (−/−) mice embryos, heart development is curtailed at E 9,5 with severely reduced and akinetic myocardial and endocardial structures. Fibroblasts isolated from mutant embryos have a reduced adhesion to FN, laminin and collagen compared with wild-type levels. In addition, both cell migration rate on theses substrates and the level of focal adhesion kinase activity were two and three fold higher respectively [60].

In mouse, the heart is already functional as a contractile organ before the appearance of the dystrophin transcripts, which are detectable from about E9 and accumulate initially in the outflow tract and at later stages in the myocytes of both the ventricular system and atria [61]. In human fetus, the protein is, with its associated proteins, expressed in the heart as soon as at 8 weeks of age [62]. At this stage, the protein is seen discontinuously at the sarcolemma and then evenly expressed by 15 weeks [63]. In rabbit, dystrophin is observed at earliest stages, mainly in the peripheral sarcolemma and then in the T-tubules as soon as they develop (1 week) [64]. The two muscle and brain dystrophin isoforms are transcribed in parallel from very early stages of cardiac muscle development [63]. In adult myocytes the protein is distributed as a uniform layer at the cytoplasmic surface of sarcolemma at both costameric and noncostameric regions of the cardiomyocytes and in the T-tubules, the association with sarcomeric apparatus at the level of Z discs being controversial

[58,65]. It has been recently proposed that a subpopulation of dystrophin molecules interacts with cardiac myocyte caveolae, some dystrophins being engaged in linking caveolin-3 with the dystroglycan complex [66]. The caveolin-3 is specific of the cardiomyocyte and is associated with the dystrophin-glycoprotein complex that serves as a link between the ECM, sarcoplasm and actin filaments. The receptor (erbB4) of a neuregulin (NRG1), that has been shown to be essential for normal cardiac development and growth of ventricular myocytes, is dynamically targeted to caveolar microdomains after NRG1 binding. After agonist binding, the m2-muscarinic cholinergic receptor is also rapidly translocated into caveolar microdomains where, among other effects, it activates the endothelial NOS isoform [67].

Main components of the cytoskeleton, such as the intermediate filaments of desmin, are involved in myocyte growth [68] and in impaired cardiac function during fetal or postnatal development [69,70]. Desmin, the muscle-specific intermediate filament constitutive protein is one of the earliest known myogenic makers in both heart and somites. However, mice with null mutation in desmin gene develop and reproduce normally, showing that desmin is need for neither the formation of the heart nor the alignment of functioning myofibrils [71,72]. These transgenic mice develop concentric cardiomyocyte hypertrophy, that is accompanied by induction of embryonic gene expression, then ventricular dilatation, and compromised systolic function [73]. Myocyte ultrastructural defects and cell death lead to supercontraction of myofibrils, fibrosis and calcification of the myocardium, which suggests that intermediate filaments are required to maintain the basic integrity of cardiomyocytes [74]. Thus desmin appears essential for normal cardiac function and the absence of an intact desmin filament network may be responsible for desmin associated cardiomyopathies. Indeed, in mice with null mutation in desmin, mitochondrial abnormalities and degeneration, already appear in two week old animals, in the absence of any other noticeable structural defects, such as loss of contractile materials and myofibrillar alignment, that occur later [75].

DISCUSSION AND CONCLUSION

Heart organogenesis and development requires migration, differentiation and precise interactions among multiple cell types that appear to depend, in part, on the interactions between ECM and cytoskeleton. The various molecules implicated in cell-ECM interactions are differently expressed along the main stages of cardiac development, notably depending they favor cell-substrate adhesion or not. Abnormalities or arrest in their expression may be responsible for some defects. However, proteins constitutive of main components of the cytoskeleton, such as desmin, or dystrophin, do not appear as essential during embryonic organogenesis but be more involved in maintaining myofibrillar structure in adult contracting muscle, by linking myofibrils to sarcolemma and via integrins or dystroglycans to ECM. The role of integrins as anchoring proteins for cytoskeleton and interacting with different intracellular signaling cascades appears more and more prominent [1]. It is of interest to compare these data to a recently proposed sequential model for the formation of an integrin-dependent adhesive link, using mutations in worm and drosophila muscles [76]. The first step would be the polarisation of the cytoskeleton in the muscles, resulting in the specific accumulation of ECM components. Then, integrins would attach to the ECM, by interactions with cytoskeleton and/or ECM and would recruit additional proteins to the muscle attachment site, such as talin and vinculin. These proteins would strengthen the interaction between the contractile apparatus and the membrane and contribute to the ordered assembly of the muscle sarcomeres. In fact, numerous dilated cardiomyopathies have been associated to molecular defects that implicate the linkage between the myocyte cytoskeleton and the extracellular matrix, see for review [70,77]. Elucidation of the precise nature, role and regulation of these multiple interactions may lead to a better understanding of cardiovascular diseases and malformations of the heart and form the basis for future therapeutic interventions.

ACKNOWLEDGEMENTS

The authors are grateful to C. Chassagne for critical review of the manuscript and to K. Chabane for assistance. P. Ratajczak is supported by an MRT training grant. Research was supported by Inserm and CNRS.

REFERENCES

1. Giancotti FG, Ruoslahti E. 1999. Integrin signaling. Science 285:1028–1032.
2. Tryggvason K. 1993. The laminin family. Curr Opin Cell Biol 5:877–882.
3. Hsueh WA, Law RE, Do YS. 1998. Integrins, adhesion, and cardiac remodeling. Hypertension 31:176–180.
4. Juliano RL, Haskill S. 1993. Signal transduction from the extracellular matrix. J Cell Biol 120:577–585.
5. Hynes RO. 1992. Integrins: versatility, modulation, and signaling in cell adhesion. Cell 69:11–25.
6. Ruoslahti E, Yamaguch IY. 1991. Proteoglycans as modulators of growth factor activities. Cell 64:867–869.
7. Borg TK, Raso DS, Terracio L. 1990. Potential role of the extracellular matrix in postseptation development of the heart. Ann NY Acad Sci 588:87–92.
8. Liu X, Wu H, Byrne M, Krane S, Jaenisch R. 1997. Type III collagen is crucial for collagen I fibrillogenesis and for normal cardiovascular development. Proc Natl Acad Sci USA 94:1852–1856.
9. Pickering JG, Chow LH, Li S, Rogers KA, Rocnik EF, Zhong R, Chan BM. 2000. alpha5beta1 integrin expression and luminal edge fibronectin matrix assembly by smooth muscle cells after arterial injury. Am J Pathol 156:453–465.
10. Samuel JL, Farhadian F, Sabri A, Marotte F, Robert V, Rappaport L. 1994. Expression of fibronectin during rat fetal and postnatal development: an in situ hybridisation and immunohistochemical study. Cardiovasc Res 28:1653–1661.
11. Kim H, Yoon CS, Kim H, Rah B. 1999. Expression of extracellular matrix components fibronectin and laminin in the human fetal heart. Cell Struct Funct 24:19–26.
12. Farhadian F, Barrieux A, Lortet S, Marotte F, Oliviero P, Rappaport L, Samuel JL. 1994. Differential splicing of fibronectin pre-messenger ribonucleic acid during cardiac ontogeny and development of hypertrophy in the rat. Lab Invest 71:552–559.
13. George EL, Georges-Labouesse EN, Patel-King RS, Rayburn H, Hynes RO. 1993. Defects in mesoderm, neural tube and vascular development in mouse embryos lacking fibronectin. Development 119:1079–1091.
14. Campbell KP. 1995. Three muscular dystrophies: loss of cytoskeleton-extracellular matrix linkage. Cell 80:675–679.
15. Koch M, Olson PF, Albus A, Jin W, Hunter DD, Brunken WJ, Burgeson RE, Champliaud MF. 1999. Characterization and expression of the laminin gamma3 chain: a novel, non-basement membrane-associated, laminin chain. J Cell Biol 145:605–618.

16. Oliviero P, Chassagne C, Salichon N, Corbie RA, Hamon G, Marotte F, Charlemagne D, Rappaport L, Samuel JL. 2000. Expression of laminin alpha2 chain during normal and pathological growth of myocardium in rat and human. Cardiovasc Res 46:346–355.

17. Kortesmaa J, Yurchenco P, Tryggvason K. 2000. Recombinant laminin-8 (alpha(4)beta(1)gamma(1)). Production, purification, and interactions with integrins. J Biol Chem 275:14853–14859.

18. Glukhova M, Koteliansky V, Fondacci C, Marotte F, Rappaport L. 1993. Laminin variants and integrin laminin receptors in developing and adult human smooth muscle. Dev Biol 157:437–447.

19. Bardy N, Merval R, Benessiano J, Samuel JL, Tedgui A. 1996. Pressure and angiotensin II synergistically induce aortic fibronectin expression in organ culture model of rabbit aorta. Evidence for a pressure-induced tissue renin-angiotensin system. Circ Res 79:70–78.

20. Hedin U, Bottger BA, Forsberg E, Johansson S, Thyberg J. 1988. Diverse effects of fibronectin and laminin on phenotypic properties of cultured arterial smooth muscle cells. J Cell Biol 107:307–319.

21. Hedin UL, Daum G, Clowes AW. 1997. Disruption of integrin alpha 5 beta 1 signaling does not impair PDGF-BB-mediated stimulation of the extracellular signal-regulated kinase pathway in smooth muscle cells. J Cell Physiol 172:109–116.

22. MacKenna DA, Dolfi F, Vuori K, Ruoslahti E. 1998. Extracellular signal-regulated kinase and c-Jun NH2-terminal kinase activation by mechanical stretch is integrin-dependent and matrix-specific in rat cardiac fibroblasts. J Clin Invest 101:301–310.

23. DiMilla PA, Stone JA, Quinn JA, Albelda SM, Lauffenburger DA. 1993. Maximal migration of human smooth muscle cells on fibronectin and type IV collagen occurs at an intermediate attachment strength. J Cell Biol 122:729–737.

24. Lundgren E, Gullberg D, Rubin K, Borg TK, Terracio MJ, Terracio L. 1988. In vitro studies on adult cardiac myocytes: attachment and biosynthesis of collagen type IV and laminin. J Cell Physiol 136:43–53.

25. Chiquet-Ehrismann R. 1995. Tenascins, a growing family of extracellular matrix proteins. Experientia 51:853–862.

26. Matsumoto K, Saga Y, Ikemura T, Sakakura T, Chiquet-Ehrismann R. 1994. The distribution of tenascin-X is distinct and often reciprocal to that of tenascin-C. J Cell Biol 125:483–493.

27. Burch GH, Bedolli MA, McDonough S, Rosenthal SM, Bristow J. 1995. Embryonic expression of tenascin-X suggests a role in limb, muscle, and heart development. Dev Dyn 203:491–504.

28. Yamamoto K, Dang QN, Kennedy SP, Osathanondh R, Kelly RA, Lee RT. 1999. Induction of tenascin-C in cardiac myocytes by mechanical deformation. Role of reactive oxygen species. J Biol Chem 274:21840–21846.

29. Corless CL, Mendoza A, Collins T, Lawler J. 1992. Colocalization of thrombospondin and syndecan during murine development. Dev Dyn 193:346–358.

30. Mann DL, Spinale FG. 1998. Activation of matrix metalloproteinases in the failing human heart: breaking the tie that binds. Circulation 98:1699–1702.

31. Shapiro SD. 1998. Matrix metalloproteinase degradation of extracellular matrix: biological consequences. Curr Opin Cell Biol 10:602–608.

32. Nakagawa M, Terracio L, Carver W, Birkedal-Hansen H, Borg TK. 1992. Expression of collagenase and IL-1 alpha in developing rat hearts. Dev Dyn 195:87–99.

33. Kim HE, Dalal SS, Young E, Legato MJ, Weisfeldt ML, D. Armiento J. 2000. Disruption of the myocardial extracellular matrix leads to cardiac dysfunction. J Clin Invest 106:857–866.

34. Howe A, Aplin AE, Alahari SK, Juliano RL. 1998. Integrin signaling and cell growth control. Curr Opin Cell Biol 10:220–231.

35. Schoenwaelder SM, Burridge K. 1999. Bidirectional signaling between the cytoskeleton and integrins. Curr Opin Cell Biol 11:274–286.

36. Fassler R, Rohwedel J, Maltsev V, Bloch W, Lentini S, Guan K, Gullberg D, Hescheler J, Addicks K, Wobus AM. 1996. Differentiation and integrity of cardiac muscle cells are impaired in the absence of beta 1 integrin. J Cell Sci 109 (Pt 13):2989–2999.

37. Volk T, Fessler LI, Fessler JH. 1990. A role for integrin in the formation of sarcomeric cytoarchitecture. Cell 63:525–536.

38. Maitra N, Flink IL, Bahl JJ, Morkin E. 2000. Expression of alpha and beta integrins during terminal differentiation of cardiomyocytes. Cardiovasc Res 47:715–725.

39. Ross RS, Pham C, Shai SY, Goldhaber JI, Fenczik C, Glembotski CC, Ginsberg MH, Loftus JC. 1998. Beta1 integrins participate in the hypertrophic response of rat ventricular myocytes. Circ Res 82:1160–1172.

40. Belkin AM, Zhidkova NI, Balzac F, Altruda F, Tomatis D, Maier A, Tarone G, Koteliansky VE, Burridge K. 1996. Beta 1D integrin displaces the beta 1A isoform in striated muscles: localization at junctional structures and signaling potential in nonmuscle cells. J Cell Biol 132:211–226.
41. Sharp WW, Simpson DG, Borg TK, Samarel AM, Terracio L. 1997. Mechanical forces regulate focal adhesion and costamere assembly in cardiac myocytes. Am J Physiol 273:H546–H556.
42. Belkin AM, Retta SF, Pletjushkina OY, Balzac F, Silengo L, Fassler R, Koteliansky VE, Burridge K, Tarone G. 1997. Muscle beta1D integrin reinforces the cytoskeleton-matrix link: modulation of integrin adhesive function by alternative splicing. J Cell Biol 139:1583–1595.
43. Baudoin C, Goumans MJ, Mummery C, Sonnenberg A. 1998. Knockout and knockin of the beta1 exon D define distinct roles for integrin splice variants in heart function and embryonic development. Genes Dev 12:1202–1216.
44. Brancaccio M, Cabodi S, Belkin AM, Collo G, Koteliansky VE, Tomatis D, Altruda F, Silengo L, Tarone G. 1998. Differential onset of expression of alpha 7 and beta 1D integrins during mouse heart and skeletal muscle development. Cell Adhes Commun 5:193–205.
45. Terracio L, Gullberg D, Rubin K, Craig S, Borg TK. 1989. Expression of collagen adhesion proteins and their association with the cytoskeleton in cardiac myocytes. Anat Rec 223:62–71.
46. Schober S, Mielenz D, Echtermeyer F, Hapke S, Poschl E, von der Mark H, Moch H, von der Mark K. 2000. The role of extracellular and cytoplasmic splice domains of alpha7-integrin in cell adhesion and migration on laminins. Exp Cell Res 255:303–313.
47. Thorsteinsdottir S, Roelen BA, Goumans MJ, Ward-van Oostwaard D, Gaspar AC, Mummery CL. 1999. Expression of the alpha 6A integrin splice variant in developing mouse embryonic stem cell aggregates and correlation with cardiac muscle differentiation. Differentiation 64:173–184.
48. Velling T, Collo G, Sorokin L, Durbeej M, Zhang H, Gullberg D. 1996. Distinct alpha 7A beta 1 and alpha 7B beta 1 integrin expressionpatterns during mouse development: alpha 7A is restricted to skeletal muscle but alpha 7B is expressed in striated muscle, vasculature, and nervous system. Dev Dyn 207:355–371.
49. Shyy JY, Chien S. 1997. Role of integrins in cellular responses to mechanical stress and adhesion. Curr Opin Cell Biol 9:707–713.
50. Yamada KM, Miyamoto S. 1995. Integrin transmembrane signaling and cytoskeletal control. Curr Opin Cell Biol 7:681–689.
51. Magnusson MK, Zhang Q, Mosher DF. 1998. Fibronectin matrix: cellular regulations. In: S. A. Moussa, ed. Cell adhesion molecules and matrix proteins: role in health and diseases: Springer-Verlag and R.G. Landes Company, 221–240.
52. Giancotti FG. 2000. Complexity and specificity of integrin signalling. Nat Cell Biol 2:E13–E14.
53. Liu S, Thomas SM, Woodside DG, Rose DM, Kiosses WB, Pfaff M, Ginsberg MH. 1999. Binding of paxillin to alpha 4 integrins modifies integrin-dependent biological responses. Nature 402:676–681.
54. Takahashi N, Seko Y, Noiri E, Tobe K, Kadowaki T, Sabe H, Yazaki Y. 1999. Vascular endothelial growth factor induces activation and subcellular translocation of focal adhesion kinase (p125FAK) in cultured rat cardiac myocytes. Circ Res 84:1194–1202.
55. Jones PL, Crack J, Rabinovitch M. 1997. Regulation of tenascin-C, a vascular smooth muscle cell survival factor that interacts with the alpha v beta 3 integrin to promote epidermal growth factor receptor phosphorylation and growth. J Cell Biol 139:279–293.
56. Cowan KN, Jones PL, Rabinovitch M. 2000. Elastase and matrix metalloproteinase inhibitors induce regression, and tenascin-C antisense prevents progression, of vascular disease. J Clin Invest 105:21–34.
57. Hornberger LK, Singhroy S, Cavalle-Garrido T, Tsang W, Keeley F, Rabinovitch M. 2000. Synthesis of extracellular matrix and adhesion through beta(1) integrins are critical for fetal ventricular myocyte proliferation. Circ Res 87:508–515.
58. Stevenson S, Rothery S, Cullen MJ, Severs NJ. 1997. Dystrophin is not a specific component of the cardiac costamere. Circ Res 80:269–280.
59. Shiraishi I, Simpson DG, Carver W, Price R, Hirozane T, Terracio L, Borg TK. 1997. Vinculin is an essential component for normal myofibrillar arrangement in fetal mouse cardiac myocytes. J Mol Cell Cardiol 29:2041–2052.
60. Xu W, Baribault H, Adamson ED. 1998. Vinculin knockout results in heart and brain defects during embryonic development. Development 125:327–337.
61. Houzelstein D, Lyons GE, Chamberlain J, Buckingham ME. 1992. Localization of dystrophin gene transcripts during mouse embryogenesis. J Cell Biol 119:811–821.

62. Mora M, Di Blasi C, Barresi R, Morandi L, Brambati B, Jarre L, Cornelio F. 1996. Developmental expression of dystrophin, dystrophin-associated glycoproteins and other membrane cytoskeletal proteins in human skeletal and heart muscle. Brain Res Dev Brain Res 91:70–82.

63. Torelli S, Ferlini A, Obici L, Sewry C, Muntoni F. 1999. Expression, regulation and localisation of dystrophin isoforms in human foetal skeletal and cardiac muscle. Neuromuscul Disord 9:541–551.

64. Frank JS, Mottino G, Chen F, Peri V, Holland P, Tuana BS. 1994. Subcellular distribution of dystrophin in isolated adult and neonatal cardiac myocytes. Am J Physiol 267:C1707–C1716.

65. Meng H, Leddy JJ, Frank J, Holland P, Tuana BS. 1996. The association of cardiac dystrophin with myofibrils/Z-disc regions in cardiac muscle suggests a novel role in the contractile apparatus. J Biol Chem 271:12364–12371.

66. Doyle DD, Goings G, Upshaw-Earley J, Ambler SK, Mondul A, Palfrey HC, Page E. 2000. Dystrophin associates with caveolae of rat cardiac myocytes: relationship to dystroglycan. Circ Res 87:480–488.

67. Zhao YY, Feron O, Dessy C, Han X, Marchionni MA, Kelly RA. 1999. Neuregulin signaling in the heart. Dynamic targeting of erbB4 to caveolar microdomains in cardiac myocytes. Circ Res 84:1380–1387.

68. Watkins SC, Samuel JL, Marotte F, Bertier-Savalle B, Rappaport L. 1987. Microtubules and desmin filaments during onset of heart hypertrophy in rat: a double immunoelectron microscope study. Circ Res 60:327–336.

69. Eble DM, Spinale FG. 1995. Contractile and cytoskeletal content, structure, and mRNA levels with tachycardia-induced cardiomyopathy. Am J Physiol 268:H2426–H2439.

70. Chien KR. 1999. Stress pathways and heart failure. Cell 98:555–558.

71. Li Z, Mericskay M, Agbulut O, Butler-Browne G, Carlsson L, Thornell LE, Babinet C, Paulin D. 1997. Desmin is essential for the tensile strength and integrity of myofibrils but not for myogenic commitment, differentiation, and fusion of skeletal muscle. J Cell Biol 139:129–144.

72. Milner DJ, Weitzer G, Tran D, Bradley A, Capetanaki Y. 1996. Disruption of muscle architecture and myocardial degeneration in mice lacking desmin. J Cell Biol 134:1255–1270.

73. Milner DJ, Taffet GE, Wang X, Pham T, Tamura T, Hartley C, Gerdes AM, Capetanak IY. 1999. The absence of desmin leads to cardiomyocyte hypertrophy and cardiac dilation with compromised systolic function. J Mol Cell Cardiol 31:2063–2076.

74. Thornell L, Carlsson L, Li Z, Mericskay M, Paulin D. 1997. Null mutation in the desmin gene gives rise to a cardiomyopathy. J Mol Cell Cardiol 29:2107–2124.

75. Milner DJ, Mavroidis M, Weisleder N, Capetanaki Y. 2000. Desmin cytoskeleton linked to muscle mitochondrial distribution and respiratory function. J Cell Biol 150:1283–1298.

76. Brown NH. 2000. An integrin chicken and egg problem: which comes first, the extracellular matrix or the cytoskeleton? Curr Opin Cell Biol 12:629–633.

77. Towbin JA. 1998. The role of cytoskeletal proteins in cardiomyopathies. Curr Opin Cell Biol 10: 131–139.

B. Ostadal, M. Nagano and N.S. Dhalla (eds.).
CARDIAC DEVELOPMENT. Copyright © 2002.
Kluwer Academic Publishers. Boston.
All rights reserved.

A DISINTEGRIN AND METALLOPROTEASE (ADAMS) FAMILY: EXPRESSION AND POTENTIAL ROLES IN THE DEVELOPING HEART

THOMAS K. BORG, ANGELA DE ALMEIDA, MELISSA JOY LOFTIS, ALEX McFADDEN, and WAYNE CARVER

Department of Developmental Biology and Anatomy, School of Medicine, University of South Carolina, Columbia, SC 29208

Summary. The A Disintegrin And Metalloproteases (ADAMs) are a rather recently identified family of cell surface molecules which have a characteristic multidomain structure. The multiple domains found in these proteins include a metalloprotease domain that has been shown to proteolytically cleave extracellular matrix and cell surface proteins. These domains also include a disintegrin region which has been shown to participate in cell-cell binding in some cell types. Through these multiple functional domains, ADAMs have been shown to play roles in diverse developmental processes including cell-cell fusion and cell migration. The roles of these proteins in the developing cardiovascular system have not been examined. In the following discussion, we will summarize the current knowledge of these molecules in other systems and present novel data regarding their expression and potential function in the developing heart.

Key words: Disintegrin, Metalloprotease, Extracellular matrix, Integrin

INTRODUCTION

Cardiovascular development requires the precise orchestration of cellular processes including migration, proliferation, differentiation and apoptosis. These processes are modulated, in part, by cell-cell and cell-extracellular matrix (ECM) interactions. Essential to these interactions are: the composition and organization of the extra-

Address Correspondence to: Wayne Carver, Department of Developmental Biology and Anatomy, University of South Carolina, School of Medicine, Columbia, SC, 29208. Phone: (803) 733-3214; Fax: (803) 733-1533; e-mail: carver@med.sc.edu

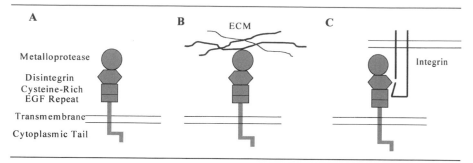

Figure 1. This schematically illustrates proposed models of transmembrane ADAM structure and function in modulating the ECM or in cell-cell adhesion. The typical domain structure of a membrane-anchored ADAM is shown in Fig. A. The metalloprotease domain is postulated to modify ECM components (Fig. B). For instance, collagen type IV has recently been demonstrated to be a substrate for ADAM 10. ADAMs also mediate cell-cell interactions by binding integrins on adjacent cells through the ADAM disintegrin domain (Fig. C).

cellular ligands; the cell surface receptors that these ligands bind; and the intracellular signaling molecules activated in response to these interactions. The A Disintegrin And Metalloproteases (ADAMs) represent a recently identified family of proteins that are thought to be important mediators of cell-cell interactions as well as proteolytic cleavage of ECM and cell surface components [1,2]. The ADAMs are cell surface proteins that are characterized by a multidomain structure including metalloprotease, disintegrin, cysteine-rich, epidermal growth factor-like, transmembrane and cytoplasmic regions. ADAMs have been shown to mediate cell-cell interactions imperative to developmental events including fertilization (ADAM 2) and skeletal myocyte fusion (ADAM 12). Several of the ADAM family members also are active proteases targeting ECM components or cell surface molecules. We have recently determined that multiple ADAMs are expressed in the developing myocardium; however, little is known about their potential function in cardiogenesis. The goals of this chapter are to discuss the current literature on the ADAM proteins and the roles that they may play during cardiac development. Due to the relative novelty of these proteins, most of the functional data in the cardiovascular system is still very speculative.

THE A DISINTEGRIN AND METALLOPROTEASES (ADAMs)

The ADAMs are a relatively novel family of proteins consisting of approximately 30 members that are thought to have important roles in embryogenesis [2]. The typical ADAMs are cell surface proteins that consist of: pro-metalloprotease, disintegrin, cysteine-rich, epidermal growth factor-like, transmembrane and cytoplasmic (signaling) domains (Fig. 1; [3]). The distinctive domains composing the ADAM proteins suggest that these molecules may modulate a number of important processes in embryonic development including proteolysis, cell adhesion, cell fusion and signaling [2,4]. The framework for the following discussion will be formed around the different functional aspects of the ADAM proteins.

THE ADAMs AS METALLOPROTEASES

The ADAMs, like the snake venom metalloproteases are part of a large family termed reprolysins that are zinc-dependent metalloproteases. The reprolysins are characterized by the consensus metalloprotease active site amino acid sequence HEXGHXXG XXHD. The ADAMs can be divided into two groups: those that contain this sequence and are thought to be active metalloproteases and others that lack this sequence and are likely catalytically inert. Regulation of metalloprotease activity occurs through a cysteine switch mechanism in which a cysteine residue in the prodomain binds to the active site zinc thereby maintaining it in an inactive state. Removal of the prodomain allows zinc binding and thereby activates the metalloproteases. Active ADAMs are thought to cleave ECM and/or cell surface substrates; however, little is known regarding the substrate-specificity of these metalloproteases.

In vitro studies have indicated that several of the ADAMs are indeed functional metalloproteases. Initial studies showed that ADAM 10 could cleave myelin basic protein and more recently this ADAM has been shown to proteolytically cleave collagen type IV [5]. A rather unique ADAM containing a thrombospodin motif (ADAM TS-1) has recently been identified as an aggrecanase [6]. ADAM 12 has been shown to be a functional metalloprotease using an α macroglobulin assay *in vitro* [6]; however, the substrate(s) of this ADAM have not been determined. While many questions remain about the ECM substrates of specific ADAMs, these studies suggest that ADAMs, being located on the cell surface, may play a role in local modification of the extracellular environment. In this context, ADAMs could be in an ideal position to influence directed cellular migration, changes in cell shape and a variety of other cellular events.

The composition and organization of the ECM have been shown to profoundly influence adhesion and organization of cardiac myocytes. The composition of the ECM substratum can influence differentiation of cardiac myocytes *in vitro* [7,8]. That is, plating of isolated myocytes onto different ECM components dramatically affects the rate of assembly and the organization of contractile proteins [8,9]. Studies have also shown that the organization of these ECM components affects the cardiomyocyte phenotype [10]. Heart myocytes plated onto aligned collagen assume a rod-shaped, *in vivo*-like morphology while those plated on random collagen attain a stellate, flattened shape. The formation of the rod-like shape is dependent on collagen-binding receptors of the integrin family [11]. These results clearly indicate that the organization of the ECM plays an important modulatory role in cardiomyocyte development and differentiation; however, the mechanisms whereby a rounded myocyte attains a rod shape and a precise 3-dimensional organization relative to surrounding cells is not known. It is easy to envision that local modification of the ECM by proteases on the surface of the myocyte may play a role in this process. Studies with generic metalloprotease inhibitors (zinc chelators) suggest that protease activity is required for myocyte spreading and elongation (unpublished observations). It is conceivable that localized modification of ECM components like laminin and collagen is required for changes in myocyte shape during heart development and maturation. Whether this involves the ADAMs members or other proteases has not been determined.

THE ADAMs AS "SHEDDASES"

A diverse range of cell surface proteins also occur as circulating forms which are generated by proteolysis of their ectodomains from the cell membrane [12]. In some cases, such as demonstrated with several growth factors, cytokines and adhesion molecules, this cleavage releases a physiologically active protein. Ectodomain cleavage could also be a mechanism for modulating levels of proteins at the cell surface. Interest in the ADAM proteins mounted considerably with the discovery that several members of the ADAM family cleave the ectodomains of other cell surface components [13–15]. Several lines of evidence now have attributed to ADAMs an exciting novel role as "sheddases" [16,17]. Initial evidence for this was obtained when it was determined that Tumor Necrosis Factor α-Converting Enzyme (TACE) is a member of the ADAM family [13,14]. Since that time, ADAMs have been shown to cleave other cell surface molecules including L-selectin [18], β amyloid precursor protein [19] and heparin binding-epidermal growth factor [20]. These studies suggest that the ADAMs could play a critical role in releasing important regulatory components from the cell surface into the extracellular milieu.

As mentioned above, another potential role of ectodomain shedding is to down-regulate cell surface levels of particular proteins. Evidence for this comes from recent work illustrating that integrins are shed from the surface of cartilage cells *in vitro* [21]. The integrins are a family of proteins that are the primary receptors for extracellular matrix components such as collagen, laminin and fibronectin [22–25]. The functional integrin on the cell surface forms a heterodimeric complex composed of an α and a β chain. The integrins are loosely divided into subfamilies based upon their component β chain. Multiple α chains can typically form a complex with a given β chain. For instance, the $\beta1$ chain can form a heterodimer with at least 11 different α chains ($\alpha1$–$\alpha10$ and αv). The combination of α and β chains appears to generate binding specificity of the integrin to given extracellular matrix components. Integrin-mediated interactions are necessary for a number of cellular processes including adhesion, migration, proliferation and even survival. The repertoire of integrins expressed on the surface of a given cell probably plays a significant role in orchestrating these very diverse cell processes during development and disease.

For some time, developmental biologists have questioned how a cell that is dependent on adhesion to the ECM for survival and normal physiological functioning can modify its cell-ECM connections to change phenotypically. For instance, how does a rounded cardiomyocyte establish an elongated rod-like shape while still maintaining enough adhesion to the ECM to continue contractile activity? Recent studies indicated that alterations in myocyte growth, shape and contractility associated with aortic stenosis is accompanied by accumulation of integrins in the interstitium [26]. This observation suggests that one mechanism whereby cells alter their phenotype may be to reduce their cell-ECM contacts by shedding the ectodomain of specific integrins from the cell surface.

To begin to explore the mechanisms of this shedding process, experiments are being carried out *in vitro* with heart fibroblasts and myocytes. In these studies, culture

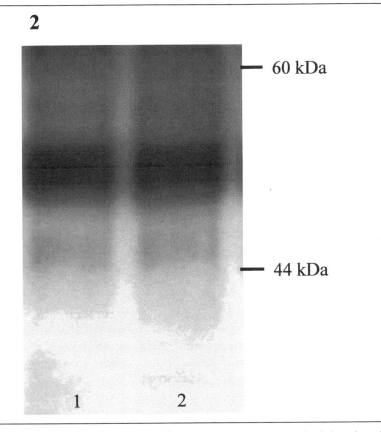

Figure 2. This shows a Western blot with anti-β1 integrin IgGs of proteins isolated from the culture medium of heart fibroblasts treated with (lane 1) or without (lane 2) insulin-like growth factor. Immuno-reactive proteins of approximately 50 kD were detected in the medium. The intact β1 integrin on the surface of cells is approximately 120 kD. These results suggest that the immuno-reactive protein in the medium may be the shed ectodmain of β1 integrin.

medium from fibroblasts and myocytes have been isolated and used for immuno-precipitation with β1 integrin antibodies. Polyacrylamide gel electrophoresis illustrates that an approximately 50 kilodaltin protein is immunoprecipitated from the culture medium with β1 integrin IgGs (Fig. 2). The intact β1 integrin on the cell surface is approximately 120 kilodaltons suggesting that the 50 kilodalton protein is a shed fragment from the cell surface. In additional experiments, cells were surface biotinylated, culture continued for varying durations and culture medium subsequently used for immunoprecipitation. In these experiments, the 50 kilodalton protein was found to be biotinylated indicating that it was present on the cell surface prior to being released into the medium. While still somewhat speculative, these experiments suggest that alterations in cellular phenotype associated with development or disease may involve changes in cell–ECM contacts through the cleavage of the ectodomain of the integrins. The mechanisms of this process have not been determined but likely involve proteases of the ADAMs family.

THE ADAMs IN CELL-CELL INTERACTIONS

Several of the ADAMs have been shown to mediate cell-cell interactions in development (Fig. 1). The most well-studied of these is the role of ADAM 1 and ADAM 2 (the α and β chains of fertilin) in sperm-egg fusion [27–30]. Fertilin was isolated initially through functional screens of monoclonal antibodies directed against the sperm surface. A monoclonal (PH-30) antibody was produced that blocked fusion of sperm to the egg surface [31]. Due to the sequence homology between the disintegrin domains of the fertilin subunits (α and β) and the snake venom integrin ligands (disintegrins), it was originally proposed that sperm-egg fusion may involve binding of fertilin to an integrin on the egg surface [32]. Several experiments have validated this hypothesis. Peptides mimicking the predicted binding region of fertilin inhibit sperm-egg binding in a dose-dependent manner [33]. More recently, significant defects have been found in the ability of sperm from ADAM 2 knockout mice to fertilize eggs from normal mice [34]. Sperm-egg fusion is, at least in part, mediated by the binding of ADAM 2 (fertilin β) on the sperm to the α6β1 integrin on the surface of the egg [35,36].

Most of the current knowledge regarding the involvement of ADAMs in cell-cell interactions has arisen from studies with ADAM 1 and 2 in fertilization. Recent studies have indicated that ADAM 15 (MDC 15) mediates cell-cell binding via interactions with the αvβ3 integrin in CHO cells [37]. ADAM 12 has also recently been shown to play a critical role in the fusion of skeletal myoblasts into myotubes [38]. However, the binding partner for ADAM 12 has not been determined.

As mentioned above, the ADAM disintegrin domain has a high degree of similarity to the disintegrin proteins discovered in the venom of viperous snakes. The snake venom disintegrins are typically 50–75 amino acid proteins that bind to platelet integrins and block fibrinogen binding, thus inhibiting platelet aggregation [2,39]. Most of these disintegrins have a 14 amino acid cell binding loop that contains an RGD sequence which mediates integrin ligation. Many of these interact specifically with the αIIBβ3 or αvβ3 integrins. Specificity in integrin binding appears to be mediated by the disintegrin loop and adjacent sequences [40]. The disintegrin domain of the ADAMs has a high degree of sequence homology to the snake venom disintegrins; however, several intriguing differences have been noted [2]. Firstly, the predicted disintegrin loops of the ADAMs are not all 14 amino acids in length. Secondly, the sequences of the disintegrin loops are much more divergent among the ADAMs than the snake venom disintegrins. The functional consequences of this divergence are not clear but it has been postulated that sequence differences within the disintegrin loop could generate cell-type or integrin-specific binding [2]. Additionally, sequence divergence within the disintegrin domain as a whole could generate differences in the structure and 3-dimensional presentation of ADAMs to integrin co-receptors. These studies suggest that the repertoire of

ADAMs expressed by a given cell during development could impact greatly on cell-cell interactions and cellular function.

POTENTIAL FUNCTIONS OF ADAMS IN HEART DEVELOPMENT

Cell migration

The ability of cells to migrate plays a crucial role in development and in disease processes including wound healing and metastasis [41]. Interactions between cells and the ECM, largely via the integrins, play important roles in migration of cells through the ECM-filled environment [42]. A number of migratory events occur during development of the heart including transformation of epithelial cells into mesenchyme and migration of these cells into the cardiac jelly of the endocardial cushions. A variety of studies have used collagen get models *in vitro* to determine the mechanisms whereby mesenchymal cells migrate into and modify the ECM [43,44]. It is clear that collagen-binding integrins, particularly $\alpha 1 \beta 1$ and $\alpha 2 \beta 1$, are essential to this process [45,46].

Several studies have shown that matrix-modifying proteases are involved in cardiac cushion formation and maturation. In order for cells to transform and migrate, they must release from adjacent cells. This involves decreased expression of cell-cell adhesion molecules such as NCAM (neural cell adhesion molecule). There is a concurrent increased expression or activation of proteases that are thought to modify the ECM as cells migrate through it. Several candidate extracellular proteases have been proposed to take part in these functions, although the substrate specificity and regulation of these molecules have not been carefully examined [47–49]. Among these are the serine protease and matrix metalloprotease families. Expression of the serine protease, urokinase, is increased in the cardiac cushions concurrent with epithelial-mesenchymal transformation [50]. Inhibition of urokinase expression by antisense oligodeoxynucleotides has profound inhibitory effects on the ability of cells from cardiac cushion explants to seed collagen gels [51].

The MMPs are a family of extracellular proteases that include at least 22 different family members (MMP 1–MMP 22). These include collagenases, stromelysins, and the type IV collagenases/gelatinases. Recent studies [52,53] indicate that mesenchymal cells within the cardiac cushions express MMP-2 (72 kD collagenase or Gelatinase A). This MMP has been localized to the leading edge of cells migrating in collagen gels *in vitro* and blocking the activity of MMP-2 inhibits the contraction of collagen gels by heart fibroblasts [54]. These studies indicate that serine proteases and MMPs play roles in ECM remodeling accompanying cardiac cushion formation and maturation.

Although the ADAMs have not been examined in migration of heart cells, it is easy to envision that cell surface proteases may modulate directed migration. It will be exciting to determine whether these proteins are involved in localized modification of the ECM within the cardiac cushions. Ongoing studies indicate that mesenhymal cells isolated from the cardiac cushions of the developing mouse heart express an array of ADAMs (Fig. 3) including ADAMs 1, 10 and 15. The roles of

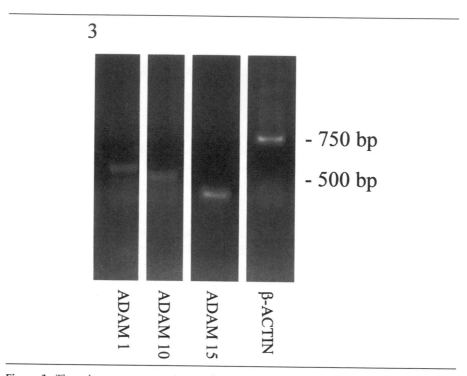

Figure 3. These show reverse transcriptase-polymerase chain reaction products obtained using RNA from mesenchymal cells and primers specific for ADAMs 1, 10 and 15 or β-actin. These results indictae that several ADAMs are expressed by mesenchymal cells isolated from the embryonic heart (12.5 days of gestation).

these ADAMs remain to be determined in the formation and maturation of the cardiac cushions of the heart.

In a variety of developmental and disease situations, cells migrate not through the ECM, but on the surface of other cells. For instance tumor cells must invade other cell populations during metastasis and leukocytes transit across the endothelium of blood vessels during inflammatory processes. A similar situation exists in the developing heart where epicardial cells migrate over the surface of the heart in contact with other heart cells [55,56]. The "driving force" for this transcellular migration appears to involve transient cell-cell adhesions. Several molecules have been identified that may be involved in these transient interactions including VCAM-1 and α4β1 integrin. Recent studies have shown that ADAM 9 (meltrin γ) mediates cell adhesion via the α6β1 integrin [57]. Interestingly, integrin-mediated binding of cells to ADAM 9 stimulated migration several-fold compared to integrin-mediated binding to laminin. These results suggest that the ADAMs on the surface of one cell may act as substrates for the migratory activity of other cells. To date, this has not been examined in migrating heart cells.

If ADAMs participate in cellular adhesion and migration, their 3-dimensional conformation and organization on the cell surface are of utmost importance. To date, it is not clear how specific domains of these proteins may be exposed for particular functions. It is tantalizing to speculate that extracellular complexes may exist similar to those described intracellularly for integrins and associated proteins. It is clear from numerous studies spanning the past decade that the integrins are associated with a variety of cytoskeletal and signaling molecules in the cytoplasm of the cell [58–61]. Few studies have been directed at elucidating the organization of components at the extracellular surface of the cell. It will be very important in terms of cell function to determine how proteases, ECM components, ADAMs, growth factors, integrins and other transmembrane or extracellular components are interrelated. It is likely that there are critical associations between these molecules that dictate a variety of cellular processes.

Cardiomyocyte development and organization

Imperative to normal development and function of the heart is the differentiation and organization of the myocyte component. Following commitment of cardiogenic cells to the myocyte lineage specific differentiation events occur transforming a rounded, noncontractile cell into an elongated beating myocyte. Efficient function of the mature heart is dependent not only on the differentiation of individual myocytes but the organization and integrated action of cells throughout the myocardium. Interactions between adjacent cardiomyocytes and between cardiomyocytes and the surrounding ECM components play critical roles in myocardial development [9,10,62]. Understanding the molecular mechanisms through which these interactions occur is imperative to determining how abnormalities in these interactions may impact upon myocardial development.

Recent studies have clearly shown that ADAM 12 (meltrin α) is essential in mediating binding and fusion of developing skeletal myoblasts [38]. However, the coreceptor or ligand for ADAM 12 has not been identified. Unlike previous work with other ADAMs, adhesion of cells to ADAM 12 appears to be mediated, at least in part, through the cysteine-rich domain [63,64]. Cell adhesion to the cysteine-rich domain of ADAM 12 appears to be mediated by syndecans and not the integrins. Due to its reported role in skeletal muscle development, we have begun studies to examine the role of ADAM 12 in developing cardiomyocytes. To test the role of ADAM 12 in mediating adhesion between adjacent cardiomyocytes, cells were isolated from neonatal rat hearts and incubated in rotation culture (72 rotations per minute) for 24 hours in the presence of antisense ADAM 12 or control oligodeoxynucleotides. Cells cultured in control oligodeoxynucleotides formed compact aggregates (Fig. 4) while cells incubated in the presence of antisense ADAM 12 oligodeoxynucleotides failed to aggregate. Studies with ADAM 12 disintegrin peptides suggest that ADAM 12-mediated cardiomyocyte interactions may occur via the binding of the disintegrin domain to a laminin receptor on adjacent cells. These studies suggest that ADAM 12 may play important roles in cell-cell interactions

4

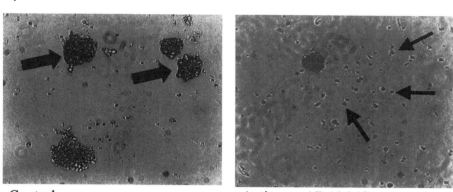

Control   Antisense ADAM 12

Figure 4. These show micrographs of myocytes that were cultured with rotation in the presence of control or antisense ADAM 12 oligodeoxynucleotides. In the presence of control oligodeoxynucleotides, myocytes formed beating aggregates of cells approximately 0.5–1.0 mm in diameter (block arrows). In the presence of the antisense ADAM 12 oligonucleotides, many small clusters of cells formed (arrows) while few large aggregates formed.

between cardiomyocytes; however, the mechanisms of these interactions are currently unknown. Experiments are underway to dissect the molecular mechanisms whereby ADAMs may be involved in interactions between adjacent cardiomyocytes.

CONCLUSIONS

As discussed above, development of the vertebrate heart involves a number of cellular processes. As multidomain, cell surface proteins, the ADAMs are in a prime position to modulate a number of these morphogenetic processes. To date, it is clear that ADAMs are involved in cell-cell fusion, migration and differentiation in various systems. Exciting work is ongoing to determine the mechanisms of these functions. To date, little work has been carried out with ADAMs in the developing or diseased cardiovascular system. While these proteins can be postulated to be important in heart development, future experimentation will be required to elucidate their actual roles in cardiogenesis.

REFERENCES

1. Wolfsberg TG, Primakoff P, Myles DG, White JM. 1995. ADAM, a novel family of membrane proteins containing A Disintegrin And Metalloprotease domain: multipotential functions in cell-cell and cell-matrix interactions. J Cell Biol 131:275–278.
2. Wolfsberg TG, White JM. 1996. ADAMs in fertilization and development. Devel Biol 180:389–401.
3. Kuno K, Kanada N, Nakashima E, Fujiki F, Ichimura F, Matsushima K. 1997. Molecular cloning of a gene encoding a new type of metalloproteinase-disintegrin family protein with thrombospondin motifs as an inflammation associated gene. J Biol Chem 272:556–562.
4. Gilpin BJ, Loechel F, Mattei MG, Engvall E, Albrechtsen R, Wewer UM. 1998. A novel, secreted

form of human ADAM 12 (meltrin alpha) provokes myogenesis *in vivo*. J Biol Chem 273:157–166.

5. Millichip MI, Dallas DJ, Wu E, Dale S, McKie N. 1998. The metallo-disintegrin ADAM 10 (MADM) from bovine kidney has type IV collagenase activity *in vitro*. Biochem Biophys Res Commun 245:594–598.

6. Loechel F, Gilpin BJ, Engvall E, Albrechtsen R, Wewer UM. 1998. Human ADAM 12 (meltrin α) is an active metalloprotease. J Biol Chem 273:16993–16997.

7. Hilenski LL, Terracio L, Sawyer R, Borg K. 1989. Effects of extracellular matrix on cytoskeletal and myfibrilar organization in vitro. Scan Microscopy 535.

8. Hilenski L, Terracio L, Borg TK. 1991. Myofibriliar and cytoskeletal assembly in neonatal rat cardiac myocytes cultured on laminin and collagen. Cell Tissue Res 264:577–587.

9. Fassler R, Rohwedel J, Maltsev V, Bloch W, Lentini S, Guan K, Gullberg D, Hescheler J, Addicks K, Wobus AM. 1996. Differentiation and integrity of cardiac muscle cells are impaired in the absence of beta 1 integrin. J Cell Science 109:2989–2999.

10. Simpson DG, Terracio L, Terracio M, Price RL, Turner DC, Borg TK. 1994. Modulation of cardiac myocyte phenotype *in vitro* by the composition and orientation of the extracellular matrix. J Cell Physiol 161:89–105.

11. Simpson DG, Reaves T, Shih ST, Burgess W, Borg TK, Terracio L. 1998. Cardiac integrins: The ties that bind. Cardiovasc Pathol 7:135–143.

12. Hooper NM, Karran EH, Turner AJ. 1997. Membrane protein secretases. Biochem J 321:265–279.

13. Black RA, Rauch CT, Kozlosky CJ, Peschon JJ, Slack JL, Wolfson MF, Castner BJ, Stocking KL, Reddy P, Srinivasan S, Nelson N, Boiani N, Schooley KA, Gerhart M, Davis R, Fitzner JN, Johnson RS, Paxton RJ, March CJ, Cerretti DP. 1997. A metalloproteinase disintegrin that releases tumour-necrosis factor-alpha from cells. Nature 385:729–733.

14. Moss ML, Jin SL, Milla ME, Bickett DM, Burkhart W, Carter HL, Chen WJ, Clay WC, Didsbury JR, Hassler D. 1997. Nature 385:729–733.

15. Peschon JJ, Slack JL, Reddy P, Stocking KL, Sunnarborg SW, Lee DC, Russel WE, Castner BJ, Johnson RS, Fitzner JN, Boyce RW, Nelson N, Kozlosky CJ, Wolfson MF, Rauch CT, Cerretti DP, Paxton RJ, March CJ, Black RA. 1998. An essential role for ectodomain shedding in mammalian development. Science 282:1281–1284.

16. Blobel C. 1997. Metalloprotease-disintegrins: Links to cell adhesion and cleavage of TNF-α and Notch. Cell 90:589–592.

17. Black RA, White JM. 1998. ADAMs: Focus on the protease domains. Curr Opin Cell Biol 10:654–659.

18. Borland G, Murphy G, Ager A. 1999. Tissue inhibitor of metalloproteinases-3 inhibits shedding of L-selectin fromleukocytes. J Biol Chem 274:2810–2815.

19. Lammich S, Kojro E, Postina R, Gilbert S, Pfeiffer R, Jasionowski M, Haass C, Fahrenholz F. 1999. Constitutive and regulated α-secretase cleavage of Alzheimer's amyloid precursor protein by a disintegrin and metalloprotease. Proc Natl Acad Sci USA 96:3922–3927.

20. Izumi Y, Hirata M, Hasuwa H, Iwamoto R, Umata T, Miyado K, Tamai Y, Kurisaki T, Sehara-Fujisawa A, Ohno A, Mekada E. 1998. A metalloprotease-disintegrin, MDC 9/meltrin-γ/ADAM 9 and PKC δ are involved in TPA-indiuced ectodomain shedding of membrane-anchored heparin-binding EGF-like growth factor. EMBO J 17:7260–7272.

21. Shakibaei M, Marker H-J. 1999. β1-integrins in the cartilage matrix. Cell Tissue Res 296:565–573.

22. Albelda AM, Buck CA. 1990. Integrins and other cell adhesion molecules. FASEB J 4:2868–2880.

23. Humphries MJ. 1990. The molecular basis and specificity of integrin-ligand interactions. J Cell Sci 97:585–592.

24. Hynes RO. 1992. Integrins: Versatility, modulation and signaling in cell adhesion. Cell 69:11–25.

25. Baldwin HS, Buck CA. 1994. Integrins and other cell adhesion molecules in cardiac development. Trends Cardiovasc Med 4:178–187.

26. Ding B, Price RL, Goldsmith EC, Borg TK, Yan X, Douglas MD, Weinberg EO, Thielen T, Didenko VV, Lorell BH. 2000. Left ventricular hypertrophy in ascending aortic stenosis mice: Anoikis and the progression to early failure. Circulation 101:2854–2862.

27. Blobel CP, Wolfsberg TG, Turk CW, Myles DG, Primakoff P, White JM. 1992. A potential fusion peptide and an integrin ligand domain in a protein active in sperm-egg fusion. Nature 356:248–252.

28. Evans J, Schwartz R, Kopf G. 1995. Mouse sperm-egg plasma membrane interactions: Analysis of roles of egg integrins and the mouse sperm homologue of PH-30 (fertilin). J Cell Sci 108:3267–3278.

29. Snell WJ, White JM. 1996. The molecules of mammalian fertilization. Cell 85:629–637.

30. Evans JP, Schultz RM, Kopf GS. 1998. Roles of the disintegrin domains of mouse fertilins alpha and beta in fertilization. Biol Reprod 59:145–152.
31. Primakoff P, Hyatt H, Tredick-Kline J. 1987. Identification and purification of a sperm surface protein with a potential role in sperm-egg membrane fusion. J Cell Biol 104:141–149.
32. Blobel CP, White JM. 1992. Structure, function and evolutionary relationship of proteins containing a disintegrin domain. Curr Opin Cell Biol 4:760–765.
33. Myles DG, Kimmel LH, Blobel CP, White JM, Primakoff P. 1994. Identification of a binding site in the disintegrin domain of fertilin required for sperm-egg fusion. Proc Natl Acad Sci USA 91:4195–4198.
34. Cho C, Bunch DO, Faure JE, Goulding EH, Eddy EM, Primakoff P, Myles DG. 1998. Fertilization defects in sperm from mice lacking fertilin β. Science 281:1857–1859.
35. Almeida E, Huovila A-P, Sutherland AE, Stephens L, Calaraco P, Shaw L, Mercurio A, Sonnenberg A, Primakoff P, Myles DG. 1999. Mouse egg integrin α6β1 functions as a sperm receptor. Cell 81:1095–1104.
36. Chen MS, Almeida EA, Huovila A, Takahashi Y, Shaw LM, Mercurio AM, White JM. 1999. Evidence that distinct states of the integrin α6β1 interact with laminin and an ADAM. J Cell Biol 144: 549–561.
37. Zhang XP, Kamamata T, Yokoyama K, Puzon-McLaughlin W, Takada Y. 1998. Specific interaction of the recombinant disintegrin-like domain of MDC-15 (metargidin, ADAM-15) with integrin alphav-beta 3. J Biol Chem 273:7345–7350.
38. Yagami-Hiromasa T, Sato T, Kurisaki T, Kamijo K, Nabeshima Y, Fujisawa-Sehara A. 1995. A metalloprotease-disintegrin participating in myoblast fusion. Nature 377:652–656.
39. Bjarnason JB, Fox JW. 1995. Snake venom metalloendopeptidases: Reprolysins. Methods Enzymol 248:345–368.
40. Tselepis VH, Green LJ, Humphries MJ. 1997. An RGD to LDV conversion within the disintegrin kistrin generates an integrin antagonist that retains potency but exhibits altered receptor specificity. J Biol Chem 272:21341–21348.
41. Thiery JP, Duband JL, Trucker GC. 1985. Cell migration in the vertebrate embryo: Role of cell adhesion and tissue environment in pattern formation. Annu Rev Cell Biol 1:91–113.
42. Rees DA, Couchman JR, Smith CG, Woods A, Wilson G. 1983. Cell-substratum interactions in the adhesion and locomotion of fibroblasts. Philosophical Trans Royal Soc London 299:169–176. 11-4-82.
43. Potts JD, Dagle JM, Walder JA, Weeks DL, Runyan RB. 1991. Epithelial-mesenchymal transformation of embryonic cardiac endothelial cells is inhibited by a modified antisense oligodeoxynucleotide to transforming growth factor beta 3. Proc Nat Acad Sci USA 88:1516–1520.
44. Potts JD, Vincent EB, Runyan RB, Weeks DL. 1992. Sense and antisense TGF beta 3 mRNA levels correlate with cardiac valve induction. Devel Dynamics 193:340–345.
45. Schiro JA, Chan BMC, Roswit WT, Kassner PD, Pentland AP, Hemler ME, Eisen AZ, Kupper TS. 1991. Integrin α2β1 (VLA-2) mediates reorganization and contraction of collagen matrices by human cells. Cell 67:403–410.
46. Carver W, Molano I, Reaves T, Borg TK, Terracio L. 1995. Role of the α1β1 integrin complex in collagen gel contraction in vitro by heart fibroblasts. J Cell Physiol 165:425–437.
47. Woessner JF. 1991. Matrix metalloproteinases and their inhibitors in connective tissue remodeling. FASEB J 5:2145–2154.
48. Werb Z. 1993. Proteinases and matrix degradation. Textbook of Rheumatology. pp 248–264.
49. Birkedal-Hansen H, Moore WE, Bodden MK, Windsor LJ, Birkedal-Hansen B, DeCarlo A, Engler JA. 1993. Matrix metalloproteinases: A review Crit Rev Oral Biol Med 4:197–250.
50. McGuire PG, Orkin RW. 1992. Urokinase activity in the developing avian heart: a spatial and temporal analysis. Devel Dynamics 193:24–33.
51. McGuire PG, Alexander SM. 1993. Inhibition of urokinase synthesis and cell surface binding alters the motile behavior of embryonic endocardial-derived mesenchymal cells in vitro. Development 118:931–939.
52. Nakagawa W, Terracio L, Carver W, Birkedal-Hansen H, Borg TK. 1992. Expression of collagenase and IL-1 alpha in developing rat hearts. Devel Dynamics 195:87–99.
53. Alexander SM, Jackson KJ, Bushnell KM, McGuire PG. 1997. Spatial and temporal expression of the 72-kDa type IV collagenase (MMP-2) correlates with development and differentiation of valves in the embryonic avian heart. Devel Dynamics 209:261–268.

54. Borg K, Burgess W, Terracio L, Borg TK. 1998. Expression of metalloproteases by cardiac myocytes and fibroblasts in vitro. Cardiovasc Pathol 6:261–269.
55. Dettman RW, Denetclaw WJ, Ordahl CP, Bristow J. 1998. Common epicardial origin of coronary vascular smooth muscle, perivascular fibroblasts, and intermyocardial fibroblasts in the avian heart. Devel Biol 193:169–181.
56. Gittenberger-de Groot AC, Vrancken PM, Mentink MM, Gourdie RG, Poelmann RE. 1998. Epicardium-derived cells contribute a novel population to the myocardial wall and the atrioventricular cushions. Circ Res 82:1043–1052.
57. Nath D, Slocombe PM, Webster A, Stephens PE, Docherty AJP, Murphy G. 2000. Meltrin γ (ADAM-9) mediates cell adhesion through α6β1 integrin, leading to a marked induction of fibroblast cell motility. J Cell Sci 113:2319–2328.
58. Horwitz A, Duggan K, Buck C, Becherle MC, Burridge K. 1986. Interaction of plasma membrane fibronectin receptor with talin- a transmembrane linkage. Nature 320:531–533.
59. Otey CA, Pavalko FM, Burridge K. 1990. An interaction between α-actinin and the β1 integrin subunit *in vitro*. J Cell Biol 111:721–729.
60. Liliental J, Chang DD. 1998. Rack 1, a receptor for activated protein kinase C, interacts with integrin β subunit. J Biol Chem 273:2379–2383.
61. Hemler MN. 1998. Integrin associated proteins. Curr Opin Cell Biol 10:578–585.
62. Borg TK, Terracio L. 1990. Interaction of the extracellular matrix with cardiac myocytes during development and disease. In: (Robinson T, ed.) Issues in Biomedicine. Basel, Karger.
63. Iba K, Albrechtsen R, Gilpin BJ, Loechel F, Wewer UM. 1999. Cysteine-rich domain of human ADAM 12 (meltrin α) supports tumor cell adhesion. Amer J Pathol 154:1489–1501.
64. Iba K, Albrechtsen, Gilpin B, Frohlich C, Loechel F, Zolkiewska A, Ishguro K, Kojima T, Liu W, Langford K, Sanderson RD, Brakebusch C, Fassler R, Wewer DM. 2000. The cysteine-rich domain of human ADAM 12 supports cell adhesion through syndecans and triggers signaling events that lead to β1 integrin-dependent cell spreading. J Cell Biol 149:1143–1155.

B. Ostadal, M. Nagano and N.S. Dhalla (eds.).
CARDIAC DEVELOPMENT. Copyright © 2002.
Kluwer Academic Publishers. Boston.
All rights reserved.

CARDIAC FIBROSIS DURING THE DEVELOPMENT OF HEART FAILURE: NEW INSIGHTS INTO SMAD INVOLVEMENT

JIANMING HAO, BAIQIU WANG, STEPHEN C. JONES, and IAN M.C. DIXON*

Laboratory of Molecular Cardiology, Institute of Cardiovascular Sciences, St. Boniface General Hospital Research Centre, Faculty of Medicine, University of Manitoba, 351 Tache Avenue, Winnipeg, Manitoba, Canada R2H 2A6

Summary. Angiotensin II (angiotensin) and transforming growth factor-β_1 (TGF-β_1) play an important role in cardiac fibrosis and infarct scar remodeling after myocardial infarction (MI). We characterized 8 week post-MI rat hearts for altered expression of Smad proteins with and without losartan treatment. AT$_1$ blockade was associated with attenuated activation of the latent form of TGF-β_1 in remnant (viable) myocardium and infarct scar. Immunofluorescence (IF) studies revealed Smad 2 localization to myofibroblasts in target tissues with less intense staining in cardiac myocytes. Losartan administration (15 mg/kg/day) for 8 weeks was associated with normalization of total cellular Smad 2 and Smad 4 overexpression in the infarct scar as well as Smad 2 overexpression in remnant heart tissue. On the other hand, phosphorylated Smad 2 (P-Smad 2) staining was reduced in cytosolic fractions from failing experimental heart tissues *vs* controls and these trends were normalized in the presence of losartan, suggesting augmented P-Smad 2 movement into nuclei in untreated hearts. Using cultured adult primary rat fibroblasts treated with 10^{-6} M angiotensin, we noted rapid translocation (15 min) of P-Smad 2 into the cellular nuclei from the cytosol. Nuclear P-Smad 2 protein levels were increased in cultured fibroblasts following 15 min angiotensin treatment, and this response was blocked by losartan treatment. We conclude that angiotensin may influence total Smad 2 and 4 expression in post-MI heart failure, and that angiotensin treatment is associated with rapid P-Smad 2 nuclear translocation in isolated fibroblasts. This study suggests that crosstalk between angiotensin and Smad signaling are associated with fibrotic events in post-MI hearts.

* Address for correspondence: Ian M.C. Dixon, Ph.D., Institute of Cardiovascular Sciences, St. Boniface General Hospital Research Centre, University of Manitoba, 351 Tache Avenue, Winnipeg, Manitoba, Canada R2H 2A6. Tel: (204) 235-3419; Fax: (204) 233-6723; e-mail: iand@sbrc.umanitoba.ca

Key words: cardiac fibrosis, heart failure, myocardial infarction, cytokine

INTRODUCTION

After myocardial infarction (MI), the myocardium undergoes a repair process involving scar formation at the site of infarction that includes fibroblast and myofibroblast proliferation and concomitant deposition of extracellular matrix proteins [1]. During the early phase of MI, activation of these processes are critical for normal wound healing in the infarcted region. However, eventual interstitial fibrosis also occurs in remnant tissue and acts to increase myocardial stiffness. Further expansion of the extracellular matrix impairs diastolic stiffness and compromises systolic mechanics contributing to subsequent cardiac hypertrophy and heart failure [2,3]. Thus, the investigation of mechanism(s) underlying post-MI cardiac fibrosis has attracted considerable attention in recent years.

Increasing evidence supports the suggestion that transforming growth factor β_1 (TGF-β_1) stimulates the progression of cardiac fibrosis during cardiac hypertrophy and heart failure [4–6]. TGF-β_1 is known to be involved in several key cellular events during both the development and adult life of many organisms, including cell migration, adhesion, multiplication, differentiation and death [7].

TGF-β_1 signaling involves a family of membrane receptor protein kinases and a family of receptor substrates, the Smad proteins [7]. To initiate the TGF-β signaling cascade, two different transmembrane protein serine/threonine kinases, known as TGF-β_1 receptor types I and II, are brought together by the ligand, which acts as a receptor assembly factor. In the ligand-induced complex, the type I receptor kinase is activated by the phosphorylation of its GS region by receptor type II. The type I receptors specifically recognize the Smad subgroup known as receptor-activated Smads (R-Smads; Smad 2 and Smad 3) [7], which are recognized by TGF-β receptors (Fig. 1). The R-Smads consist of two conserved domains that form globular structures separated by a linker region [8,9]. The N-terminal MH1 domain has DNA-binding activity whereas the C-terminal MH2 domain drives translocation into the nucleus and possesses transcriptional regulatory activity. Receptor-mediated phosphorylation of the C-terminal SSxS sequence motif appears to relieve these two domains from a mutually inhibitory interaction and leads to R-Smad activation. Once activated, the R-Smad then binds to a common-mediator Smad (Co-Smad; Smad 4 in TGF-β signaling) and this complex translocates to the nucleus [7]. Once in the nucleus, it appears that Smad proteins can interact with a variety of nuclear factors that may act as DNA-binding proteins, transcriptional co-activators or co-repressors. Fast 2 is one such DNA-binding partner that associates with the Smad proteins in the nucleus, allowing the entire complex to assemble on a sequence-specific DNA element to strongly activate transcription [10,11]. Further enhancement of Smad-mediated transcription occurs through the direct interaction of CBP/P300 with the activated R-Smad, an interaction that is enhanced by TGF-β-induced phosphorylation [12]. Smads can also bind transcription repressors such as TGIF, c-Ski or SnoN to inhibit or down-regulate the transcription of target genes [13,14]. Thus, following activation and nuclear

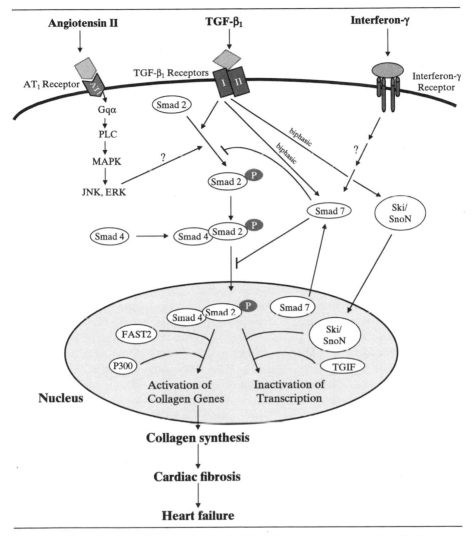

Figure 1. Schematic of putative interactions in the Smad signaling pathway in cardiac fibroblasts in response to TGF-β_1, Angiotensin II (Ang II) or Interferon-γ (INF-γ) stimulation. Activated TGF-β_1 receptor phosphorylates Smad 2, which may also be mediated by JNK or ERK downstream of Angiotensin II receptor activation. Activated Smad 2 binds to Smad 4 and the dimer translocates to the nucleus, associating with co-activators (FAST2, P300) or co-repressors (c-Ski, SnoN, TGIF). Binding of the Smad complex to co-activators may assist in the activation of collagen genes in the progression of cardiac fibrosis, and binding to co-repressors may inactivate the transcription of target genes. Smad 7 may play a role in negative feedback on the TGF-β_1 signal, regulating the phosphorylation and nuclear translocation of Smad 2 under TGF-β_1 or INF-γ stimulation. INF-γ may regulate Smad 7, Ski or SnoN to exert an inhibitory effect on the Smad signal. Blunt-ended arrows represent inhibitory effects.

translocation, the R-Smad-Co-Smad complex can regulate transcription both positively and negatively depending on the interacting partners. In this sense, the mix of Smad partners and regulators present in a given cell at the time of TGF-β stimulation may decide the ultimate cellular response.

In addition to R-Smads and Co-Smads, which carry signals from receptors to the nucleus, a third group of Smads called inhibitory Smads (I-Smads), including Smad 6 and Smad 7 may abrogate TGF-β signal transduction. Smad 7 inhibits Smad phosphorylation by occupying TGF-β type I receptors [15]. The expression of both Smad 6 and Smad 7 is increased in response to TGF-β, supporting the existence of roles in negative feedback of these pathways [16]. The expression of Smad 7 can also be regulated by other cytokines such as interferon-γ [17]. Interferon-γ stimulates the expression of Smad 7 through Jak 1 tyrosine and the Stat 1 transcription factor and thus exerts an inhibitory effect on TGF-β signaling [17].

TGF-β_1 is a powerful initiator for the synthesis of collagen and other major extracellular matrix (ECM) components in a variety of cell types [18]. The expression of TGF-β_1 is increased in the myocardium during pressure overload-induced hypertrophy [19] and early after myocardial infarction [20]. We have observed activation of TGF-β_1 and the increased expression of novel downstream Smad 2 and Smad 4 signaling proteins in infarct scar and remnant myocardium during the chronic phase of MI [21]. These events were positively correlated to ongoing cardiac fibrosis in remnant tissues as well as scar remodeling in post-MI heart, which is modulated exclusively by cardiac fibroblasts and myofibroblasts [21,22].

A significant body of literature indicates that elevated angiotensin signaling is associated with the onset of cardiac fibrosis in different models of heart failure, including myocardial infarction [5,23]. In the infarcted rat heart, local angiotensin generation is activated in the remnant myocardium and scar [23]. The predominant collagen-synthesizing cells in post-MI heart have been identified as myofibroblasts [24], and AT_1 receptor antagonism significantly attenuates fibrosis in both infarcted and non-infarcted rat myocardium [5,25]. Angiotensin-mediated modulation of the expression of TGF-β_1 ligand occurs *in vitro* [26,27] and *in vivo* [28] in various cell types including cardiac fibroblasts. However, information about crosstalk between angiotensin and TGF-β_1 in post-MI heart at the post-receptor level (Smad proteins) is lacking. Furthermore, the role of putative angiotensin/TGF-β_1 crosstalk in the development of cardiac fibrosis and heart failure is unclear. This study addressed whether chronic AT_1 receptor blockade, a known anti-fibrotic strategy, was associated with modulation of cardiac Smad expression and activation in failing rat heart post-MI.

MATERIALS AND METHODS

Experimental model

All experimental protocols for animal studies were approved by the Animal Care Committee of the University of Manitoba, Canada, following guidelines established by the Medical Research Council of Canada. MI was produced in male Sprague-Dawley rats (weighing 200–250 g) by ligation of the left coronary artery, as described previously [29]. Surviving rats from sham–operated and MI groups were divided into 3 groups: group 1, sham–operated animals; group 2, MI; and group 3, MI rats treated with losartan (15 mg/kg/day) [5,30]. All losartan treatment regimens were initiated immediately after coronary occlusion by implantation of Alzet osmotic mini-pumps consecutively to achieve the eight week treatment (Alza Corporation, La Jolla, CA; model 2002 and 2ML4 in sequence). For comparative purposes, sham–operated controls (group 1) and MI animals were administered vehicle (0.9% saline) in the same fashion. The experimental rats were sacrificed after 8 weeks, and cardiac tissue was isolated from three left ventricle regions: remnant/ viable (noninfarcted LV free wall remote from infarct and septum), border ($\approx$2 mm viable tissue and $\approx$2 mm scar tissue) and infarct scar. Tissues from these regions were used for Western blot analysis and immunohistochemistry to quantify and localize TGF-β_1 and its downstream effectors Smad 2 (both total and phosphorylated) and Smad 4.

Hemodynamic measurements

Mean arterial blood pressure (MAP) and LV function of sham-operated control, MI, and MI treated with losartan groups were measured after 8 weeks following induction of MI, as described previously [3]. Briefly, a micromanometer-tipped catheter (2-0) (Millar SPR-249) was inserted into the right carotid artery and advanced into the aorta to determine MAP, and then further advanced to the LV chamber to record LV systolic pressure (LVSP), LV end-diastolic pressure (LVEDP), the maximum rate of isovolumic pressure development (+dP/dt$_{max}$) and the maximum rate of isovolumic pressure decay (−dP/dt$_{max}$).

Determination of infarct size in experimental animals

After 8 weeks, the rats were sacrificed and the hearts were excised. The LV was fixed by immersion in 10% formalin and embedded in paraffin. Six transverse slices were cut from the apex to the base, and serial sections (5 μm) were cut and mounted. The percentage of infarcted LV was estimated at 8 weeks after coronary ligation by planimetric techniques as described previously [5]. Animals with an infarct size less than 40% of the LV free wall were excluded.

Adult cardiac fibroblast isolation and culture

Adult cardiac fibroblasts were isolated from male Sprague-Dawley rats according to the methods of Brilla et al. [31] with minor modifications [32]. The adult rat heart was subjected to Langendorff perfusion at a flow of 5 ml/min at 37°C with recirculatory Joklik's medium containing 0.1% collagenase and 2% bovine serum albumin (BSA) for 25–35 minutes. Liberated cells were collected by centrifugation at 2000 rpm for 10 minutes. Following this, the suspension of DMEM/F12 was plated on a 100 mm noncoated culture flask at 37°C with 5% CO$_2$ for 2 h. Cardiac fibroblasts attached to the bottom of the culture flask during 2 h incubation while non-adherent myocytes were removed by changing the culture medium. The cells were maintained in DMEM/F12 supplemented with 10% fetal bovine serum, 100 unit/ml penicillin and 100 µg/ml streptomycin. The cells used for the study were from the second passage (P2), and the purity of fibroblasts used in these experiments was found to be ≥95%, using routine phenotyping methods described previously [22,32]. For stimulation with angiotensin, fibroblasts were maintained in serum-free media for 24 h before administration of angiotensin (10^{-6} M) for 15 min. Equimolar losartan was added to cultured cells 1 hour before angiotensin treatment to achieve AT_1 blockade.

Immunofluorescent localization of TGF-β_1, Smad proteins in post-MI heart

A total of 12 rats with 4 rats in each group were used in these studies. Left ventricular tissue from sham and viable left ventricle remote to the infarct as well as border and scar tissues from MI rats were immersed in OCT compound (Miles Inc., Elkhart, IN). Serial cryostat sections (7 µm) of ventricular tissue were mounted on gelatin coated slides. A minimum of 6 sections from different regions of each group was processed. Indirect immunofluorescence was performed as described in detail previously [22,32]. Tissue sections were fixed in 4% paraformaldehyde for 15 minutes. Polyclonal antibodies against TGF-β_1, Smad 2, Smad 4 and phosphorylated Smad 2 (P-Smad 2) were diluted 1:20–1:40 with 1% BSA in PBS and applied as the primary antibodies. The anti-TGF-β_1 antibody recognizes both latent and active forms of TGF-β_1 and the Smad 2 antibody detects both phosphorylated and non-phosphorylated Smad 2. For double staining with vimentin, monoclonal mouse anti-vimentin clone #V9 (1:100 with 1% BSA in PBS) was added to the slides at the same time. After incubation overnight at 4°C, the sections were washed with PBS and incubated with biotinylated, anti-goat (or rabbit) IgG secondary antibody and subsequently incubated with FITC-labeled streptavidin for 90 minutes. To distinguish anti-vimentin antibody from other primary antibodies, an anti-mouse linked Texas Red conjugate (1:20 with 1% BSA in PBS) was added with streptavidin-FITC. Thus, vimentin was labelled with Texas Red and the other primary antibodies were labeled with FITC. Slides were mounted and coverslipped and tissue sections were examined under a Nikon Labophot microscope equipped with epifluorescence optics and appropriate filters. The results were photographed on Provia Fujichrome 400 color film.

Immunofluorescence assay in isolated fibroblasts

Adult cardiac fibroblasts were plated on coverslips and allowed to grow for 24 h. Cells were fixed with 1% paraformaldehyde after 15 min treatment with 10^{-6} M angiotensin. Immunofluorescent staining was performed by the indirect immunofluorescence technique [33] to detect either total Smad 2 or phosphorylated Smad 2. Cells were incubated with either of these antibodies overnight at 4°C. The primary antibodies were diluted (1:20–40) with PBS containing 1% BSA. After washing with PBS, cells were incubated with biotinylated anti-goat IgG secondary antibody followed by incubation with FITC-labelled streptavidin. After washing (3 × 5 min) with cold PBS, slides were immersed for 30 s in 10 µg/ml of Hoechst

Dye 33342 in order to stain cellular nuclei, and then subjected to an additional wash (3 × 5 min) in cold PBS. The slides were examined under a microscope equipped with epifluorescence optics, and photographed on Provia Fujichrome 400 color film.

Protein extraction and assay

Cardiac tissues from sham-operated left ventricle, viable left ventricle, border area and scar regions were homogenized in 100 mM Tris (pH 7.4) containing 1 mM EDTA, 1 mM PMSF, 4 μM leupeptin, 1 μM pepstatin A, and 0.3 μM aprotinin. Samples were sonicated for five seconds three times. Cytosolic fractions were isolated as described elsewhere [34]. Briefly, after homogenization, samples were centrifuged at 3000 × g at 4°C for 10 minutes to remove unbroken cells and nuclei. The resulting supernatant was further subjected to centrifugation at 48000 × g for 20 minutes at 4°C. The supernatant fraction was used for the protein determination of TGF-β_1 and phosphorylated Smad 2. For total cardiac Smad 2 and Smad 4 protein detection, tissues were homogenized with the above buffer containing 0.1% Triton X-100 and phosphatase inhibitors (10 mM NaF, 1 mM NaOV and β-glycorophosphate). This homogenate was sonicated for 5 seconds (repeated 5 times) to disrupt nuclear membranes. The samples were allowed to lyse for 15 minutes on ice. After centrifugation at 10000 × g for 20 min at 4°C, the supernatant was used for the cytosolic Smad protein assay. Total protein concentration of all samples was measured using the bicinchoninic acid (BCA) method as described previously [35].

Nuclear isolation from cardiac fibroblasts

Nuclei of cardiac fibroblasts were isolated using the Nuclei EZ Prep Nuclear Isolation Kit (Sigma-Aldrich, Oakville, ON, Canada) according to the manufacturer's instructions. The purity and integrity of isolated nuclei was confirmed by flow cytometry and light microscopy following trypan blue staining (data not shown). Isolated nuclei were resuspended in 100 mM Tris (pH 7.4) containing 1 mM EDTA, 1 mM PMSF, 4 μM leupeptin, 1 μM pepstatin A, and 0.3 μM aprotinin. Phosphatase inhibitor (10 mM NaF, 1 mM NaOV and 20 mM β-glycorophosphate) were also added to the solution. Samples were subjected to sonication 3 × 10 sec to further disrupt the nuclei and the nuclear protein concentration analysis was performed by BCA methods [30].

Western blot analysis of TGF-β_1, Smad 2 and Smad 4

Prestained low molecular weight marker (Bio-Rad, Hercules, CA) and 30 μg of protein from samples were separated on 10% or 12% SDS gels by SDS-PAGE. Separated protein was transferred onto 0.45 μM polyvinylidene difluoride (PVDF) membrane that was blocked at room temperature for 1 h or overnight at 4°C in Tris-buffered saline with 0.2% Tween-20 (TBS-T) containing 8% skim milk and probed with primary antibodies. Primary antibodies against TGF-β_1 (detects both latent and active TGF-β_1) and Smad 4 were diluted 1 : 250 in TBS-T. Anti-Smad 2 antibody, which recognizes both phosphorylated and nonphosphorylated Smad 2, was diluted 1 : 250 in TBS-T. To specifically detect phosphorylated Smad 2 (P-Smad 2), a polyclonal antibody against P-Smad 2 was used (1 : 500). Secondary antibodies included: (1) horseradish peroxidase (HRP)-labeled anti-rabbit IgG for detection of Smad 4 protein (2) HRP-labeled anti-goat IgG for detection of Smad 2 proteins. All secondary antibodies were diluted 1 : 10000 with TBS-T. Afterwards, blocking peptides of TGF-β_1 and Smad 2 were used to identify the band specific to each protein. These bands were visualized by enhanced chemiluminescence (ECL) or by ECL + Plus according to the manufacturer's instructions (Amersham Life Science Inc. Arlington Heights, IL). Autoradiographs from Western blots were quantified using a CCD camera imaging densitometer (Bio-Rad, model GS 670) [21].

Reagents

Primary antibodies against Smad 2, Smad 4, TGF-β_1, control peptides for TGF-β_1 and Smad 2 as well as HRP-labeled anti-goat secondary antibody were obtained from Santa Cruz Biotechnology, Inc. (Santa Cruz, CA). P-Smad 2 primary antibody was obtained from Upstate Biotechnology (Lake Placid, NY). For cell phenotyping, monoclonal antibody against procollagen type 1 (SP1.D8) was from the Developmental Studies Hybridoma Bank (University of Iowa, USA), monoclonal antibody against desmin was from Calbiochem (Cambridge, MA) and antibodies against smooth muscle myosin, α-smooth muscle actin and factor VIII (von Willebrand factor) were from Sigma-Aldrich (Oakville, ON, Canada). Monoclonal mouse anti-vimentin antibody (clone #V9) was obtained from Sigma. Biotinylated anti-rabbit and anti-goat secondary antibodies, anti-mouse linked Texas Red conjugate, FITC-labeled streptavidin, and HRP-labeled anti-rabbit secondary antibody were purchased from Amersham Life Science Inc. (Arlington Heights, IL). Losartan was a kind gift from the Merck & Co., Inc. (Rahway, NJ).

Statistical analysis

All values are expressed as mean ± SEM. One way analysis of variance (ANOVA) followed by Student-Newman-Keuls method was used for comparing the differences among multiple groups (SigmaStat). Significant differences among groups were defined by a probability less than 0.05.

RESULTS

General observations: cardiac hypertrophy, total cardiac collagen concentration and heart failure

Hearts of experimental animals were characterized by significant cardiac hypertrophy as reflected by an increase in the mass of the viable left ventricular tissue (LV) and also by the increased LV to body mass (BW) ratio in experimental animals compared to control values (data not shown). The incidence and magnitude of left ventricular hypertrophy noted was comparable to our previous findings [22,29]. Cardiac collagen concentration in surviving myocardium remote to infarct (i.e., remnant heart: 58.2 ± 5.1 µg/mg dry wt) and border + scar tissues (126.3 ± 10.8 µg/mg dry wt) were both significantly higher than that of control value ($20.3 \pm 3.2\,\mu g/mg\,dry$ wt). Furthermore, cardiac collagen concentration in remnant heart treated with losartan ($37.4 \pm 3.4\,\mu g/mg\,dry\,wt$) was significantly reduced *vs* values from non-treated tissues. Heart failure, reflected by an increase in left ventricular end-diastolic pressure (LVEDP) and a decrease in the maximum rate of isovolumic pressure development or decay ($\pm dP/dt_{max}$) relative to their controls, along with congested lung, has been characterized in this model from our previous studies [3]. Losartan treatment was associated with normalization of indices of cardiac hypertrophy and cardiac function, in agreement with our previous findings [5].

Localization and quantification of cardiac Smads in post-MI heart

Immunofluorescent staining revealed that total Smad 2 protein was localized to the extracellular space proximal to nuclei as shown in Fig. 2. Double staining with vimentin showed that Smad 2 was mainly localized to nonmyocytes proximal to the nuclei. We observed enhanced accumulation of Smad 2 proteins in the nuclei of cells from scar tissue. Western analysis was used to determine the protein concentration of cardiac Smad 2 and Smad 4 from different groups. Cardiac Smad 2 (62 kDa) protein concentration was significantly increased in remnant and scar tissues when compared to control values, while cardiac Smad 4 (62 kDa) protein concentrations was only significantly elevated in scar tissue *vs* control. Losartan treatment was associated with a significant inhibitory effect on Smad 2 and Smad 4 accumulation in viable tissue and infarct scar tissue, respectively (Fig. 2).

Effect of losartan on the expression of cardiac TGF-β_1

Using Western blot analysis, cardiac TGF-β_1 protein concentration was quantified in control and viable left ventricular tissues as well as border and scar tissues of 8-week post-MI rats. The TGF-β_1 polyclonal antibody recognized both the latency associated peptide (LAP) and active forms of TGF-β_1 at ~40 kDa and 25 kDa, respectively. Although the LAP dimer of ~80 kDa binds TGF-β_1 *per se*, we observed the monomeric LAP band due to reducing gel conditions. The active form of TGF-β_1 was increased in both remnant and scar tissues from post-MI heart, which was significantly attenuated by the administration of losartan. Conversely, the latent form of TGF-β_1 was decreased in both remnant and scar tissues, and this decrease was partially prevented by losartan treatment (Fig. 3). Previous studies have shown that TGF-β_1 can be released from latent complexes and can be activated by cleaving an inactive high molecular weight precursor complex [36]. We observed that the conversion of TGF-β_1 from its latent to active form was augmented in remnant myocardium and infarct scar. Losartan treatment was associated with an inhibition of this conversion. Immunofluorescent staining revealed that total TGF-β_1 localized to the extracellular space in normal tissue and remnant myocardium. Furthermore, the infarct scar stained brightly for total TGF-β_1, as did myocytes bordering the infarct scar region. Cardiac myocytes remote to the infarct scar expressed comparatively moderate levels of TGF-β_1 (data not shown).

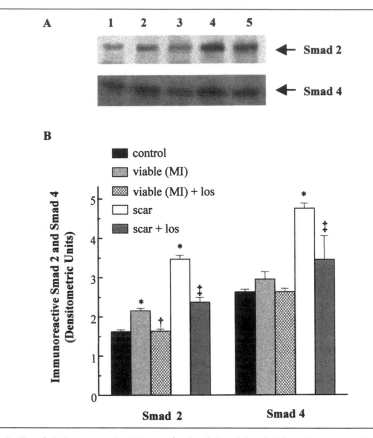

Figure 2. Panel A. Representative Westerns for Smad 2 and Smad 4 from sham-operated control hearts (lane 1) as well as viable remnant tissue (lane 2), viable remnant tissue with 8 week losartan treatment (lane 3), infarct scar tissue (lane 4) and infarct scar tissue with 8 week losartan treatment (lane 5) from 8 week post-MI left ventricular samples. **Panel B.** Histographic representation of quantified data of Smad 2 and Smad 4 expression in respective groups in **A** (quantified by densitometric scanning). The data depicted is the mean ± SEM of 4–6 experiments. P ≤ 0.05 is expressed by * *vs* sham, † *vs* viable and ‡ *vs* scar.

Total and phosphorylated Smad 2 distribution in post-MI heart and cultured cardiac fibroblasts

Immunofluorescence data indicated relatively moderate staining of phosphorylated Smad 2 (P-Smad 2) in myocytes of sham-operated, remnant and losartan-treated remnant tissues from post-MI rat heart (Fig. 4A, C, and E). Compared to control and viable tissues, the scar and treated scar sections (Fig. 4G and I, respectively) were characterized by brightly stained regions, and areas of punctate nuclear accumulation of P-Smad 2 were found in the scar (arrows). This pattern was associated with cellular nuclei in scar (Fig. 4H and J). Western analysis of cytosolic P-Smad 2 revealed a significant decrease in band intensity from cytosolic viable and scar tissue compared to sham-operated control (Fig. 5). These trends were normalized by losartan

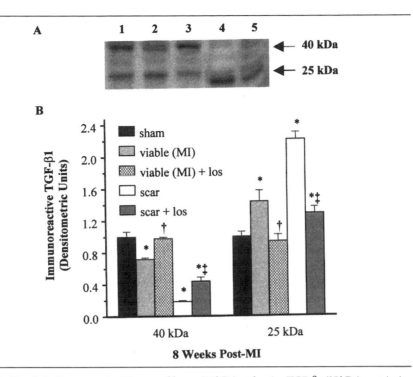

Figure 3. Panel A. Representative Western of latent (44 kDa) and active TGF-β_1 (25 kDa) protein in from sham-operated control hearts (lane 1) as well as viable remnant tissue (lane 2), viable remnant tissue with 8 week losartan treatment (lane 3), infarct scar tissue (lane 4) and infarct scar tissue with 8 week losartan treatment (lane 5) from 8 week post-MI rat heart left ventricular samples. **Panel B.** Histograms for quantified data from multiple samples from the groups in **A**. The data depicted is the mean ± SEM of 4–6 experiments. P ≤ 0.05 is expressed by * *vs* sham values; † *vs* viable values and ‡ *vs* scar values.

treatment. In studies of quiescent and unstimulated cultured cardiac fibroblasts, total Smad 2 localized to cellular nuclei and cytosol (Fig. 6a—panel A), as did P-Smad 2 (Fig. 6b—panel E). Total Smad 2 staining was elevated in intensity after stimulation with angiotensin (10^{-6} M) for 15 min *vs* unstimulated cells (Fig. 6a—panel C). Furthermore, 15 min angiotensin (10^{-6} M) stimulation was associated with marked translocation of P-Smad 2 from the cytosol to the nuclei (Fig. 6b—panel G). Western analysis of nuclei isolated from cultured cardiac fibroblasts from normal rat heart revealed that angiotensin stimulation (10^{-6} M) for 15 min was associated with a significant increase of P-Smad 2 protein, and this change was inhibited by AT$_1$ receptor blockade (Fig. 7).

DISCUSSION

Animals with a relatively large infarct 8 weeks post-MI were considered to be in moderate heart failure based on current data and previous observations [3,29]. Using this model, we have previously observed significant elevation in the deposition of

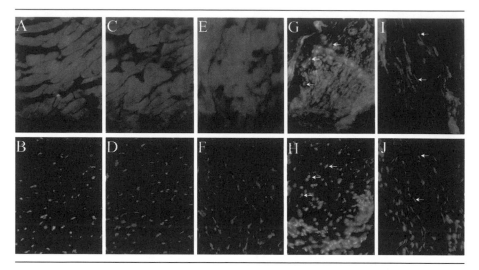

Figure 4. Smad 2 localization in untreated and losartan-treated sections of viable tissue and infarct scar in post-MI heart. Immunoreactive phosphorylated Smad 2 in sham-operated control hearts (A) as well as viable remnant tissue (C), viable remnant tissue with 8 week losartan treatment (E), infarct scar tissue (G) and infarct scar tissue with 8 week losartan treatment (I) from 8 week post-MI rat left ventricle. Fields depicted in panels A, C, E, G and I were stained for cellular nuclei with Hoescht 33342 and are shown in panels B, D, F, H and J, respectively. Arrows indicate focal bright staining for nuclei and phosphorylated Smad 2 in identical cells from corresponding panels. Experimental animals were harvested 8 weeks after surgery. Magnification ×400.

cardiac collagen, in addition to the persistence of myofibroblasts in the remnant myocardium and scar tissue [3,37]. These findings, in addition to enhanced Smad expression in these cells, provide a strong indication that infarct scar is not quiescent in 8 week post-MI hearts. In this regard, chronic scar remodeling has been shown to play a role in the functional preservation of the infarcted ventricle [38].

Fibroblasts, myofibroblasts and cardiac fibrosis

Following MI, fibroblasts arrive at the site of repair where they undergo phenotypic transformation to myofibroblasts, a process inducible by TGF-β_1 [39]. Myofibroblasts express α-smooth muscle actin (α-SMA), providing contractility and chronic mechanical tension to the remodeling scar [39]. Myofibroblasts have a high synthetic capacity for fibrillar collagens and express cytokines including angiotensin and TGF-β_1. These cells also express angiotensin receptors as well as TGF-β_1 receptors which potentiate fibroproliferative behavior [40]. In this regard, angiotensin and TGF-β_1 have been identified as contributors to cardiac fibrosis [39,41] and angiotensin is known to influence TGF-β_1 ligand expression [26], however crosstalk between the activated post-receptor mechanisms for these two systems in heart failure is unknown. We demonstrate that in heart failure, AT$_1$ blockade is associated with i) altered TGF-β_1 ligand processing in post-MI hearts, ii) normalization of both

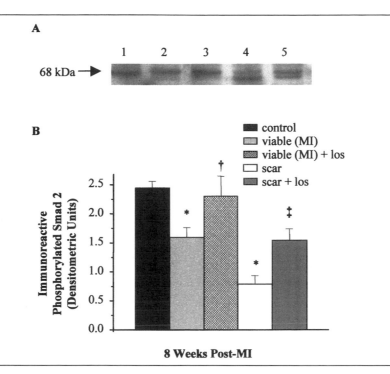

Figure 5. Panel A. Representative Western of cardiac tissue cytosolic fractions probed for phosphorylated Smad 2 in sham left ventricular tissue (lane 1), viable remnant myocardium (lane 2), viable tissue treated for 8 weeks with losartan (3), scar tissue (lane 4) and from scar tissue with 8 week losartan treatment (lane 5). Experimental animals were harvested 8 weeks after surgery. **Panel B.** Histograms for quantified data from multiple samples from the groups in **A** (quantified by densitometric scanning). The data depicted is the mean + SEM of 4–6 experiments. P ≤ 0.05 is expressed by * *vs* sham values; † *vs* viable values; ‡ *vs* scar values.

increased Smad 2 expression in remnant myocardium and infarct scar and increased Smad 4 expression in infarct scar. Furthermore, these events are positively associated with normalized cardiac function and significant reduction in cardiac fibrosis in treated experimental hearts. Finally, we show that angiotensin may elevate Smad 2 expression and nuclear accumulation in cultured adult cardiac fibroblasts, suggesting a direct mediation of this event.

Angiotensin and cardiac fibrosis

Angiotensin has been shown to stimulate cardiac fibrosis in several different models of heart failure [5,25,30,42]. Further, angiotensin stimulates collagen production in cultured cardiac fibroblasts [43], and its expression and AT_1 receptor density in myofibroblasts of the infarct scar are significantly increased [44,45]. We have demonstrated that AT_1 blockade is associated with partial attenuation of cardiac fibrosis in post-MI rats [46,47], however the precise mechanism of the antifibroproliferative effect

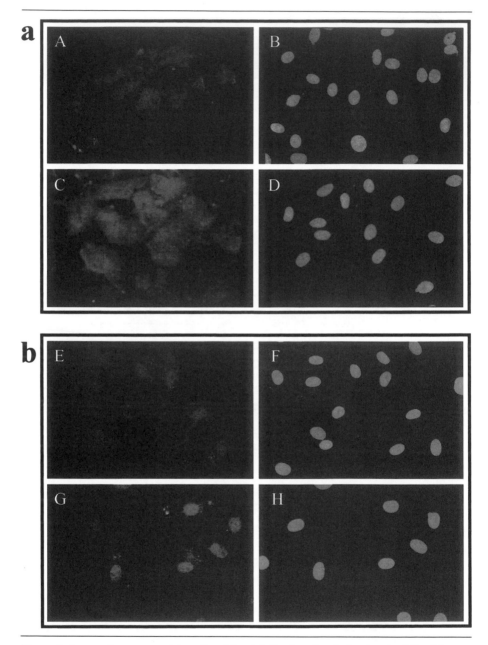

Figure 6. Immunofluorescent staining of total Smad 2 (**Section a**) and phosphorylated Smad 2 (**Section b**) from cultured cardiac fibroblasts stimulated by angiotensin (10^{-6} M) for 15 min. Panels A and E represent untreated fibroblasts showing total Smad 2 and phosphorylated Smad 2, respectively. Panels B, D, F and H represent nuclei (Hoechst 33342 staining) of identical sections corresponding to panels A, C, E and G, respectively. Magnification ×400.

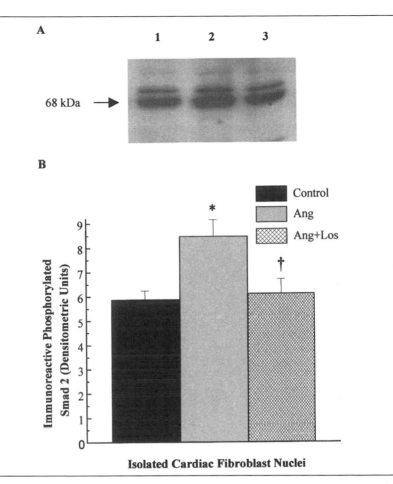

Figure 7. Panel A. Representative Western blot for phosphorylated Smad 2 in nuclei isolated from cardiac fibroblasts cultured in defined media. The 68 kDa band shown represents nuclear phosphorylated Smad 2 from untreated control cells (lane 1), 15 minute angiotensin (10^{-6} M) stimulated cells (lane 2), and 15 min angiotensin (10^{-6} M) stimulated cells with losartan (10^{-6} M) treatment (lane 3). **Panel B.** Histographic representation of quantified data from multiple samples from the groups in **A**: untreated (control), angiotensin treated (Ang) and angiotensin plus losartan treatment (Ang + Los). The data depicted is the mean ± S.E.M. of 3 experiments. $P < 0.05$ is expressed by * *vs* untreated control and † *vs* angiotensin treated values.

of this therapeutic intervention is unclear. Mounting evidence supports the existence of putative crosstalk between angiotensin and TGF-β at the level of ligand expression in cultured cells including adult primary cardiac fibroblasts [26,27]. Furthermore, AT_1 receptor blockade has been shown to be associated with increased steady-state abundance of TGF-β_1 mRNA observed in 4 weeks post–MI rat heart [28]. These findings support the hypothesis that AT_1 modulation of TGF-β_1 ligand may occur in cardiac fibroblasts. Nevertheless, a role of angiotensin at the post-receptor levels of TGF-β_1 signaling has not been identified.

AT$_1$ activation and TGF-β ligand processing/bioavailability in failing hearts

TGF-β is secreted as an inactive precursor complex containing a signal peptide, the active TGF-β_1 molecule, and the cleaved propeptide known as the latency associated peptide (LAP) [48]. Following removal of the signal peptide, the gene product undergoes proteolytic cleavage to produce mature TGF-β_1 (residues 279–390) and LAP (residues 30–278) [36,48]. We found that the active form of TGF-β_1 (25 kDa) is significantly elevated in remnant (viable) and scar tissues, whereas the LAP (~40 kDa in monomeric form as seen in a reducing gel) latent form of TGF-β_1 is decreased vs control in heart failure. This indicates a redistribution in expression of active TGF-β_1/LAP ratio in the remnant myocardium and infarct scar. As losartan treatment led to a normalization of this trend, AT$_1$ activation may play a role in relative activation of TGF-β_1 in experimental hearts, and thus regulate the bioavailability of the active TGF-β_1 molecule.

Effect of angiotensin on phosphorylation and translocation of Smad 2 in cultured cardiac fibroblasts

In recent years, Smad 2 has been well characterized as a key downstream effector of TGF-β signaling in mammalian cells, and it is clear that the phosphorylation of Smad 2 is required for nuclear translocation and subsequent regulation of transcription. Our previous data have shown that Smad 2 is upregulated in the infarct scar 8 weeks after MI. However, the effect of angiotensin on the phosphorylation and nuclear translocation of Smad 2 in cardiac fibroblasts and post MI heart has not been reported. In this study we noted increased total Smad 2 and decreased P-Smad 2 in cytosol sections from viable and scar tissues post-MI, suggesting an increased nuclear accumulation of P-Smad 2. In vivo, these trends were normalized by AT$_1$ receptor blockade. Our in vitro study demonstrated that angiotensin (10^{-6} M) stimulation of cultured adult cardiac fibroblasts is associated with an elevation of total Smad 2 protein. Furthermore, the presence of angiotensin caused an increased nuclear accumulation of P-Smad 2 in fibroblasts, as indicated by immunofluorescent staining and Western analysis. The protein level of P-Smad 2 in nuclei isolated from cardiac fibroblasts increased following angiotensin stimulation, an effect that was blocked by AT$_1$ receptor blockade. Taken together, these results indicate a possible link between angiotensin and the phosphorylation and nuclear translocation of Smad 2. The molecular mechanism underlying this link is not yet clear, and it is currently unknown whether this action is dependent or independent of TGF-β_1 ligand. It has been reported that Smad 2 activation may not be restricted to TGF-β receptors [49], and our data suggest a direct role for angiotensin in this regard. Recently Janus N-terminal kinase (JNK) activity has been shown to cause phosphorylation of the C-terminal tyrosines on receptor-activated Smads [50]. Furthermore, AT$_1$ activation causes a rapid increase (5 min) in JNK activity in cardiac cells in dose-dependent manner [8]. Additionally, Smad nuclear accumulation can by inhibited by Ras-activated Erk kinases [51]. Together these findings support a novel angiotensin-mediated pathway for phosphorylation/activation of cardiac Smad 2 proteins that is independent of TGF-β_1 receptor activation. Our data indicating rapid nuclear translocation of Smad 2 in cultured fibroblasts in the presence of angiotensin support this hypothesis, however further investigation is required in the heart to prove the existence of a direct angiotensin-Smad 2 interaction.

In conclusion, these results indicate that elevated Smad expression in experimental heart failure is normalized by long-term AT_1 receptor blockade and that these changes are paralleled by modulation of fibroproliferative events in these hearts. Further, AT_1 activation is associated with augmented nuclear accumulation of phosphorylated Smad 2 in failing hearts and with angiotensin stimulation of cultured cardiac fibroblasts. The current results also provide a link between angiotensin receptor activation and potentiation of Smad protein function in cardiac fibroblasts.

ACKNOWLEDGMENTS

This study was supported by funding from the Medical Research Council of Canada (IMCD). IMCD is a scholar of the Medical Research Council of Canada/PMAC health program with funding provided by Astra-Zeneca, Inc (Canada). JH is a recipient of the traineeship of Heart and Stroke Foundation of Canada. We thank Dr. A. Junaid for his thoughts and comments addressing this study and Dr. E. Kardami for her kind technical assistance. Losartan was a kind gift from Merck & Co., Inc.

REFERENCES

1. Weber KT, Sun Y, Katwa LC. 1996. Wound healing following myocardial infarction. Clin Cardiol 19:447–455.
2. Pfeffer JM, Fischer TA, Pfeffer MA. 1995. Angiotensin-converting enzyme inhibition and ventricular remodeling after myocardial infarction. Annu Rev Physiol 57:805–826.
3. Ju H, Zhao S, Tappia PS, Panagia V, Dixon IMC. 1998. Expression of Gqalpha and PLC-beta in scar and border tissue in heart failure due to myocardial infarction. Circulation 97:892–899.
4. Weber KT. 1997. Extracellular matrix remodeling in heart failure: a role for de novo angiotensin II generation. Circulation 96:4065–4082.
5. Ju H, Zhao S, Davinder SJ, Dixon IM. 1997. Effect of AT1 receptor blockade on cardiac collagen remodeling after myocardial infarction. Cardiovasc Res 35:223–232.
6. Lijnen PJ, Petrov VV, Fagard RH. 2000. Induction of cardiac fibrosis by transforming growth factor-beta(1) [In Process Citation]. Mol Genet Metab Sep–Oct;71(1–2):418–435.
7. Massague J. 1998. TGF-beta signal transduction. Annu Rev Biochem 67:753–791.
8. Kudoh S, Komuro I, Mizuno T, Yamazaki T, Zou Y, Shiojima I, Takekoshi N, Yazaki Y. 1997. Angiotensin II stimulates c Jun NH2-terminal kinase in cultured cardiac myocytes of neonatal rats. Circ Res 80:139–146.
9. Chenf YG, Hata A, Lo RS, Wotton D, Shi Y, Pavletich N, Massague J. 1998. Determinants of specificity in TGF-beta signal transduction. Genes Dev 12:2144–2152.
10. Chen X, Weisberg E, Fridmacher V, Watanabe M, Naco G, Whitman M. 1997. Smad4 and FAST-1 in the assembly of activin-responsive factor. Nature 389:85–89.
11. Labbe E, Silvestri C, Hoodless PA, Wrana JL, Attisano L. 1998. Smad2 and Smad3 positively and negatively regulate TGF beta-dependent transcription through the forkhead DNA-binding protein FAST2. Mol Cell 2:109–120.
12. Derynck R, Zhang Y, Feng XH. 1998. Smads: transcriptional activators of TGF-beta responses. Cell 95:737–740.

13. Wotton D, Lo RS, Lee S, Massague J. 1999. A Smad transcriptional corepressor. Cell 97:29–39.
14. Massague J, Chen YG. 2000. Controlling TGF-beta signaling. Genes Dev Mar 15;14(6):627–644.
15. Itoh S, Landstrom M, Hermansson A, Itoh F, Heldin CH, Heldin NE, ten Dijke P. 1998. Transforming growth factor beta1 induces nuclear export of inhibitory Smad7. J Biol Chem 273: 29195–29201.
16. Nakao A, Afrakhte M, Moren A, Nakayama T, Christian JL, Heuchel R, Itoh S, Kawabata M, Heldin NE, Heldin CH, ten Dijke, P. 1997. Identification of Smad7, a TGFbeta-inducible antagonist of TGF-beta signalling. Nature 389:631–635.
17. Ulloa L, Doody J, Massague J. 1999. Inhibition of transforming growth factor-beta/SMAD signalling by the interferon-gamma/STAT pathway. Nature 397:710–713.
18. Massague J. 1990. The transforming growth factor-beta family. Annu Rev Cell Biol 6:597–641.
19. Li JM, Brooks G. 1997. Differential protein expression and subcellular distribution of TGF beta1, beta2 and beta3 in cardiomyocytes during pressure overload-induced hypertrophy. J Mol Cell Cardiol 29:2213–2224.
20. Thompson NL, Bazoberry F, Speir EH, Casscells W, Ferrans VJ, Flanders KC, Kondaiah P, Geiser AG, Sporn MB. 1988. Transforming growth factor beta-1 in acute myocardial infarction in rats. Growth Factors 1:91–99.
21. Hao J, Ju H, Zhao S, Junaid A, Scammell-LaFleur T, Dixon IM. 1999. Elevation of expression of Smads 2, 3, and 4, decorin and TGF-beta in the chronic phase of myocardial infarct scar healing. J Mol Cell Cardiol 31:667–678.
22. Peterson D, Ju H, Jianming Hao PM, Chapman D, Dixon IMC. 1998. Expression of Gia2 and Gsa in myofibroblasts localized to the infarct scar in heart failure due to myocardial infarction. Cardiovasc Res 41:575–585.
23. Fabris B, Jackson B, Kohzuki M, Perich R, Johnston CI. 1990. Increased cardiac angiotensin-converting enzyme in rats with chronic heart failure. Clin Exp Pharmacol Physiol 17:309–314.
24. Sun Y, Weber KT. 1996. Angiotensin converting enzyme and myofibroblasts during tissue repair in the rat heart. J Mol Cell Cardiol 28:851–858.
25. Hanatani A, Yoshiyama M, Kim S, Omura T, Toda I, Akioka K, Teragaki M, Takeuchi K, Iwao H, Takeda T. 1995. Inhibition by angiotensin II type 1 receptor antagonist of cardiac phenotypic modulation after myocardial infarction. J Mol Cell Cardiol 27:1905–1914.
26. Campbell SE, Katwa LC. 1997. Angiotensin II stimulated expression of transforming growth factor-beta1 in cardiac fibroblasts and myofibroblasts. J Mol Cell Cardiol 29:1947–1958.
27. Gray MO, Long CS, Kalinyak JE, Li HT, Karliner JS. 1998. Angiotensin II stimulates cardiac myocyte hypertrophy via paracrine release of TGF-beta 1 and endothelin-1 from fibroblasts. Cardiovasc Res 40:352–363.
28. Sun Y, Zhang JQ, Zhang J, Ramires FJ. 1998. Angiotensin II, transforming growth factor-beta1 and repair in the infarcted heart. J Mol Cell Cardiol 30:1559–1569.
29. Dixon IMC, Lee SL, Dhalla NS. 1990. Nitrendipine binding in congestive heart failure due to myocardial infarction. Circ Res 66:782–788.
30. Smits JF, van Krimpen C, Schoemaker RG, Cleutjens JP, Daemen MJ. 1992. Angiotensin II receptor blockade after myocardial infarction in rats: effects on hemodynamics, myocardial DNA synthesis, and interstitial collagen content. J Cardiovasc Pharmacol 20:772–778.
31. Brilla CG, Zhou G, Matsubara L, Weber KT. 1994. Collagen metabolism in cultured adult rat cardiac fibroblasts: response to angiotensin II and aldosterone. J Mol Cell Cardiol 26:809–820.
32. Ju H, Hao J, Zhao S, Dixon IMC. 1998. Antiproliferative and antifibrotic effects of mimosine on adult cardiac fibroblasts. Biochim Biophys Acta 1448:51–60.
33. Polak JM, van Noorden S. 1984. An introduction to immunocytochemistry: current techniques and problems. Polak J.M. 1–49. Oxford, Oxford University Press. Microscopy Handbooks. Polak J.M.
34. Gettys TW, Sheriff Carter K, Moomaw J, Taylor IL, Raymond JR. 1994. Characterization and use of crude alpha-subunit preparations for quantitative immunoblotting of G proteins. Anal Biochem 220:82–91.
35. Smith PK, Krohn RI, Hermanson GT, Mallia AK, Gartner FH, Provenzano MD, Fujimoto EK, Goeke NM, Olson BJ, Klenk DC. 1985. Measurement of protein using bicinchoninic acid. Anal Biochem 150:76–85.
36. Harpel JG, Metz CN, Kojima S, Rifkin DB. 1992. Control of transforming growth factor-beta activity: latency vs. activation. Prog Growth Factor Res 4:321–335.
37. Sun Y, Cleutjens JP, Diaz-Arias AA, Weber KT. 1994. Cardiac angiotensin converting enzyme and myocardial fibrosis in the heart. Cardiovasc Res 28:1423–1432.

38. Holmes JW, Nunez JA, Covell JW. 1997. Functional implications of myocardial scar structure. Am J Physiol 272:H2123–H2130.
39. Weber KT. 1997. Fibrosis, a common pathway to organ failure: angiotensin II and tissue repair. Semin Nephrol 17:467–491.
40. Powell DW, Mifflin RC, Valentich JD, Crowe SE, Saada JI, West AB. 1999. Myofibroblasts. I. Paracrine cells important in health and disease. Am J Physiol 277:C1–C9.
41. Weber KT, Swamynathan SK, Guntaka RV, Sun Y. 1999. Angiotensin II and extracellular matrix homeostasis. Int J Biochem Cell Biol 31:395–403.
42. Schieffer B, Wirger A, Meybrunn M, Seitz S, Holtz J, Riede UN, Drexler H. 1994. Comparative effects of chronic angiotensin-converting enzyme inhibition and angiotensin II type 1 receptor blockade on cardiac remodeling after myocardial infarction in the rat. Circulation 89:2273–2282.
43. Chua CC, Chua BH, Zhao ZY, Krebs C, Diglio C, Perrin E. 1991. Effect of growth factors on collagen metabolism in cultured human heart fibroblasts. Connect Tissue Res 26:271–281.
44. Yamagishi H, Kim S, Nishikimi T, Takeuchi K, Takeda T. 1993. Contribution of cardiac renin-angiotensin system to ventricular remodelling in myocardial-infarcted rats. J Mol Cell Cardiol 25:1369–1380.
45. Sun Y, Weber KT. 1996. Cells expressing angiotensin II receptors in fibrous tissue of rat heart. Cardiovasc Res 31:518–525.
46. Dixon IMC, Ju H, Jassal DS, Peterson DJ. 1996. Effect of ramipril and losartan on collagen expression in right and left heart after myocardial infarction. Mol Cell Biochem 165:31–45.
47. Makino N, Hata T, Sugano M, Dixon IMC, Yanaga T. 1996. Regression of hypertrophy after myocardial infarction is produced by the chronic blockade of angiotensin type 1 receptor in rats. J Mol Cell Cardiol 28:507–517.
48. Miyazono K, Hellman U, Wernstedt C, Heldin CH. 1988. Latent high molecular weight complex of transforming growth factor beta 1. Purification from human platelets and structural characterization. J Biol Chem 263:6407–6415.
49. Zhang Y, Derynck R. 1999. Regulation of Smad signalling by protein associations and signalling crosstalk. Trends Cell Biol 9:274–279.
50. Engel ME, McDonnell MA, Law BK, Moses HL. 1999. Interdependent SMAD and JNK signaling in transforming growth factor-beta-mediated transcription. J Biol Chem 274:37413–37420.
51. Kretzschmar M, Doody J, Timokhina I, Massague J. 1999. A mechanism of repression of TGFbeta/Smad signaling by oncogenic Ras. Genes Dev 13:804–816.

B. Ostadal, M. Nagano and N.S. Dhalla (eds.).
CARDIAC DEVELOPMENT. Copyright © 2002.
Kluwer Academic Publishers. Boston.
All rights reserved.

DEVELOPMENTAL CHANGES IN CALCIUM CHANNEL LOCALIZATION IN RAT HEART: INFLUENCE OF THYROID HORMONE AND PRESSURE OVERLOAD

MAURICE WIBO and FRANTISEK KOLAR[1]

Laboratoire de Pharmacologie, Université catholique de Louvain, UCL 54.10, Avenue Hippocrate 54, B-1200 Brussels, Belgium, and [1] Institute of Physiology, Academy of Sciences of the Czech Republic, Videnska 1083, CZ-14220 Prague, Czech Republic

Summary. To better understand the developmental changes in cardiac excitation-contraction coupling, we analyzed the early postnatal changes in myocardial density, subsarcolemmal localization and isoform expression of dihydropyridine receptors (DHPRs) in rat ventricle and the influence of thyroid status and aortic constriction on these changes. Newborn rats were made hypo- or hyperthyroid, or were subjected to aortic constriction on day 2. As shown by radioligand binding and density gradient centrifugation techniques, the myocardial density of DHPRs increased 3-fold from day 1 to day 14 in control rats, and this increase occurred predominantly in junctional structures (dyadic couplings). This maturation was delayed in hypothyroid rats and in severely hypertrophied ventricles after aortic banding, and somewhat accelerated by hyperthyroidism. DHPR $\alpha 1$ subunit isoform expression was analyzed by reverse transcription-polymerase chain reaction and restriction enzyme analysis. The proportion of $\alpha 1$ subunit mRNA variants typical of foetal heart decreased with age in control rats, and this reduction was delayed by hypothyroidism. In conclusion, hypothyroidism and pressure overload impaired the postnatal concentration of DHPRs into junctional structures; hypothyroidism also delayed the postnatal decrease in the expression of $\alpha 1$ subunit variants typical of foetal heart.

Key words: Thyroid hormone, Aortic constriction, Junctional structures, Dihydropyridine receptor, Ryanodine receptor

Corresponding author: Dr Maurice Wibo, Laboratoire de pharmacologie, UCL 54.10, Université catholique de Louvain, Avenue Hippocrate 54, B-1200 Brussels (Belgium). Tel: 322 764 54 17; Fax: 322 764 54 60; e-mail: wibo@farl.ucl.ac.be

INTRODUCTION

Postnatal growth of mammalian heart is characterized by marked changes in excitation-contraction coupling and Ca^{2+} handling [1], supported by important modifications in gene expression of major Ca^{2+} transport systems [2,3]. In particular, the sarcoplasmic reticulum (SR) progressively assumes a predominant role in the Ca^{2+} fluxes associated with contraction and relaxation. Ca^{2+} release from SR occurs through ryanodine-sensitive channels and is driven by a local increase of the Ca^{2+} concentration, which results predominantly from Ca^{2+} entry through the dihydropyridine (DHP)-sensitive voltage-dependent Ca^{2+} channels of the sarcolemma. During maturation of ventricular tissue, most dihydropyridine receptors (DHPRs) appear to concentrate into specialized areas of the sarcolemma that are physically associated with SR structures containing the ryanodine receptors (RYRs) [4–6]. This junctional localization favors the process of Ca^{2+}-induced Ca^{2+} release from the SR and is consistent with a "local control" model of excitation-contraction coupling, in which one L-type channel triggers a regenerative cluster of a few SR release channels [4,7]. Refilling of the SR Ca^{2+} stores is ensured by the SERCA2 ATPase, which is up-regulated during postnatal maturation, while the sarcolemmal Na^+-Ca^{2+} exchanger is down-regulated in a reciprocal manner [8].

Thyroid hormone is essential for normal cardiac growth and modulates postnatal changes in cardiac excitation-contraction coupling at the level of contractile function and calcium handling [9]. In particular, hypothyroidism induced after birth results in decreased calcium uptake by the sarcoplasmic reticulum and increased sensitivity to the negative inotropic effect of the calcium channel blocker verapamil, suggesting that hypothyroid heart remains more dependent on trans-sarcolemmal Ca^{2+} fluxes than age-matched euthyroid heart. Therefore, we investigated the influence of thyroid status on the developmental changes in the properties of the sarcolemmal and SR Ca^{2+} channels. In a subsequent study, we examined whether a pathological growth stimulus, that is, pressure overload induced by aortic banding, could influence the postnatal maturation of cardiac Ca^{2+} channels.

POSTNATAL CHANGES IN SUBSARCOLEMMAL DISTRIBUTION AND ISOFORM EXPRESSION OF RAT CARDIAC DHPRS: MODULATION BY THYROID HORMONE

Newborn rats were treated from postnatal day 2 with L-triiodothyronine (T3) or 6-n-propyl-2-thiouracil (PTU) as described previously [9] and ventricles were collected on day 1, 7 and 14. First, we examined the effect of age and thyroid status on receptor properties in total particulate fractions prepared from left ventricles [10]. Receptors were identified by specific radioligands (DHPR, [^{3}H](+)-PN200-110; RYR, [^{3}H]ryanodine; α-adrenoceptor, [^{3}H]prazosin; β-adrenoceptor, [^{3}H](−)-CGP-12177) and we did not detect any difference in affinity related to age or thyroid status. As shown in Fig. 1, control hearts showed an increase by a factor of about 3 in the tissue density of receptors (expressed as pmol per gram tissue) from day 1 to day 14. Postnatal hypothyroidism induced some reduction in the tissue density of DHPRs and RYRs at day 14, while hyperthyroidism had only a marginal effect on

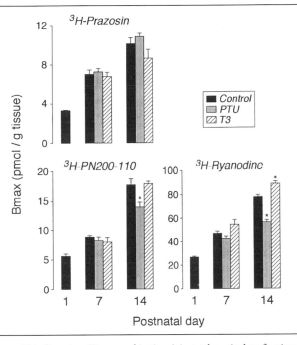

Figure 1. Numbers of binding sites (B_{max}, pmol/g tissue) in total particulate fractions from ventricles. Data are means from 4 preparations (each from at least 5 hearts), except for Control/day 1 and T3/day 7 (2 preparations). S.e.m. values are indicated by vertical bars. Significant differences between age-matched groups are indicated: PTU- or T3-treated vs Control (*), $P < 0.01$, except for [^{3}H](+)-PN200-110 binding, PTU/day 14 vs Control/day 14 ($P < 0.02$).

RYRs at day 14. The thyroid status had no significant influence on α-adreno-ceptors but (not shown on the Figure), it markedly decreased the number of β-adrenoceptors even at day 7 [10].

Profound structural modifications are known to take place in the rat ventricular myocyte during the postnatal period, in particular the growth of the SR and the development of t-tubules, which are rich in dyadic couplings with terminal SR cisternae [11]. We reasoned that those modifications could give rise to time-dependent differences in distribution patterns of receptors after density gradient centrifugation. We used an analytical approach [12], in which microsomal fractions are layered on top of a linear sucrose density gradient and thereafter subjected to prolonged centrifugation to bring the constituent particles to an equilibrium position. Some 10 to 15 subfractions are then collected from the gradient and assayed for the receptors of interest, which allows to reconstruct their density distribution patterns.

Figure 2 shows the effect of age on the density distributions of α-adrenoceptors, DHPRs and RYRs [10]. As previously found, the total number of binding sites in the gradient, which corresponds to the area under the curve, increases by a factor of about

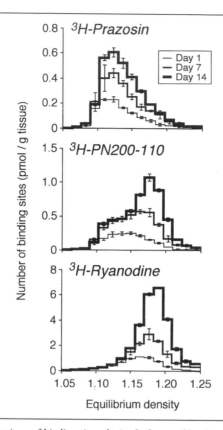

Figure 2. Density distributions of binding sites obtained after equilibration of microsomal fractions from control ventricular tissue (day 1, 7 and 14) in sucrose gradient. Each histogram was constructed from average number of binding sites (B_{max}) calculated from two gradient experiments. Vertical bars indicate values obtained in individual gradient experiments.

3 from day 1 to day 14. Age does not influence the shape of the distribution of α-adrenoceptors, which are recovered predominantly at low densities, below 1.15. Similarly, age has little effect upon the shape of the distribution in the case of RYRs, which are recovered essentially at high densities, above 1.15. The behavior of DHPRs is unique, in that the distribution at day 1 is similar to that of α-adrenoceptors, whereas the distribution at day 14 resembles more that of RYRs. Clearly, from day 7 to day 14, DHPRs increase in number only in high-density subfractions, that is, in the same subfractions in which the additional RYRs are also found.

Figure 3 shows the situation at day 21, which is almost identical to that found in adult tissue [13]. Now it is quite clear that the vast majority of DHPRs are distributed like the RYRs and are associated with structural elements that differ from those bearing β- (and α-) adrenoceptors. In agreement with the immuno-

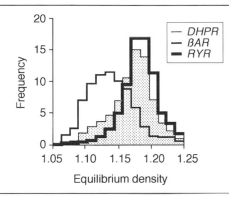

Figure 3. Density distributions of binding sites obtained after equilibration of microsomal fractions from control ventricular tissue (day 21) in sucrose gradient. Number of binding sites is expressed as frequency, which corresponds to the fraction of total numbers recovered over a given density interval. βAR, β-adrenoceptor.

localization data obtained by others [5], we had concluded that most of the DHPRs in adult ventricle are linked to junctional structures between t-tubules and terminal SR cisternae [4]. Ca^{2+} entry through DHP-sensitive channels of dyadic couplings is thus especially suited to induce Ca^{2+} release from the SR. In these dyadic couplings, we estimate that RYRs outnumber DHPRs by a factor of 5 to 10 [4], in agreement with the cluster bomb model proposed by Stern and Lakatta [7].

Let us now turn to the influence of the thyroid status on the density distributions of receptors at day 14 (Fig. 4). Abnormal levels of thyroid hormone do not change the shape of the distributions of α-adrenoceptors and RYRs. In contrast, in the case of DHPRs, the distribution pattern is flat and bimodal in hypothyroid ventricle, whereas, in hyperthyroid ventricle, it shows a sharp peak at high densities, similar to that found at day 21 in control rats. Therefore, hypothyroidism seems to delay the maturation of dyadic couplings and thus the evolution towards an adult pattern of excitation–contraction coupling, whereas hyperthyroidism has the opposite effect [10,13].

We also examined the effect of age and thyroid status on the expression of variants of the DHPR α1-subunit, using reverse transcription and polymerase chain reaction (RT-PCR) analysis of mRNA, combined with restriction enzyme analysis [10]. In newborn heart, two variants can be detected in motif IV of the α1-subunit [14]. In particular, at the level of the third trans-membrane segment (IVS3), there are two variants produced by alternative splicing, the IVS3B variant being the only one present in adult tissue. The IVS3A variant is typical of foetal heart and its proportion decreases after birth. As shown in Table 1, we found this variant in higher proportion in hypothyroid ventricle at postnatal days 7 and 14, indicating again a delay in the maturation of DHPRs [10].

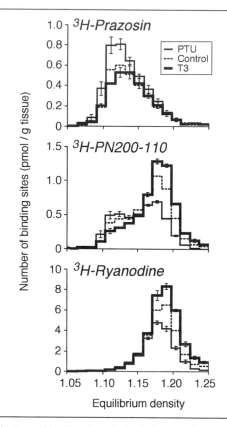

Figure 4. Density distributions of binding sites obtained after equilibration in sucrose gradient of microsomal fractions from control, PTU-treated and T3-treated rats at postnatal day 14. Each histogram was constructed from average numbers of binding sites (B_{max}) calculated from two gradient experiments. Vertical bars indicate values obtained in individual gradient experiments. Except for vertical bars, which were omitted, control histograms are identical to those shown in Fig. 2.

Table 1. Effect of age and thyroid status on frequency of a foetal variant of the DHPR α1 subunit

	Control	PTU-treated	T3-treated
Day 1	15.4 ± 2.8		
Day 7	3.6 ± 1.0★	31.8 ± 4.8†	4.7 ± 2.6‡
Day 14	0.2 ± 0.2★	7.6 ± 1.9†	1.4 ± 1.4§

Frequency of the IVS3A (foetal) variant is expressed in percent of total variants. Values are mean ± s.e.m. from 3 preparations [10].
★ Significantly different from Day 1, $P < 0.01$.
† Significantly different from Control, $P < 0.01$.
‡ Significantly different from PTU-treated, $P < 0.01$.
§ Significantly different from PTU-treated, $P < 0.02$.

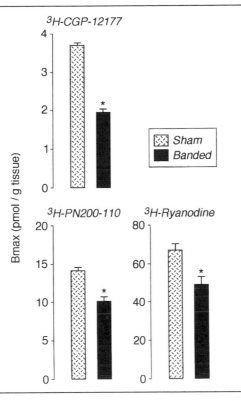

Figure 5. Numbers of binding sites (B_{max}, pmol/g tissue) in total particulate fractions from ventricles at postnatal day 10, obtained from sham-operated rats and from rats with aortic constriction (banded). Data are means from 4 preparations. S.e.m. values are indicated by vertical bars. Significant differences are indicated by asterisks.

EFFECT OF AORTIC CONSTRICTION ON THE POSTNATAL CHANGES IN SUBSARCOLEMMAL DISTRIBUTION OF RAT CARDIAC DHPRS

In this study [15], aortic constriction (banding) was applied at day 2, as described previously [16], and rats were killed at day 10. Only severely hypertrophied left ventricles were included in the banded group; their average weight was almost doubled with respect to sham-operated rats. As shown in Fig. 5, the number of β-adrenoceptors per gram tissue was halved in total particulate fractions prepared from left ventricles of rats with aortic constriction. There was also a significant reduction (25–30%) of the tissue density of DHPRs and RYRs with respect to sham-operated rats.

Particulate fractions from sham and banded rats were subfractionated by density gradient centrifugation (Fig. 6). β-Adrenoceptors were found mainly at low densities and RYRs receptors at high densities and the shape of their distributions was not appreciably modified after aortic constriction. In contrast, the shape of the

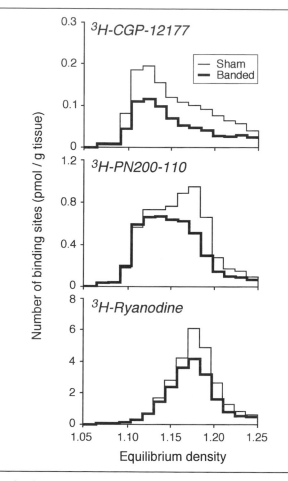

Figure 6. Density distributions of binding sites obtained after equilibration in sucrose gradient of particulate fractions from ventricles at postnatal day 10, obtained from sham-operated rats and from rats with aortic constriction (banded). Each histogram was constructed from average numbers of binding sites (B_{max}) calculated from 3 gradient experiments.

distribution of DHPRs was modified after banding: whereas, in the case of sham animals, there was a distinct peak at high densities, in the subfractions enriched with RYRs, such a peak was not observed in the DHPR distribution obtained from rats with aortic constriction. The shape of the DHPR distribution obtained at day 10 from banded rats is strikingly similar to that obtained from control rats at day 1 (see Fig. 2). Thus, severe pressure overload appears to delay the normal maturation of DHPRs in left ventricle.

The ultrastructure of those hearts at day 10 has been examined by Dr. D. Jarkowska (personal communication). Transverse tubules are still undetectable in ventricular cardiomyocytes, but, in tissue samples from sham, dyadic couplings with feet structures are easily recognizable at the periphery of the myocyte. In contrast, the frequency of couplings and the number of feet in each coupling are lower after banding. This is in agreement with the decrease in the association of DHPRs with RYRs induced by aortic constriction, as suggested by the density gradient studies.

CONCLUSION

In conclusion, we have shown that both neonatal hypothyroidism and neonatal aortic constriction impair the postnatal maturation of DHPRs in rat ventricle, by decreasing their tissue density and by reducing the proportion of receptors associated with junctional structures. In the hypothyroid model, we have also shown that the disappearance of foetal variants of the DHPR $\alpha 1$ subunit is delayed. Therefore, our data suggest that hypothyroidism, a condition that impairs normal cardiac growth, and severe pressure overload, a condition that leads to pathological hypertrophy, both delay the maturation of dyadic couplings in the developing rat ventricle.

ACKNOWLEDGEMENTS

The authors thank O. Feron, L. Zheng, M. Maleki, V.M.N. Cunha. and D. Jarkowska for their valuable collaboration.

REFERENCES

1. Mahony L. 1996. Regulation of intracellular calcium concentration in the developing heart. Cardiovasc Res 31:E61–E67.
2. Arai M, Otsu K, MacLennan DH, Periasamy M. 1992. Regulation of sarcoplasmic reticulum gene expression during cardiac and skeletal muscle development. Am J Physiol 262:C614–C620.
3. Brillantes A-MB, Besprozvannaya S, Marks AR. 1994. Developmental and tissue-specific regulation of rabbit skeletal and cardiac muscle calcium channels involved in excitation-contraction coupling. Circ Res 75:503–510.
4. Wibo M, Bravo G, Godfraind T. 1991. Postnatal maturation of excitation-contraction coupling in rat ventricle in relation to the subcellular localization and surface density of 1,4-dihydropyridine and ryanodine receptors. Circ Res 68:662–673.
5. Lewis Carl S, Kelly F, Caswell AH, Brandt NR, Ball WJ Jr, Vaghy PL, Meissner G, Ferguson DG. 1995. Immunolocalization of sarcolemmal dihydropyridine receptor and sarcoplasmic reticular triadin and ryanodine receptor in rabbit ventricle and atrium. J Cell Biol 129:673–682.
6. Sun X-H, Protasi F, Takahashi M, Takeshima H, Ferguson DG, Franzini-Armstrong C. 1995. Molecular architecture of membranes involved in excitation-contraction coupling of cardiac muscle. J Cell Biol 129:659–671.
7. Stern MD, Lakatta EG. 1992. Excitation-contraction coupling in the heart: the state of the question. FASEB J 6:3092–3100.
8. Vetter R, Studer R, Reinecke H, Kolar F, Ostadalova I, Drexler H. 1995. Reciprocal changes in the postnatal expression of the sarcolemmal Na^+-Ca^{2+}-exchanger and SERCA2 in rat heart. J Mol Cell Cardiol 27:1689–1701.
9. Kolar F, Seppet EK, Vetter R, Prochazka J, Grünermel J, Zilmer K, Ostadal B. 1992. Thyroid control of contractile function and calcium handling in neonatal rat heart. Pflügers Arch 421:26–31.
10. Wibo M, Feron O, Zheng L, Maleki M, Kolar F, Godfraind T. 1998. Thyroid status and postnatal changes in subsarcolemmal distribution and isoform expression of rat cardiac dihydropyridine receptors. Cardiovasc Res 37:151–159.
11. Olivetti G, Anversa P, Loud AV. 1980. Morphometric study of early postnatal development in the left and right ventricular myocardium of the rat. II. Tissue composition, capillary growth, and sarcoplasmic alterations. Circ Res 46:503–512.

12. Beaufay H, Amar-Costesec A. 1976. Cell fractionation techniques. In: Methods in Membrane Biology. Ed ED Korn 6:1–100. New York: Plenum Press.
13. Wibo M, Kolar F, Zheng L, Godfraind T. 1995. Influence of thyroid status on postnatal maturation of calcium channels, β-adrenoceptors and calcium transport ATPases in rat ventricular tissue. J Mol Cell Cardiol 27:1731–1743.
14. Feron O, Octave J-N, Christen M-O, Godfraind T. 1994. Quantification of two splicing events in the L-type calcium channel α-1 subunit of intestinal smooth muscle and other tissues. Eur J Biochem 222:195–202.
15. Cunha VMN, Kolar F, Godfraind T, Wibo M. 1998. Delayed maturation of cardiac calcium channels after aortic constriction in newborn rats. Br J Pharmacol 123:58P.
16. Kolar F, Papousek F, Pelouch V, Ostadal B, Rakusan K. 1998. Pressure overload induced in newborn rats: effects on left ventricular growth, morphology and function. Pediatr Res 43:521–526.

B. Ostadal, M. Nagano and N.S. Dhalla (eds.).
CARDIAC DEVELOPMENT. Copyright © 2002.
Kluwer Academic Publishers. Boston.
All rights reserved.

T-TYPE AND L-TYPE CALCIUM CURRENTS MODULATE FORCE IN EMBRYONIC CHICK MYOCARDIUM

ELIZABETH A. SCHRODER,[1] JONATHAN SATIN,[2]
SERGEI ROUTKEVITCH,[3] PAVEL TSYVIAN,[3] and
BRADLEY B. KELLER[1]

University of Kentucky, [1]Department of Pediatrics, [2]Department of Physiology, 800 Rose Street, Room MN472, Lexington, KY 40536, USA; [3]Yekaterinburg Branch, Physiological Institute of the Russian Academy of Sciences, Mother and Child Institute Yekaterinburg, Russia

Summary. We used T-type and L-type Ca^{2+} channel blocking agents and the sarcoplasmic reticulum Ca^{2+} release blocker ryanodine to determine the relative contribution of these Ca^{2+} flux pathways on contractile force. We used isolated, perfused embryonic cardiac muscle strips from stage 24 and stage 31 chick embryos to assess isometric twitch force amplitude and duration, steady-state force interval relations (FIR), poststimulation potentiation (PSP), and postextrasystolic potentiation (PESP). Active force and all FIR increased with development. Nifedipine (1.0 nM), 0.1 μM ryanodine, or 100 μM nickel reduced twitch force, PSP and PESP in all preparations. In addition, T-type Ca^{2+} channel blockers inhibited spontaneous contractile activity. Specimens displayed a positive staircase in normal buffer solutions which was diminished in the presence of sarcolemmal Ca^{2+} channel blockers. Patch clamp experiments in isolated cells revealed both nifedipine sensitive (L-type) and nifedipine insensitive but nickel sensitive (T-type) Ca^{2+} currents. Thus, Ca^{2+} entry via T-type and L-type Ca^{2+} channels and intracellular Ca^{2+} storage influence active force generation and FIR during cardiac development.

Key words: chick embryo, cardiac development, sarcolemmal Ca^{2+} channels, sarcoplasmic reticulum, force-interval relations

INTRODUCTION

Calcium transport across the sarcolemma and the sarcoplasmic reticulum (SR) directly regulates cardiac force production [1]. Several lines of evidence suggest that

Address for corresponding author and reprints: Elizabeth A. Schroder, Ph.D., Division of Pediatric Cardiology, 800 Rose Street, Room MN 472, Lexington, KY 40536-0298. Telephone: 859-323-5494; Fax: 859-323-3499; e-mail: eschr0@pop.uky.edu

immature cardiomyocytes have a limited reserve of exchangeable Ca^{2+} and poorly developed SR and T-tubule systems [2–4]. During myocardial development active contraction depends primarily on sarcolemmal Ca^{2+} influx via L-type Ca^{2+} channels, T-type Ca^{2+} channels and Na^+/Ca^{2+} exchange [5–8].

The majority of the existing data on Ca^{2+} handling in the embryonic myocardium focuses on mid-gestation following the completion of cardiac morphogenesis and not during the critical period of primary cardiac development [9–12]. This is particularly true for whole cell recordings. Kawano and DeHaan utilized pharmacology to identify T-type and L-type components to the current in 7 day and 14 day chicken embryos [13–15]. Separation of currents was achieved by a combination of differences in voltage thresholds and pharmacological sensitivity. They found that I_T had a greater current density than that of adult cardiac tissue and was the major contributor to I_{Ca} in the embryonic preparations. Brotto and Creazzo [16] have also focused on I_{Ca} during this midgestational period. Using a combination of whole cell recording, Ca^{2+} imaging and pharmacological blockade, they attributed as much as 25 percent of the total I_{Ca} to T-type channels in the day 11 chicken embryo [16].

Recent data in chick and mouse embryos has shown that the developing myocardium can acutely alter developed force in response to loading conditions and that changes in embryonic heart function influence cardiac morphogenesis [17]. However, it is unclear how the developing cardiomyocyte acutely regulates active force production. Therefore, the aim of the present study was to define the age-dependent role of plasma membrane and SR Ca^{2+} channels on myocardial force generation. Experiments were conducted using the L-type Ca^{2+} channel blocker nifedipine [16,18–21] in order to block an important mechanism of sarcolemmal Ca^{2+} current. Sub-millimolar nickel [22] was employed in these experiments to selectively block the T-type Ca^{2+} channel, which have been shown to be a major contributor to I_{Ca} in the early chicken embryo [13]. Ryanodine was used to block and lock the SR Ca^{2+} release channel in a stable, subconducting open state [23,24] in order to evaluate the contribution of SR Ca^{2+} storage and release on twitch force and FIR. We noted an increase in force generation was present with increasing developmental age. A positive staircase with increased pacing rate was observed in normal buffer solutions which was diminished in the presence of the sarcolemmal T-type Ca^{2+} channel blocker and became negative in the presence of the L-type Ca^{2+} channel blocker nifedipine. Ryanodine reduced active force generation but had no effect on the positive staircase. These results demonstrate the developmental maturation of Ca^{2+} handling in the chick embryonic myocardium and confirm that the embryonic myocardium is capable of regulating cardiomyocyte force generation acutely despite limited maturation of excitation-contraction coupling.

MATERIALS AND METHODS

Tissue preparation

We tested isolated myocardial preparations of stage 24 (day 4) and stage 31 (day 7) chick embryos (21-day incubation period). Fertile white Leghorn chicken eggs were incubated in a force-draft incubator at 38.5°C and 99% relative humidity. Developmental landmarks, including limb bud size, eye pigmentation, and cardiac morphology, were used to verify embryo stage [25]. At stage 24, the trabeculated embryonic ventricle has undergone partial septation and by stage 31 the embryonic ventricle has increased more than 8 fold in mass and is fully septated [26]. In addition, the onset of functional parasympathetic innervation occurs at stage 29. Our research protocols conform to the *Guide for the Care and Use of Laboratory Animals* published by the US National Institutes of Health (NIH Publication No. 85-23, revised 1985).

Embryos were removed from the surface of the egg yolk and transferred to a Petri dish containing warmed buffer solution. The buffer solution contained (in mM): NaCl, 137; KCl, 4; $MgSO_4$, 1; $CaCl_2$, 2; glucose, 10; and Trizma-HCl Trizma-base, 10. The solution was bubbled with 95% O_2, 5% CO_2 and, pH was adjusted to 7.4 at a temperature of 37°C. The ventricle was removed from the embryo by cutting along the atrioventricular groove and across the conotruncal cushions. The whole ventricle was used at stage 24. Myocardial strips (average dimensions 0.5×0.3 mm) were dissected from the left ventricle of stage 31 chick embryos in a longitudinal orientation (parallel to blood flow). Myocardial specimens were then attached between two stainless steel, bevel-tipped wires using an ultra-pure, low viscosity, fast cure, alpha-cyanoacrylate ester (model 262, Permabond International, Englewood, NJ) [27]. One wire was connected to a force transducer (model 403A, Cambridge Technology, Cambridge, MA) and the other to a micromanipulator.

Muscle stimulation protocols

Embryonic chick myocardial specimens were mounted in a small volume, Plexiglas chamber that was gravity perfused with 37°C, oxygenated buffer solution at a constant flow rate of 5 ml/min. The preparations were initially electrically paced at a frequency of 1.0 Hz by square-wave pulses of 5 ms duration at 30% over-threshold voltage (Grass Instruments, Quincy, MA model S88). All preparations were stretched to the length at which maximal twitch force was obtained (L_{max}). L_{max} was determined for each preparation. 0.95 L_{max} was used for the working preparation. Pacing continued for a 30-minute equilibrium period prior to data collection. Each myocardial preparation was stable for at least 90 minutes based on the presence of reproducible, stable peak tension wave forms and the absence of tonic contraction.

The diameter of each muscle was measured with an eyepiece reticle. Cross-sectional area was calculated assuming cylindrical geometry. Cross-sectional area was 0.377 mm^2 $\pm$ 0.012 at stage 24 and was 0.384 ± 0.018 mm^2 at stage 31. Due to the presence of a lumen at stage 24, myocardial area was assumed to be 70% of the circular cross-sectional area [27]. Isometric force was measured by the force transducer and the analog force waveform was sampled at 500 Hz by an analog-to-digital board (model AT-MIO16-E2, National Instruments, Austin, TX) and stored digitally. A custom software program was used for data acquisition and analysis. Data analysis was performed off-line. Protocols were performed in 5 different superfusion solutions: physiologic buffer with 2 mM Ca^{2+} (n = 47, stage 24; n = 33, stage 31), and 2.0 mM Ca^{2+} buffer solutions containing 0.1 µM ryanodine (n = 11, stage 24; n = 11, stage 31), 100 µM nickel (n = 21, stage 24; n = 10, or 1 nM nifedipine (n = 10, stage 24; n = 14, stage 31). Nifedipine was dissolved in DMSO. Equivalent concentrations of DMSO without the addition of Nifedipine were added to the buffer solution and showed no significant effects on the studied mechanical properties. The buffer container and muscle bath were covered to prevent light exposure during experimentation with nifedipine. All reagents were purchased from the SIGMA Chemical Company, St. Louis, MO.

Cell cultures

Ventricular specimens were harvested from stage 24 (day 4) embryos. Myocytes were isolated following two 15-minute digestions in 0.05% trypsin (GIBCO). After isolation cells were resuspended in MEM (GIBCO) containing 10% heat-inactivated fetal calf serum and 1% antibiotic-antimycotic solution (GIBCO). The media and cells were pre-plated on a polystyrene plate and allowed to settle for one hour. Myocyte containing media was then re-plated in a new dish containing glass coverslips.

Patch clamp protocols

Immediately prior to experiments culture media was replaced with a whole-cell recording bath solution (in mM): 140 NaCl, 5 CsCl, 2.5 KCl, 10 TEA-Cl, 2.5 $CaCl_2$, 1 $MgCl_2$, 5 Hepes, 5 glucose, 300 µM TTX, pH 7.4. The pipette contained (in mM): 110 K-gluconate, 40 CsCl, 1 $MgCl_2$, 3 EGTA, 5 Hepes, pH 7.4 with CsOH. Experiments were performed in the whole-cell configuration of the patch clamp technique at room temperature (20–22°C). To avoid the complexity of L-type Ca^{2+} channel run-down a separate series of experiments were performed with the nystatin, perforated patch. Pipettes were pulled from borosilicate glass with a resistance ranging from 1.5 to 2.0 MΩ. Currents were filtered at 10 kHz. Data was acquired using a Digidata 1200 A/D converter, Axopatch 200B amplifier and pClamp6 software. Current amplitudes and exponential fits were calculated using Clampfit (Axon Instruments, Inc.).

Spontaneous beating rate

The rate of spontaneous beating was measured in stage 24 ventricular specimens over a period of two minutes in control buffer (2.0 mM Ca^{2+}), nickel (100 µM), nifedipine (1 nM), and ryanodine (0.1 µM). All specimens, with exception of those in the ryanodine buffer beat continuously for the entire time period without external pacing. Specimens in ryanodine buffer displayed periods of rapid beating with intermittent quiescent periods. Beat rate was calculated during the period of spontaneous activity for the ryanodine specimens. We did not measure spontaneous beating in the stage 31 specimens because this activity was extremely inconsistent.

Data analysis

The data are summarized as mean ± SE. Single-factor ANOVA was used to analyze the difference between groups (stage 24 and stage 31) in each of the buffers. We considered differences within the ANOVA analysis to be statistically significant only if $P < 0.05$ for the entire sequence under analysis. A Tukey post-hoc procedure was used to determine the pairwise significance.

RESULTS

Twitch force and duration

We calculated tension as the maximal force divided by the cross-sectional area for each specimen. As would be expected with the progression of normal development, total tension (active + passive) in physiological buffer solution ($Ca^{2+} = 2.0$ mM) was higher at stage 31 (66.57 ± 5.77 mg/mm^2) than at stage 24 (44.84 ± 2.98 mg/mm^2) (Fig. 1A). This increase was also observed for both active tension (Fig. 1B) and passive tension (Fig. 1C) in the control buffer. At stage 24, the addition of each Ca^{2+} channel blocker diminished total tension. Peak active tension at steady-state decreased when compared to control in presence of each of the Ca^{2+} blockers at both stages studied. Because diastolic tension (passive tension) increased in the presence of ryanodine at stage 31, total tension was not affected by ryanodine at this stage. Sarcolemmal Ca^{2+} channel blockade did not effect peak diastolic tension in the stage 24 or stage 31 embryonic myocardium.

Time to peak tension (TPT) was calculated as the time from the onset of contraction to peak tension. Relaxation time (RT), an approximation of the rate of decline of ventricular pressure, was calculated as the time of relaxation from peak to 30% peak force. Figure 2A illustrates an increase in TPT with developmental age in the control, nickel and ryanodine buffers. An increase in RT was observed only in the control buffer from stage 24 to stage 31 (Fig. 2B). The addition of 100 μM nickel or 0.1 μM ryanodine to the buffer at stage 24 resulted in a decrease in TPT. Maximum dF/dt was diminished in all buffers when compared with control (Fig. 2C).

Effects of pacing frequency on steady-state force

Force-interval relations (FIR) define the relationship between stimulation pattern and contractile force and encompass such mechanisms as poststimulation potentiation (PSP) and postextrasystolic potentiation (PESP). We assessed steady-state FIR, PSP and PESP at both stages 24 and 31. The steady-state FIR of each myocardial preparation was determined by pacing at four different rates from 1.0 to 3.3 Hz in random order [28]. Figures 3A and B represent the averaged steady-state relationships between active force and frequency recorded in 2.0 mM Ca^{2+}, 0.1 μM ryanodine, 1 nM nifedipine, and 100 μM nickel. Force is normalized to cross-sectional area (expressed as active tension) and was recorded at 1.0 Hz, 1.5 Hz, 2.0 Hz, and 3.3 Hz. A positive staircase (from 1.0 to 2.0 Hz at stage 24; from 1.0 to 3.3 Hz at stage 31) was observed in all buffers, at both stages, with the exception of the buffer

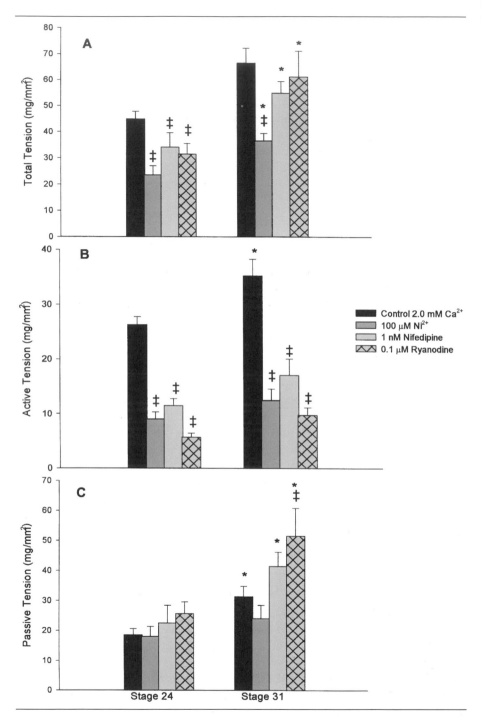

Figure 1. *A*: Total tension. *B*: Active tension. *C*: Passive tension. Force normalized to cross–sectional area (tension) during pacing at 1.0 Hz in 2.0 mM Ca^{2+} solution, and in 2.0 mM Ca^{2+} solution with 100 μM Ni^{2+}, 1 nM Nifedipine, or 0.1 μM Ryanodine. All values are mean ± SE. *P < 0.05 vs Stage 24; ‡P < 0.05 vs 2.0 mM Ca^{2+} buffer.

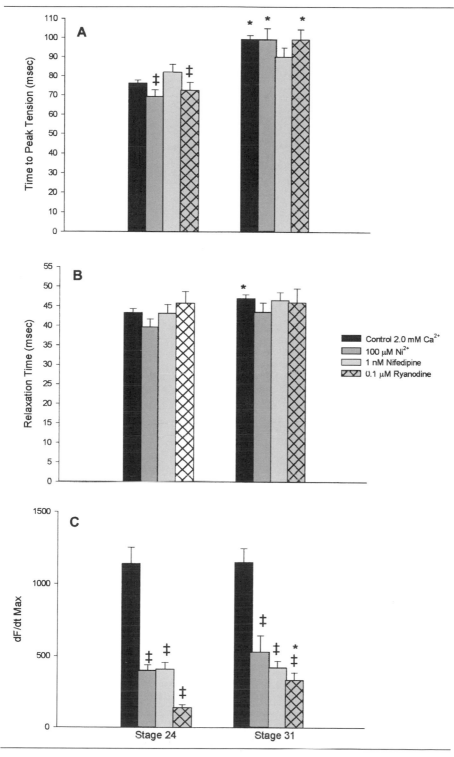

Figure 2. *A*: Time to Peak Tension for stage 24 and stage 31 chick myocardium in the 5 buffer solutions. *B*: Relaxation Time for stage 24 and stage 31 chick myocardium in the 5 buffer solutions. *C*: The maximal rate of rise of force/sec (dF/dt_{max}) determined from the dynamic force tracings at 1.0 Hz pacing in the stage 24 and stage 31 chick myocardium. All values are mean ± SE. *$P < 0.05$ vs Stage 24; ‡$P < 0.05$ vs 2.0 mM Ca^{2+} buffer.

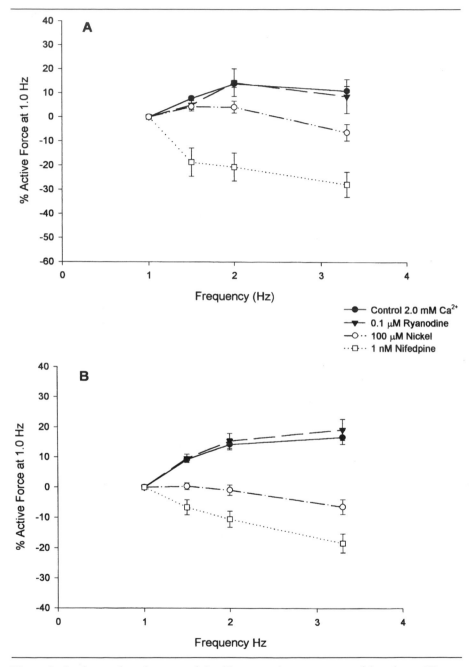

Figure 3. Steady-state force-frequency relationship expressed as a percentage of the value at 1 Hz pacing in 2.0 mM Ca²⁺ solution, and in 2.0 mM Ca²⁺ solution with 100 μM Ni²⁺, 1 nM Nifedipine, or 0.1 μM Ryanodine. *A*: Stage 24. *B*: Stage 31. All values are mean ± SE.

containing the L-type Ca^{2+} channel blocker nifedipine. $100\,\mu M$ nickel produced a moderate decrease in the observed staircase.

PSP and PESP provide indirect information on dynamic changes in SR Ca^{2+} content. PSP was determined by pacing from $1.0\,Hz$ to $3.3\,Hz$ followed by a return to baseline pacing at a rate of $1.0\,Hz$. The absolute value of PSP was calculated as the increase in active tension (mg/mm^2) above baseline of the first regular beat after the period of increased pacing (Fig. 4A). Figure 4B compares the absolute values of the PSP in the stage 24 and stage 31 embryonic myocardium. PSP increased from $5.10 \pm 0.41\,mg/mm^2$ at stage 24 to $8.64 \pm 0.94\,mg/mm^2$ at stage 31 in the control buffer. All Ca^{2+} channel blockers significantly reduced PSP.

PESP is influenced both by the basal stimulation rate and the extrasystolic interval. We therefore made all PESP measurements at a baseline pacing frequency of $0.5\,Hz$. During steady-state pacing, we introduced a premature test beat at intervals varying from 120 to $500\,ms$. The interval was then adjusted until maximal PESP was observed (Fig. 5A). PESP was calculated as the increase in amplitude (active tension (mg/mm^2)) of the postextrasystolic beat over the amplitude at the baseline pacing frequency. Similar to PSP, the absolute value of PESP increased significantly from stage 24 to stage 31 in the control buffer (Fig. 5B). As with PSP, Ca^{2+} channel blockers diminished PESP at both stages.

Effect of Ca^{2+} channel blockers

Embryonic chick ventricular myocytes express both T- and L-type Ca^{2+} channels [13–16]. To assess the efficacy of T-type and L-type Ca^{2+} current blockade we used the same concentrations of Ni^{2+} or nifedipine as tested in the force experiments. Whole-cell patch clamp recordings reveal a low density Ca^{2+} current. To improve the signal/noise ratio we tested tail current through Ca^{2+} channels elicited by large hyperpolarizations (inset, Fig. 6). This data was fit using a double exponential which was comprised of a fast and a slow component. Based on the relative time course of deactivation we attribute this slow current to the T-type Ca^{2+} channel [29,30]. $100\,\mu M$ Ni^{2+} caused 100% blockade of I_T in 3 out of 4 cells and a 60% blockade in the fourth (Fig. 6A). The current density of the nickel sensitive component for these cells was $9.84 \pm 2.94\,pA/pF$. Figure 6B shows the nickel sensitive component of this current. $1\,nM$ nifedipine had no effect on this slowly deactivating current (Fig. 6C). The lack of a nifedipine sensitive component of this inward current is apparent in Fig. 6D. In whole-cell configuration, L-type Ca^{2+} current is sometimes prone to run-down whereas T-type is not [30]. Therefore we used the nystatin perforated-patch configuration to assess nifedipine blockade of L-type current. Nifedipine selectively blocked the rapid-deactivation component of tail current (Figs. 6C, 6D).

Spontaneous beating rate

I_T is often correlated with spontaneously excitable cells [31]. Embryonic ventricular myocytes uniquely display spontaneous contractions *in vitro* at stage 24. Nifedipine

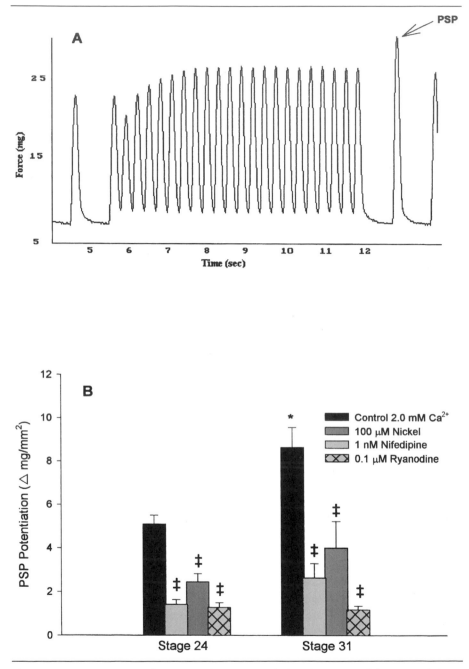

Figure 4. *A*: A representative force tracing for a stage 31 chick embryo myocardial specimen (2.0 mM Ca^{2+} control buffer) displaying a positive staircase during increased pacing frequency from 1 Hz to 3 Hz and post-stimulation potentiation (PSP). *B*: Poststimulation potentiation (PSP), the percentage increase in active force of the first regular beat after a period of increased pacing and return to steady-state. Twitch force potentiation expressed as active tension (mg/mm²) above baseline in 2.0 mM Ca^{2+} solution, and in 2.0 mM Ca^{2+} solution with 100 μM Ni^{2+}, 1 nM Nifedipine, or 0.1 μM Ryanodine. All values are mean ± SE $\star P < 0.05$ vs Stage 24; $^{\ddagger}P < 0.05$ vs 2.0 mM Ca^{2+} buffer.

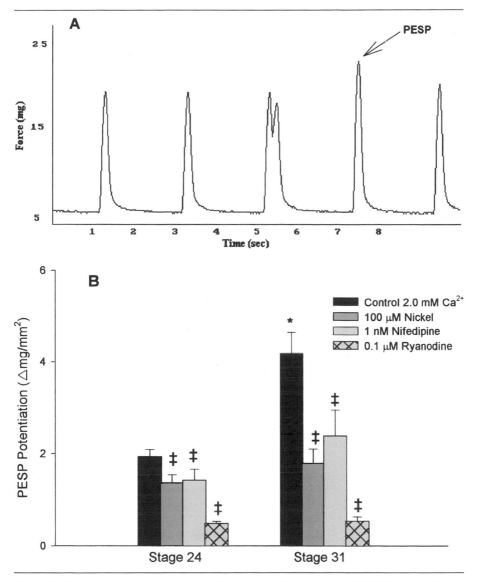

Figure 5. *A*: A representative force tracing of post-extrasystolic potentiation (PESP) in a stage 31 chick embryo myocardial specimen in control buffer (2.0 mM Ca^{2+}). *B*: Post-extrasystolic potentiation (PESP), the percentage increase in active force of the maximal post-extrasystolic beat versus active force at baseline frequency. Twitch force potentiation expressed as active tension (mg/mm^2) above baseline in 2.0 mM Ca^{2+} solution, and in 2.0 mM Ca^{2+} solution with 100 μM Ni^{2+}, 1 nM Nifedipine, or 0.1 μM ryanodine. All values are mean ± SE *P < 0.05 vs Stage 24; ‡P < 0.05 vs 2.0 mM Ca^{2+} buffer.

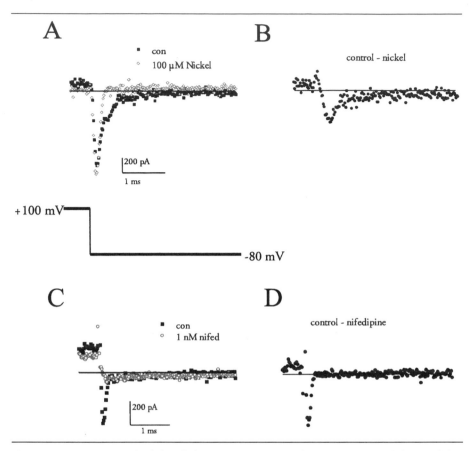

Figure 6. *A*: Superimposed whole-cell data at −80 mV in control and in 100 μM nickel. *B*: Nickel sensitive component of current produced by the subtraction of nickel data from control. *C*: Superimposed whole-cell data at −80 mV in control and in 1 nM nifedipine. *D*: Nifedipine sensitive component of current produced by the subtraction of nifedipine data from control.

addition did not significantly alter spontaneous beat rate (Fig. 7). Buffer containing ryanodine increased this spontaneous activity. The only solution which completely suppressed spontaneous contraction at 37°C was the buffer containing 100 μM nickel.

DISCUSSION

Twitch force and duration

When examining total tension we most consider both the active and passive components. Both active and passive tension increased with developmental stage. This occurs in concert with maturation of intracellular excitation-contraction coupling and both cell-cell and cell-matrix relations [2,12,19,32,33]. All Ca^{2+} channel block-

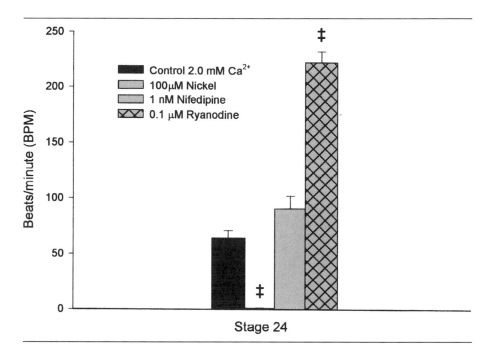

Figure 7. Spontaneous activity measured in beats per minute (BPM) in 2.0 mM Ca^{2+} solution, and in 2.0 mM Ca^{2+} solution with 100 μM Ni^{2+}, 1 nM Nifedipine, or 0.1 μM ryanodine. All values are mean ± SE, $^{‡}P < 0.05$ vs 2.0 mM Ca^{2+} buffer.

ers had negative inotropic effects. This reduction in active tension can be explained by the decreased availability of Ca^{2+} to the developing myofibers as has been previously observed in the developing heart [11,19,34,35]. In the adult myocardium ryanodine has no effect on diastolic tension [36–38]. The observed increase in diastolic tension in the embryonic myocardium may reflect the immaturity of intracellular mechanisms to buffer, sequester or extrude Ca^{2+} from the cell in order to sufficiently decrease cytosolic Ca^{2+} concentrations during relaxation. Because the immature cardiomyocyte is not able to remove Ca^{2+} at a sufficient pace, Ca^{2+} cannot completely dissociate from troponin C [39] and therefore fewer cross-bridges can be generated during the contraction. This accounts for the reduced active force observed in the ryanodine experiments. Because of this increase in diastolic tension and decrease in active tension, ryanodine buffers had the smallest effect on total tension. Changes in active and passive tension support the increased role of sarcolemmal Ca^{2+} channels early in development when compared to adult but still shows a functional contribution of the SR at these early stages.

Altered L-type Ca^{2+} channel activity has been associated with diminished contractility in the chick embryo experimental model of neural crest ablation associated with conotruncal heart defects [9] and in the Splotch mouse that contains an altered *pax3* gene and structural heart defects [40]. Creazzo noted altered L-type

Ca^{2+} channel activity in malformed chick embryos following neural crest ablation, however it is not clear if the altered Ca^{2+} channel activity was responsible for producing the malformations or was a consequence of altered cardiomyocyte proliferation and maturation [9].

In atrial subsidiary pacemaker cells I_T may have the dual role of providing inward cation current for action potential initiation, and trigger Ca^{2+} for EC coupling [31]. Differences in the spatial distribution of T and L-type Ca^{2+} channels influence their role in myocyte EC coupling. Zhou and January [41] demonstrated that both T and L-type Ca^{2+} current could contribute to EC coupling in adult canine purkinje cells containing a simple T tubule system. They found that L-type Ca^{2+} channels were more effective in initiating contraction and hypothesized that this was due to the close proximity of the L-type Ca^{2+} channels to the SR Ca^{2+} release mechanism. T-type Ca^{2+} channels located at greater distances would have diminished effectiveness in triggering contraction due to longer diffusion distances. They suggested that this distance was an explanation for their observed increase in TPT in T-type Ca^{2+} channel activated contraction. Although chicken ventricular cells lack a T-tubule system, it is a more difficult argument to make in a $10\,\mu M$ diameter embryonic heart cell. We observed a decrease in TPT in the nickel and ryanodine buffers at stage 24. T-type Ca^{2+} channel blockade greatly diminishes a major source of Ca^{2+} entry for embryonic myocardium [13]. Reduced Ca^{2+} influx also reduced the time required to reach peak tension. Brotto and Creazzo [16] saw a decrease in TPT in the presence of ryanodine at 11 days incubation in the chicken embryo that they attributed to an immature CICR mechanism. The slight increase in TPT and RT with developmental age may have less to do with maturation of Ca^{2+} handling machinery and more with myofiber maturation and isoform switching.

The maximum rate of rise of force $(+dF/dt)$ was significantly reduced in the presence of all Ca^{2+} channel blockers utilized in this study at both stages, consistent with diminished Ca^{2+} available for contraction. A slower entry or release of Ca^{2+} provides explanation for the observed decrease in the rate of force generation (dF/dt) in all buffers at both stages.

Force–interval relations

A positive FIR was observed in all buffers with the exception of nifedipine, at both stages 24 and 31. A similar relationship has been demonstrated in chicken embryonic myocytes at later developmental stages [16,42] and in the mature heart in several species [43–45]. This increase in force generation at higher pacing frequencies results from increased I_{Ca}, increased diastolic (passive) Ca^{2+}, and increased SR Ca^{2+} available for release. Diastolic Ca^{2+} increases from Ca^{2+} loading due to the increased pacing rate. Ca^{2+} enters the cell but the time for extrusion is diminished. Higher concentrations of Na^+ also accumulate during increased pacing. This increase favors reverse Na^+/Ca^{2+} exchange which further accumulates Ca^{2+} in the cytoplasm and SR [39]. Because the positive staircase is presumably due to a net increase in Ca^{2+} across the sarcolemma at increased pacing rates, it would follow that sarcolemmal Ca^{2+} channel blockers would most effectively diminish this staircase. This indeed was the case at both stages. Nifedipine buffer produced a negative staircase. Nickel lessened the positive staircase and ryanodine cause no significant changes. These results highlight the importance of sarcolemmal Ca^{2+} channels at pacing rates similar to that observed *in vivo* [46].

PSP and PESP are important FIR measures of SR function that allow us to glean information about SR functional maturation. Hoffman first described PESP in 1956 [47]. During PESP an extrasystolic contraction occurs prior to restitution. This contraction is usually smaller in force generation because it occurs while the SR release channel is refractory to further Ca^{2+} release. During this extrasystolic contraction some Ca^{2+} will enter the cell across the sarcolemma which is then stored in the SR. Potentiation of the subsequent contraction results from the increased Ca^{2+} available to be released from the SR. PSP also depends somewhat on SR storage but shows a greater dependence on Ca^{2+} loading across the sarcolemma.

SR development is first evident in the 5–6 somite stage chick embryo as a small number of SR-like segments near the sarcolemma. Complete meshworks of SR surround myofibrils by embryonic day 9 [19]. Our experimental results show a marked increase in PSP and PESP from stage 24 to stage 31 which coincides with SR maturation. At both stages PSP and PESP were dramatically decreased in the presence of the Ca^{2+} channel blockade. The effects of Ca^{2+} channel blockade on PSP and PESP were slightly different because PSP is more dependent upon sarcolemmal Ca^{2+} for potentiation. During the period of increased pacing the cytoplasm and SR are loaded with Ca^{2+} from across the plasma membrane which is stored for release with the return to baseline pacing. Thus, sarcolemmal Ca^{2+} channel blockade could be predicted to have a greater effect on PSP than PESP when compared to their values in control buffer.

Differential effect of T and L-type Ca^{2+} channel blockers

Both T- and L-type Ca^{2+} channels are present in embryonic chick ventricular myocytes [13–16]. Whole-cell patch clamp recordings were used to test the effectiveness of the pharmacological blockade used in the force experiments. $100\,\mu M$ Ni^{2+} caused 100% blockade of I_T in 3 out of 4 cells and a 60% block in the fourth. This result is similar to that observed by Kawano and DeHaan [13] in 14 day chick embryos. They found that $120\,\mu M$ Ni^{2+} reduced I_T 86.4% when compared to control.

In contrast, $1\,nM$ nifedipine had no effect on this slowly deactivating current. Nifedipine effects on FFR suggest for a significant L-type channel component, even in the earliest embryonic stages tested. However, we could not detect $I_{Ca,L}$ using whole-cell recordings. This may be due to small current amplitudes, or to current run-down in the whole-cell conditions optimized to measure I_T. Although nystatin, perforated patch recordings have higher series resistance, this configuration has the advantage of preserving the intracellular milieu. Similar to recordings from the whole-cell configuration, perforated patch recordings revealed two distinct kinetic components of inward tail currents for potentials hyperpolarized to $+20\,mV$.

Nifedipine had no effect on the slow component with the well-established prevalent component I_T as a significant fraction of the total Ca^{2+} current in early embryonic cardiac myocytes [13–16]. These results are consistent with the well-established prevalence of I_T in early embryonic development [13–16].

Spontaneous contractility

Embryonic ventricular myocardium spontaneously contracts *in vitro* [48,49] and as development progresses this spontaneous contractile activity diminishes. This decrease in spontaneous activity occurs concomitant with a progressive hyperpolarization of the maximum diastolic potential [50–52], and an increase in the maximal upstroke velocity (dV/dt_{max}) of the action potential. The relatively slow dV/dt_{max} in the stage 14–24 chick embryo (5–20 V/s) and the action potential insensitivity to TTX suggest a Ca^{2+} channel mediated rapid upstroke [49]. T-type Ca^{2+} channels activate in a more hyperpolarized voltage range than Na^+ or L-type Ca^{2+} channels, thus they may influence both excitation and contraction. In spontaneously beating adult mammalian atrial myocytes 50 μM nickel selectively inhibited the late diastolic slope of the action potential [53]. T-type Ca^{2+} channels contribute to spontaneous contractile activity in mature mammalian SA node cells [54]. Our observation that 100 μM nickel inhibited spontaneous activity suggests that T-type Ca^{2+} channel contribute to the pacemaker depolarization in the early embryonic myocardium.

The addition of 1 nM nifedipine to the buffer did not significantly alter the spontaneous beating rate when compared to control. L-type Ca^{2+} channels activate in a more depolarized range than T-type Ca^{2+} channels. As a result, L-type channels would require depolarization prior to their activation and therefore would not act as a trigger for spontaneous activity. Thus, blocking these channels with nifedipine would have no effect on the spontaneous contraction of the cell.

Summary and conclusions

Utilizing various Ca^{2+} channel blockers we investigated the roles of Ca^{2+} channels on the sarcolemmal and SR contributions to force generation and force-interval regulation of embryonic chick myocardium at stages 24 and 31. These results demonstrate the significant role of sarcolemmal T-type and L-type Ca^{2+} channels in the development of force at early stages of development. A positive staircase in the presence of all but nifedipine illustrated the greater role of L-type Ca^{2+} channels (sarcolemmal) in Ca^{2+} entry for force generation. Spontaneous contractions were completely suppressed in the presence of the T-channel blocker, nickel, highlighting the potential role of T-channels in pacemaker activity. SR ryanodine-sensitive Ca^{2+} channels were also noted to play a role in regulating force generation in embryonic myocardium as early as stage 24. Recent work from our group demonstrated the presence of T-type Ca^{2+} channels in the developing mouse ventricle [55]. Ongoing experiments with the addition of simultaneous Ca^{2+} imaging will enable us to more fully understand the role of Ca^{2+} channels in regulating force production during normal and altered cardiovascular development.

ACKNOWLEDGEMENTS

This research was supported by (1) Fogarty International Research Collaboration Award #R03-TW00527, (2) Civilian Research and Development Foundation #5270, and (3) National Institutes of Health, Individual NRSA, #l F32 HL10200-01 (4) National Institutes of Health, RO1 HL64626.

REFERENCES

1. Weiss JN. 1997. Ion Channels in Cardiac Muscle. In: The Myocardium (2 ed.). Ed. GA Langer, 81–133. San Diego, CA: Academic Press.
2. Protasi F, Sun X-H, Franzini-Armstrong C. 1996. Formation and Maturation of the Calcium Release Apparatus in Developing and Adult Avian Myocardium. Dev Biol 173:265–278.
3. Tanaka H, Takagi N, Shigenobu K. 1993. Inotropic effects of ryanodine and calcium antagonists on embryonic and hatched chick myocardium. J Dev Physiol 19:235–240.
4. Vetter R, Will H, Kuttner I, Kemsies C, Will-Shahab L. 1986. Developmental changes of Ca^{++} transport systems in chick heart. Biomed Biochim Acta 45:S219–S222.
5. Chin TK, Christiansen GA, Caldwell JG, Thorbum J. 1997. Contribution of the sodium–calcium exchanger to contractions in immature rabbit ventricular myocytes. Ped Res 41:480–485.
6. Davies MP, An RH, Doevendans P, Kubalak S, Chien KR, Kass RS. 1996. Developmental changes in ionic channel activity in the embryonic murine heart. Circ Res 78:15–25.
7. Haddock PS, Artman M, Coetzee WA. 1998. Influence of postnatal changes in action potential duration on Na-Ca exchange in rabbit ventricular myocytes. Pflugers Archiv—Euro J Physiol 435:789–795.
8. Nakanishi T, Seguchi M, Takao A. 1988. Development of the myocardial contractile system. Experentia 44:936–943.
9. Creazzo TL. 1990. Reduced L-Type Calcium Current in the Embryonic Chick Heart with Persistent Truncus Anteriosus. Circ Res 66:1491–1498.
10. Creazzo TL, Brotto MAP, Burch J. 1997. Excitation-contraction coupling in the day 15 embryonic chick heart with persistent truncus anteriosus. Ped Res 42:731–737.
11. Godt RE, Fogaca RTH, Nosek TM. 1990. Changes in force and calcium sensitivity in the developing avian heart. *Can J Physiol Pharmacol* 69:1692–1697.
12. Godt RE, Fogaca RTH, Silva IK, Nosek TM. 1993. Contraction of Developing Avian Heart Muscle. Comp Biochem Physiol 105A: 213–218.
13. Kawano S, DeHaan RL. 1989. Low-threshold current is major calcium current in chick ventricle cells. Am J Physiol 256:H1505–H1508.
14. Kawano S, DeHaan RL. 1990. Analysis of T-Type Calcium Channel in Embryonic Chick Ventricular Myocytes. J Membrane Biol 116:9–17.
15. Kawano S, DeHaan RL. 1991. Developmental Changes in the Calcium Currents in Embryonic Chick Ventricular Myocytes. J Membrane Biol 120:17–28.
16. Brotto MADP, Creazzo TL. 1996. Ca^{2+} transients in embryonic chick heart: contributions from Ca^{2+} channels and the sarcoplasmic reticulum. Am J Physiol 270:H518–H525.
17. Burggren WW, Keller BB. 1997. Development of Cardiovascular Systems: Molecules to Organisms. New York: Cambridge University Press.
18. Dutro SM, Airey JA, Beck CF, Sutko JL, Trumble WR. 1993. Ryanodine receptor expression in embryonic avian cardiac muscle. Dev Biol 155:431–441.
19. Komazaki S, Hiruma T. 1997. Development of Mechanisms Regulating Intracellular Ca^{2+} Concentration in Cardiac Muscle Cells of Early Chick Embryos. Dev Biol 186:177–184.
20. Renaud JF, Kazazoglou T, Schmid A, Romey G, Lazdunski M. 1986. Differentiation of receptor sites for [^{3}H] nitrendipine in chick hearts and physiological relation to the slow Ca^{2+} channel and to excitation-contraction coupling. Euro J Biochem 139:673–681.
21. Yao A, Su Z, Nonaka A, Zubair I, Lu L, Philipson KD, Bridge JH, Barry WH. 1998. Effects of overexpression of the Na^+-Ca^{2+} exchanger on [Ca^{2+}] transients in murine ventricular myocytes. Circ Res 82:657–665.
22. Hille B. 1992. Ionic Channels of Excitable Membranes. Sunderland, MA: Sinauer Associates.
23. Meissner G. 1986. Ryanodine activation and inhibition of the Ca^{2+} release channel of sarcoplasmic reticulum. J Biol Chem 261:6300–6306.

24. Rousseau E, Smith JS, Meissner G. 1987. Ryanodine modifies conductance and gating behavior of single Ca^{2+} release channel. Am J Physiol 253:C364–C368.
25. Hamburger V, Hamilton HL. 1951. A series of normal stages in the development of the chick embryo. J Physiol 88:49–92.
26. Sedmera D, Pexieder T, Hu N, Clark EB. 1997. Developmental changes in the myocardial architecture of the chick, Anat Rec 248:421–432.
27. Miller CE, Vanni MA, Taber LA, Keller BB. 1997. Passive stress-strain measurements in the stage-16 and stage-18 embryonic chick heart. J Biomech Eng 119:445–451.
28. Toyota H, Matsumura M. 1989. Relationship between contraction strength and stimulation frequency in cultured chick embryonic heart cells. Jap J Physiol 39:87–100.
29. Cribbs LL, Lee JH, Yang J, Satin J, Zhang Y, Daud A, Barclay J, Williamson MP, Fox M, Rees M, Perez-Reyes E. 1998. Cloning and characterization of alphaIH from human heart, a member of the T-type Ca^{2+} channel gene family. Circ Res 83:103–109.
30. Satin J, Cribbs LL. 2000. Identification of a T-Type Ca^{2+} Channel Isoform in Murine Atrial Myocytes (AT-1 Cells). Circ Res 86:636–642.
31. Huser J, Blatter LA, Lipsius SL. 2000. Intracellular Ca^{2+} release contributes to antomaticity in cat atrial pacemaker cells. J Physiol 524(2):415–422.
32. Fischman DA, Bader D, Obinata T. 1985. Regulating expression of protein isoforms. Overview. Ad Exp Med Biol 182:203–214.
33. Simpson DG, Terracio L, Terracio M, Price RL, Turner DC, Borg TK. 1994. Modulation of cardiac myocyte phenotype in vitro by the composition and orientation of the extracellular matrix. J Cell Physiol 161:89–105.
34. Fabiato A, Fabiato F. 1979. Use of Chlorotetrcycline flourescence to demonstrate Ca^{2+}-induced release of Ca^{2+} from the sarcoplasmic reticulum of skinned cardiac cells. Nature 281:146–159.
35. Hensley J, Billman GE, Johnson JD, Hohl CM, Altschuld RA. 1997. Effects of calcium channel antagonists on Ca^{2+} transients in rat and canine cardiomyocytes. J Mol Cell Cardiol 29:1037–1043.
36. Benijamali HS, Gao WD, Macintosh BR, ter Keurs HEDJ. 1991. Force-interval relations of twitches and cold contractures in rat cardiac trabeculae. Circ Res 69:937–948.
37. Cooper IC, Fry CH. 1990. Mechanical Restitution in Isolated Mammalian Myocardium: Species Differences and Underlying Mechanisms. J Mol Cell Cardiol 22:439–452.
38. Ezzaher A, Bouanani NEH, Crozatier B. 1992. Force-frequency relations and response to ryanodine in failing rabbit. Am J Physiol 263:H1710–H1715.
39. Bers DM. 1993. Excitation-Contraction Coupling and Cardiac Contractile Force. Ed. AH Dordrecht. The Netherlands: Kluwer Academic Publishers.
40. Conway SJ, Henderson DJ, Copp AJ. 1997. *Pax3* is required for cardiac neural crest migration in the mouse: evidence from the *splotch* (Sp^{2H}) mutant. Dev 124:505–514.
41. Zhou Z, January CT. 1998. Both T- and L-Type Ca^{2+} Channels Can Contribute to Excitation-Contraction Coupling in Cardiac Purkinje Cells. Biophys J 74:1830–1839.
42. Lee HC, Clusin WT. 1987. Cytosolic calcium staircase in cultured myocardial cells. Circ Res 61:934–939.
43. Allen DG, Kurihara S. 1981. The effects of muscle length on intracellular calcium transients in mammalian cardiac muscle. J Physiol 327:79–94.
44. Bers DM. 1991. Species differences and the role of sodium-calcium exchange in cardiac muscle relaxation. Annals of the New York Academy of Sciences 639:375–385.
45. Layland J, Kentish JC. 1999. Positive Force and $[Ca^{2+}]_i$-frequency relationships in rat ventricular trabeculae at physiological frequencies. Am J Physiol 276:H9–H18.
46. Clark EB, Hu N, Dummett JL, Vandekeift GK, Olson C, Tomanek R. 1986. Ventricular Function and Morphology in Chick Embryo from Stages 18–29. Am J Physiol 250:H407–H413.
47. Hoffman BF, Bindler E, Suckling EE. 1956. Postextrasystolic Potentiation of Contraction in Cardiac Muscle. Am J Physiol 185:95–102.
48. Kamino K. 1991. Optical Approaches to Ontongeny of Electrical Activity and Related Functional Organization During Early Heart Development. Physiol Rev 71:53–91.
49. Satin J, Fujii S, DeHaan RL. 1988. Development of Cardiac Beat Rate in Early Chick Embryos is Regulated by Regional Cues. Dev Biol 129:103–113.
50. DeHaan, R.L. 1980. Differentiation of Excitable Membranes. Current Topics in Dev Biol 16:117–164.
51. McDonald TF, DeHaan RL. 1973. Ion Levels and Membrane Potential in Chick Heart Tissue and Cultured Cells. J Gen Physiol 61:89–109.

52. Sperelakis N. 1984. Developmental Changes in Membrane Electric Properties of the Heart. In: Physiology and Pathophysiology of the Heart. Ed. N Sperelakis. 543–573. Boston, MA: M. Nijhoff.
53. Wu JY, Lipsius SL. 1990. Effects of Extracellular Mg^{-2+} on T-Type and L-Type Ca^{2+} Currents in Single Atrial Myocytes. Am J Physiol 259:H1842–H1850.
54. Hagiwara N, Irisawa H., Kameyama M. 1988. Contribution of Two Types of Calcium Currents to the Pacemaker Potentials of Rabbit Sino-Atrial Node Cells. J Physiol 395:223–253.
55. Cribbs LL, Martin BL, Schroder EA, Keller BB, Delisle BP, Satin J. 2001. Identification of the T-type Calcium Channel ($Ca_v3.ld$) in Developing Mouse Heart. Circ Res 88:403–407.

B. Ostadal, M Nagano and N.S. Dhalla (eds.).
CARDIAC DEVELOPMENT. Copyright © 2002.
Kluwer Academic Publishers. Boston.

DEVELOPMENTAL CHANGES IN REGULATION OF CARDIAC CONTRACTILE FUNCTION

YING-YING ZHOU, WILLIAM A. COETZEE,
TOMOE Y. NAKAMURA, and MICHAEL ARTMAN

Pediatric Cardiology, New York University Medical School, New York, New York, USA

Summary. Molecular and cellular aspects of excitation-contraction (EC) coupling and relaxation have been well characterized in the adult heart. Modulation of these processes by various signaling pathways provides the mechanisms whereby contraction and relaxation are modified in response to various pharmacological interventions. The developing heart undergoes profound changes in the molecular and cellular pathways involved in the transport of calcium to and from the contractile proteins. In contrast to the mature heart, relatively little is known regarding the cellular mechanisms involved in the regulation of contractile function in the immature heart. We propose that a thorough understanding of the fundamental processes of calcium transport in the developing heart is necessary in order to formulate rational therapeutic strategies for manipulating contraction and relaxation during development. The purpose of this review is to provide an overview of the current concepts of EC coupling and calcium regulation in the immature heart. We hope that this information will be helpful in designing future experimental to address the existing gaps in our current knowledge and explore novel approaches to the pharmacological manipulation of contractile function in the developing heart.

Key words: EC coupling, development, calcium regulation, pharmacology

Corresponding authors: Ying-Ying Zhou, MD, PhD, Pediatric Cardiology, TH 501, 560 First Avenue, New York University Medical Center, New York, NY10016, USA. Phone: 212-263-8518; Fax: 212-263-1393; e-mail: Zhouy01@med.nyu.edu   Michael Artman, MD, Pediatric Cardiology, TWR Suite 9-V, 540 First Avenue, New York University Medical Center, New York, NY10016, USA. Phone: 212-263-5993; Fax: 212-263-5808; e-mail: Michael.Artman@mcd.nyu.edu

I. OVERVIEW OF ADULT CARDIAC MYOCYTE EC COUPLING: CENTRAL ROLE OF SARCOPLASMIC RETICULUM

Cardiac excitation-contraction (EC) coupling is initiated during the action potential by Ca^{2+} influx via sarcolemmal Ca^{2+} channels. In adult cardiac myocytes, the Ca^{2+} influx itself is not sufficient to produce a contraction but triggers ~10 fold more Ca^{2+} release from the sarcoplasmic reticulum (SR). The increase in intracellular cytosolic Ca^{2+} (Ca_i) promotes Ca^{2+} binding to the contractile myofilaments and induces cell shortening (contraction). Cardiac relaxation occurs when Ca_i is recycled into the SR by SR Ca^{2+} pumps, and to a lesser extent, extruded from the cell via sarcolemmal Na^+-Ca^{2+} exchangers and Ca^{2+} pumps (for review see [1]).

In mature mammalian ventricular myocardium, Ca^{2+} released from the SR contributes up to 90% of the Ca_i transient and plays a central role in cardiac EC coupling (for review see [2]). It has been well established that the opening of specific SR Ca^{2+} release channels (ryanodine receptors) is triggered by an influx of Ca^{2+} across the sarcolemma mainly through L-type Ca^{2+} channels in a process known as Ca^{2+}-induced Ca^{2+} release (CICR) [3]. The structural basis for CICR is the co-localization of sarcolemmal L-type Ca^{2+} channels (predominantly in the T-tubules) and junctional SR ryanodine receptors in the diadic junction [4,5] (Fig. 1). The close physical relationship of L-type Ca^{2+} channels and ryanodine receptors (~10 nm) in this region allows a single or a small cluster of ryanodine receptors to open in response to a local, spatially restricted, microdomain of elevated Ca^{2+} that results from the nearby influx of Ca^{2+} through an L-type Ca^{2+} channel. In this way, instead of a regenerative CICR (as predicted by the "common pool" model), SR Ca^{2+} release is graded as a function of L-type Ca^{2+} currents ("local control" model) [6]. Although L-type Ca^{2+} channels have "privileged access" to the ryanodine receptors of the SR [7,8], Ca^{2+} influx from Na^+-Ca^{2+} exchangers [9–11] and T-type Ca^{2+} channels [12,13] may also play a role in CICR under certain conditions. However, whether SR Ca^{2+} release in cardiac muscle can be triggered by membrane depolarization alone is still controversial [14–16].

II. DIMINISHED ROLE OF THE SARCOPLASMIC RETICULUM IN IMMATURE HEART AND THE MECHANISMS

Each of the mechanisms of EC coupling discussed above for the adult heart relies upon the release of Ca^{2+} from intracellular stores to activate contractions. In contrast, a large body of literature indicates that immature myocytes depend much less on SR Ca^{2+} release for the initiation of contraction. The profound differences between contraction and relaxation processes in the developing and mature heart [17–19] are likely to be explained by fundamental developmental differences in the key cellular components involved in producing the mature EC coupling phenotype, including the SR and T-tubules. The concept that the SR plays a lesser role in EC coupling in the developing heart is supported by results from experiments employing ultrastructural [20,21], pharmacological [22,23], biochemical [24,25], electrophysiological [26,27] or molecular biological [28] approaches. Despite this abundance of indirect information, we [29] and Miller et al. [30] have shown that,

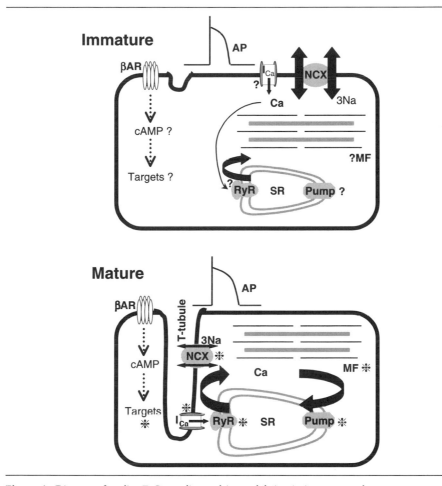

Figure 1. Diagram of cardiac E-C coupling and its modulation in immature and mature myocytes. Lower panel: SR plays a central role in adult cardiac myocyte E-C coupling. The dyadic junction of T-tubules makes I_{Ca}-mediated Ca^{2+}-induced Ca^{2+} release from junctional SR the major source of Ca^{2+} to activate the myofilament. Ca^{2+} influx through "reverse" NCX may only contributes a small portion under physiological condition. During repolarization, intracellular Ca^{2+} is mainly recycled back to SR by SR Ca^{2+} pumps and in part extruded via sarcolemmal NCX. βAR stimulation modulates all major constituents of the cardiac EC coupling cascade including L-type Ca^{2+} channels, RyR, NCX and MF via a cAMP-dependent pathway. In contrast, as shown in the upper panel, the immature cardiac myocyte has no well-developed T-tubules but a greater surface area-to-volume ratio, so the transsarcolemmal Ca^{2+} influx mainly via NCX acts as the predominant source of activator Ca^{2+}. The action potential configuration and the intracellular Na^+ concentration may regulate Ca^{2+} transport via NCX. How βAR activation modulates cardiac E-C coupling in developing heart has not been fully characterized. The solid line and arrow indicates the direction of ionic (such as Ca^{2+} and Na^+) flow, while the size of the line depicts the relative magnitude of the contribution from each of the various components. The dotted line and arrow indicates the signal transduction pathways for βAR stimulation. The star symbol indicates the targets for βAR stimulation and the question mark indicates it is not clear for the signal transduction pathway of βAR stimulation and involvement of SR in immature cardiac E-C coupling. Abbreviations: AP, action potential; βAR, β-adrenergic receptor; I_{Ca}, L-type Ca^{2+} channel current; RyR, ryanodine receptor; NCX, Na^+-Ca^{2+} exchanger; MF, myofilament; Pump, SR Ca^{2+} pump; SR, sarcoplasmic reticulum.

in contrast to our expectations, caffeine-induced Ca^{2+} release from the SR in immature cells is comparable to that observed in adult myocytes. We interpreted the observation that steady-state twitch amplitudes and Ca^{2+} transients are much lower than those during a caffeine contracture [29] as indicative of diminished fractional SR Ca^{2+} release during normal EC coupling in newborns. However, this approach cannot distinguish between *lower* fractional release and a *total absence of SR Ca^{2+} release*. Thus, the question of whether SR Ca^{2+} release occurs at all during normal EC coupling in immature cells remains to be answered.

The major structural components of EC coupling in mature ventricular myocardium are (i) sarcolemmal L-type Ca^{2+} channels (mostly clustered in the T-tubules), (ii) Ca^{2+} release channels (ryanodine receptors) in the junctional SR and (iii) the diadic junction of T-tubules with the junctional SR which makes the coupling of sarcolemmal L-type Ca^{2+} channels and SR Ca^{2+} release channels possible. Our recent findings of a lower fractional Ca^{2+} release in EC coupling of immature rabbit ventricular myocytes (see above) indicate a discontinuity between one or more of these processes.

(i) Ontogeny of cardiac L-type Ca^{2+} channel. Purified L-type Ca^{2+} channels are oligomeric complexes consisting of a pore-forming α_1-subunit along with an accessory β subunit and disulphide-linked $\alpha 2/\delta$ subunits. At least 6 different genes for α_1-subunits (α_{1S}, α_{1A-E}), 4 for β subunits (β_{1-4}) and one for α_2/δ subunit have been identified by molecular cloning [31]. In addition, alternative splicing may also add structural diversity to the multitude of L-type Ca^{2+} channels. In cardiac myocytes, α_{1C^-} and β_2-subunits are preferentially expressed. Quantitative immunoblotting reveals that in embryonic mouse and rat hearts, α_{1C} expression is observed at fetal day 12, peaks around birth and declines shortly after birth. In contrast, β_2 is not detected until fetal day 20 and persists during maturation. Furthermore, in addition to the adult isoforms (250 kDa full-length α_{1C} and 85 kDa β_2), in fetal and neonatal hearts, several other isoforms such as 220 kDa α_{1C} and 90/100 kDa β_2 as well as β_4 isoforms are also present [32].

Expressed L-type Ca^{2+} channels are characterized by their sensitivity to dihydropyridines (DHPs). Most DHPs (e.g. nifedipine and nitrendipine) act as antagonists (L-type Ca^{2+} channel blockers), while some (e.g. BAY K 8644) serve as agonists. Functional L-type Ca^{2+} channels have been observed in embryonic stem cell-derived cardiac precursor cells before the myocytes start to contract [33]. The amplitude of L-type Ca^{2+} currents ($I_{Ca,L}$), recorded using the whole cell voltage-clamp technique, increased during myogenesis [26,34–39]. Similarly, α_{1C}-subunit mRNA levels [28] and the number of DHPR binding sites increases during the perinatal and postnatal periods [37]. Since there is a dramatic developmental change in cell size and capacitance among different species, the $I_{Ca,L}$ density (i.e., $I_{Ca,L}$ current amplitude normalized by cell capacitance) has been reported to be either increased [27,40], decreased [39] or not changed with maturation [41–43].

In summary, L-type Ca^{2+} channels are functionally mature during fetal stages, so the location of L-type Ca^{2+} channels might be responsible for the uncoupling of L-type Ca^{2+} channels with SR Ca^{2+} release channels in immature heart. This notion is supported by the observation that after birth, along with the development of T tubules, up to 3-fold more abundant DHPR are located in T-tubules than in external sarcolemma, which is consistent with the postnatal maturation of cardiac EC coupling [37].

(ii) **Development of SR Ca^{2+} release channels.** The SR Ca^{2+} release channel is a homotetramer which has a high affinity for the neutral plant alkaloid, ryanodine, and thus is also known as the ryanodine receptor (RyR). So far, three different isoforms of RyR (RyR1, RyR2, RyR3) have been identified. RyR2, the so-called cardiac RyR, is detected in developing heart tube as early as embryonic day 8.5 [44], whereas RyR3 accumulated around the time of birth [45]. Both RyR2 density and mRNA level [28,37,45,46] increase during the development, but RyR3 is only abundant in adult Purkinje myocytes. Another type of Ca^{2+} release channel, IP3 receptor (IP3R) which is usually present in endoplasmic reticulum, is also abundant at early developing cardiac myocytes, but decreases and is prominent in conduction tissues after birth [44,45]. Thus, IP3R might be more important in the development of heart and specialized conduction function, while RyR2 is mainly responsible for cardiac EC coupling.

In murine embryonic stem cell-derived cardiac precursor cells, ryanodine-sensitive Ca^{2+} release is detected later (embryonic day 10) than I_{Ca} (embryonic day 7). Interestingly, the appearance of functional RyR coincides with the initiation of contraction. Caffeine can induce Ca^{2+} release in hearts isolated from mouse embryos as early as day 8.5 [44]. However, ryanodine or other SR Ca^{2+} release inhibitors produce a greater negative inotropic effect in adult than in immature hearts [29,42,47,48]. While SR inhibition can largely abolish Ca^{2+} transients or contraction in mature hearts, it only inhibits Ca^{2+} transient or contraction in the immature heart by ~50% in rat [49], 30% in chicken [50] and has almost no effect in rabbit [30,48]. It is also noteworthy that in RyR2 knockout mice [51], the heart still starts to spontaneously contract at embryonic day 9.5. However, severe morphological change in SR and mitochondria were detected at embryonic day 10 when the mice die. These results suggest that even though RyR may not play an important role in EC coupling at early developmental stage, it might be crucial for Ca^{2+} homeostasis during cardiogenesis [51].

(iii) **Formation of T-tubules.** As discussed above both L-type Ca^{2+} channels and SR Ca^{2+} release channels are present and quite mature before birth, so a lack of diadic junctional coupling may be a key factor in the inadequate coupling of Ca^{2+} influx pathways with SR Ca^{2+} release in the neonatal heart. In most species (such as rat, rabbit, dog and hamster), T-tubules do not appear until approximately 2 weeks—2 months after birth [17]. Thus, the relative paucity of T-tubules may limit the close physical relation between sarcolemmal Ca^{2+} channels and SR Ca^{2+} release channels, resulting in functional isolation of the SR from participation in EC coupling under physiological conditions. The developmental morphogenesis of T-tubules and the temporal relationship between the postnatal acquisition of T-tubules and the appearance of an adult EC coupling phenotype remains to be determined in the human heart.

III. TRANSSARCOLEMMAL INFLUX AS AN ALTERNATIVE TO SR RELEASE AS THE PREDOMINANT SOURCE OF ACTIVATOR Ca^{2+}

As described above, under normal physiological conditions in adult ventricular myocytes, transsarcolemmal Ca^{2+} influx does not participate directly in activating the myofilaments, but instead functions to trigger SR Ca^{2+} release as the source of activator Ca^{2+}. In contrast, morphological considerations in immature myocytes support the feasibility of transsarcolemmal Ca^{2+} influx serving as a direct source of activator Ca^{2+}. Fetal and newborn myocytes are relatively small and, despite a lack of T-tubules, have a much higher cell surface area-to-volume ratio than adult myocytes [39,52]. A high surface area-to-volume ratio and the subsarcolemmal position of myofibrils in fetal and newborn myocytes [21,53] might support direct transsarcolemmal Ca^{2+} delivery to (and from) the contractile proteins. By comparison, in cells that lack a well developed SR or T-tubule network (such as atrial or Purkinje fiber myocytes or myocytes isolated from frogs, fish and birds) sarcolemmal Ca^{2+} influx can potentially lead to measurable subsarcolemmal Ca^{2+} gradients that are quite different from the uniform Ca_i transient induced by SR Ca^{2+} release in adult ventricular cells [54–56]. Our recent results showed that subcellular Ca^{2+} gradients indeed occur in newborn rabbit ventricular myocytes [48], suggesting that neonatal cardiac myocytes also depend predominantly on transsarcolemmal Ca^{2+} influx and are less reliant on Ca^{2+} release from SR stores. It therefore becomes essential to determine the possible sources of activator Ca^{2+} for contraction in immature myocytes.

(i) Calcium currents. In developing myocardium, the comparatively greater negative inotropic response to calcium channel blockers in a variety of species [17] suggests a strong dependence upon I_{Ca} for contraction. However, this is difficult to reconcile with electrophysiological studies which describe I_{Ca} density (compared with adults) to be smaller in neonatal rabbits [27,40], greater in neonatal rats [39] or not different in human newborns [41–43]. One possible explanation for the greater sensitivity of immature myocardium to the negative inotropic effects of L-type calcium channel blockers may be due to age-related differences in the contractile responses to shortening of the action potential ([52,57,58] and see below). In addition, in rat cardiomyocytes, the slower inactivation rate of $I_{Ca,L}$ in newborn than in adult contributes to a 6-fold higher sarcolemmal Ca^{2+} influx, which provide the basis for the strong dependence of neonatal heart on extracellular Ca^{2+} for contractile activation [39,59].

Recently, it was found that T-type Ca^{2+} channels may also contribute to CICR in adult myocytes (particularly at more negative membrane potentials) [13]. Although the density of T-type Ca^{2+} channels appears to be low in developing rabbit heart [27], their exact role in immature EC coupling in human heart remains to be established. Further, although P, Q and N type Ca^{2+} channels are not thought to be abundantly expressed in adult heart, the possibility that they may contribute to Ca^{2+} influx and EC coupling in immature myocytes cannot be discounted. Thus, a more detailed study to systematically characterize the role of Ca^{2+} entry though different types of Ca^{2+} channels as a trigger of SR Ca^{2+} release or as a direct source of activator Ca^{2+} in immature hearts is necessary.

(ii) **Na$^+$-Ca^{2+} exchange (NCX).** There is general agreement that the main functional role of NCX in mature cardiac cells is to extrude calcium during relaxation [1,60,61]. However, Ca^{2+} entry via "reverse" NCX can trigger SR Ca^{2+} release during depolarization; either directly [62] or as a result of subsarcolemmal Na$^+$ accumulation resulting from the Na$^+$ current [63]. The importance of this phenomenon has recently been underscored by experiments performed at near-physiological conditions (~37°C and/or without the use of cesium in the pipette solution used for voltage clamp experiments) [9,10].

Three genes (NCX1, NCX2 and NCX3) encode the Na$^+$-Ca^{2+} exchanger. NCX1 is primarily present in the heart. NCX1 expression is detected within 7.5–8 dpc cardiogenic plate before the first heart beat and initially in a heart-restricted pattern [64]. We previously demonstrated that NCX activity in sarcolemmal vesicles, sarcolemmal NCX protein content and steady-state mRNA levels were highest in late fetal and early newborn rabbits and declined postnatally to adult levels by two to three weeks of age [65,66]. Subsequent immunohistochemical studies in intact myocytes confirmed that NCX protein expression is high at birth in rabbits and that the exchanger is homogeneously distributed over the cell surface [48,67]. In addition, I$_{NaCa}$ density is high at birth and declines during the first 3 weeks after birth in rabbit ventricular myocytes [52,68]. Similar results were obtained from other species, including human [69,70]. Furthermore, our initial mathematical modeling studies suggested that Ca^{2+} fluxes via NCX during an action potential can account for the subsarcolemmal Ca^{2+} gradients observed in newborn rabbit myocytes [48].

Interestingly, during the first few weeks after birth, while NCX is down-regulated, the sarco(endo)plasmic reticulum Ca^{2+}-ATPase (SERCA2) is up-regulated [71,72], consistent with a postnatal transition from the sarcolemma to the SR as the predominant source of activator calcium. The time course of the down-regulation of NCX and up-regulation of SERCA2 coincides with that of the postnatal acquisition of T-tubules. Figure 1 illustrates these general concepts. These findings lend support to the concept that *NCX is a major route for sarcolemmal Ca^{2+} entry in the immature heart.* Thus, a role for NCX-mediated Ca^{2+} influx in contributing to EC coupling can easily be visualized either by (a) triggering SR Ca^{2+} release or (b) by directly activating contractile myofilaments. The relative roles of these postulated pathways in immature human myocytes remain to be elucidated.

(iii) **Voltage-activated Ca^{2+} release.** As described above, under certain specific conditions (e.g. with cAMP$_i$) voltage-activated Ca^{2+} release (VACR) has been reported to occur in mature cardiac myocytes [14,15]. The potential role of VACR under physiological conditions remains unclear at present, but it is intriguing to speculate that age-related changes in this mechanism might be involved in the developmental differences in EC coupling that have been previously observed. Presently, however, the presence and relevance of this mechanism remain highly controversial [16].

IV. MODULATION OF CA^{2+} TRANSIENTS IN THE IMMATURE HEART

In mature ventricular myocytes, graded control of SR Ca^{2+} release and contraction amplitude is achieved largely by changes in the magnitude of I$_{Ca}$, by virtue of its role in triggering SR Ca^{2+} release (as briefly reviewed above). Under physiologically relevant conditions, I_{Ca} is regulated by membrane potential and phosphorylation state [1,60]. The evidence accumulated to date suggests that coupling of I_{Ca} with SR Ca^{2+} release *does not* control contraction amplitude in immature myocytes. However, since contraction in immature myocytes is not an all-or-none phenomenon, there must be alternative mechanisms for exerting graded control of contraction amplitude in developing cells. If these overall concept are correct, then graded control of $[Ca^{2+}]_i$ and contraction amplitude is predicted to be achieved in immature myocytes predominantly by factors that modulate NCX activity. NCX activity may be influenced by a number of factors (e.g. ATP, pH, PIP_2, PKC, redox state) [61,73,74], but the extent and duration of membrane depolarization and the transsarcolemmal gradients of Na^+ and Ca^{2+} are the *primary* determinants of I_{NaCa}. More recently, β-adrenergic stimulation by isoproterenol has been shown to stimulate NCX in giunea-pig ventricular myocytes [75]. However, it is uncertain whether this is also the case in immature cardiac myocytes. Control of contractile function in the immature heart is likely to be substantially different from the mechanisms operative in the fully mature heart. Future studies will be necessary to determine the effects of other factors noted above that may also be involved in regulating NCX activity.

(i) Action potential. During a normal AP, the magnitude of Ca^{2+} entry is a complex function of the time and voltage dependence of L-type Ca^{2+} channels and NCX activity. AP configuration changes during cardiac maturation in every mammalian species examined [76–79], although the perinatal pattern of change varies by species. The molecular basis for developmental changes in the AP may be related to age-related differences in the transient outward current (I_{to}) [80], but since the pattern of postnatal change differs among various species, the underlying mechanisms are likely to be species-dependent. Regardless of the etiology of AP variation, the important implication is that age-appropriate and species-specific action potentials should be considered as the most relevant driving ionic force for experimental studies of developmental aspects of EC coupling. Furthermore, a greater dependency on NCX as the source of activator Ca^{2+} (as we propose exists in immature myocardium) predicts that graded control of Ca^{2+} influx (and hence, the force of contraction) can be achieved by subtle changes in AP duration and/or configuration.

(ii) Changes in $[Na^+]_i$. It is known that cardiac sarcolemmal sodium pump activity changes during development in a variety of different species [81–83]. Results from these studies are generally consistent in demonstrating that sodium pump activity is higher in the neonate compared to the adult within the same species (including humans [84]). It is well known that in adult myocytes, minor variations in $[Na^+]_i$ can lead to substantial changes in $[Ca^{2+}]_i$ and contraction [85,86], mediated by changes in NCX activity. If NCX plays a greater role during EC coupling in the fetus and neonate, then $[Na^+]_i$ may be an even more important regulator of contraction in these age groups.

Recently, we used the fluorescence approach to compare resting $[Na^+]_i$ in ventricular myocytes isolated from immature rabbits. Basal $[Na^+]_i$ in ventricular myocytes did not differ significantly among three different groups of immature rabbits from 3 to 21 days of age [87]. However, additional work is necessary to determine the responses to physiological and pharmacological manipulation and to relate changes in $[Na^+]_i$ to contractile function.

(iii) **Cytosolic Ca^{2+} buffering capacity.** Numerous high and low affinity Ca^{2+} binding sites are present in ventricular myocytes, including myosin, calmodulin, troponin, small mobile molecules (e.g. ATP and phosphocreatine) and Ca^{2+} transport proteins such as the SR Ca^{2+}-ATPase and the sarcolemmal Na^+-Ca^{2+} exchanger. Thus, Ca^{2+} entering the cell is tightly buffered by a variety of intracellular buffering systems. Based upon theoretical and experimental approaches, the cytosol in adult ventricular myocytes is capable of buffering Ca^{2+} 50–100 fold over the physiological range of changes in $[Ca^{2+}]_i$ ($100\,nM$ – $1\,\mu M$) [88,89]. In other words, at least $50\,\mu mole$ Ca^{2+} must be added to the cytosol in order to rapidly raise $[Ca^{2+}]_i$ from $100\,nM$ at rest to a peak of ~$1\,\mu M$. Based upon recognized age-related changes in virtually all of the intrinsic Ca^{2+} buffering systems, it is likely that cytosolic Ca^{2+} buffering power changes during development. It has recently been shown that ventricular myocytes from immature rats exhibit lower intrinsic cytosolic Ca^{2+} buffering [90], but no comparable information exists for humans.

(iv) **β-adrenergic stimulation.** Driven by sympathetic neurotransmitters and adrenal hormones, β-adrenergic activation regulates virtually all major constituents of the cardiac EC coupling cascade, e.g., L-type Ca^{2+} channels, ryanodine receptors, Na^+-Ca^{2+} exchangers, phospholamban and contractile myofilaments. These effects are mainly mediated via the classic stimulatory G protein (G_s)—adenylyl cyclase—cAMP—protein kinase A (PKA) signaling cascade and subsequent phosphorylation of the target proteins by PKA. Previously, β-adrenergic stimulation has been shown to modulate NCX in frog myocytes [91,92] but not in mammalian cardiac myocytes. Recently, Perchenet et al. [75] showed that non-selective β-adrenergic agonist isoproterenol can enhance both inward and outward NCX currents in adult guinea pig myocyte at 37°C but not 20°C, because NCX activity is highly sensitive to temperature. In addition, they showed that the NCX response to isoproterenol is mimicked by the adenylyl cyclase activator forskolin and can be totally inhibited by a β-adrenergic blocker or PKA inhibitor. It has been shown that regulation of NCX activity by PKA is isoform-specific [93]. Although the cardiac-specific isoform of NCX1 gene contains consensus PKA phosphorylation sites within the large intracellular loop [94], it has not yet been determined whether the exchanger or some unidentified regulatory proteins is phosphorylated under physiologically relevant conditions *in vivo*. At present, it is unclear whether β-adrenergic stimulation has a similar effect on NCX activity in immature myocytes.

In addition to the possibility that immature cardiac myocytes might possess qualitatively and quantitatively different NCX proteins, β-adrenergic signaling changes dramatically during development. Even though β-adrenergic receptors are detected in early fetal hearts long before postnatal sympathetic innervation, the response of I_{Ca}, Ca_i transient and cell contraction to β-adrenergic stimulation only become evident in the late gestation stage. This is due to uncoupling of the receptor from downstream signaling in the early gestation stages [38,95]. Furthermore, the signal transduction pathways of β-adrenergic receptor in the immature heart might not be identical to that in mature heart. For example, the sensitivity of neonatal cardiac myocytes to β_2-adrenergic receptor agonists is much higher as compared to that of adult cardiac myocytes [96]. Recently, the β_2-adrenergic receptor was found to be coupled to the arachidonic acid pathway in fetal chick ventricular myocytes [97]. More surprisingly, repeated β-adrenergic receptor stimulation *sensitizes* the β-adrenergic signaling pathway in neonatal rat cardiac myocytes, which is in sharp contrast to the agonist-induced desensitization in adult cardiac myocytes [98]. Thus, whether β-adrenergic receptor stimulation can modulate NCX activity in immature cardiac myocytes and its underlying cellular mechanism(s) clearly merit further investigation.

V. EXCITATION-CONTRACTION COUPLING IN IMMATURE HUMAN HEART

Much of our current understanding of developmental changes in EC coupling calcium regulation is based upon animal experiments (particularly rabbits). A few investigators have compared I_{Ca} in myocytes isolated from infants and children to adult cells [41,43] or from infants compared with young children [42]. A consistent finding has been that current amplitude, normalized for differences in cell size (I_{Ca} density; pA/pF), does not differ among the different age groups. However, important differences were observed in I_{Ca} decay kinetics [41] and in the voltage dependence of steady-state inactivation [43]. Results from a single study using atrial myocytes from young children (3 days to 4 years of age) suggested that either I_{Ca} or caffeine can trigger SR Ca^{2+} release and evoke a Ca^{2+} transient (recorded using fura-2) in immature human myocytes [42]. However, the changes in $[Ca^{2+}]_i$ were relatively small (240 ± 45 nM following depolarization and 236 ± 37 nM in response to caffeine), the time courses of the transients were quite prolonged (consistent with limited SR reuptake but also possible due to limitations of dye kinetics related to Ca^{2+} buffering) and there was no attempt to correlate these responses to cell contraction. Although inward I_{NaCa} evoked by caffeine-induced SR Ca^{2+} release was demonstrated, no attempts were made to characterize I_{NaCa} in this study. Lastly, these experiments were conducted at room temperature using a fixed concentration of $[Na^+]_i$ and a cesium-containing pipette solution, both of which limit assessment of EC coupling mechanisms in immature atrial myocytes. Consequently, it is necessary to perform more direct and detailed studies to fully define mechanisms of normal EC coupling in the immature human heart. Furthermore, the relationship between normal developmental changes in action potential configuration and EC coupling remains to be determined.

VI. IMPLICATIONS FOR MANIPULATION OF CARDIAC CONTRACTILE FUNCTION IN INFANTS AND CHILDREN

The results reviewed above suggest that entirely new approaches are necessary when considering the fundamental mechanisms of $[Ca^{2+}]_i$ regulation in the immature heart. It seems inappropriate to extrapolate from adults, since the molecular and cellular basis for EC coupling is vastly different in immature mammalian myocardial cells. Admittedly, most of the foundation for our current understanding of $[Ca^{2+}]_i$ regulation and cardiac contraction during human development is derived from animal studies. However, it is clear that many of the findings derived from immature animal models correlate with clinical observations in premature and term newborns, infants and children. Infants born at 26–28 weeks gestation are commonplace and at this stage, these human infants represent a much earlier phase of development than many of the mammalian fetal/newborn animal models that are known to exhibit profound immaturity of contractile function and inotropic responsiveness. Although infants and children with cardiac dysfunction represent a heterogeneous group, a common feature of all of these children is that the scientific foundation for understanding (and therefore, manipulating) their cardiac contractile function is markedly deficient.

We hope that this brief review will stimulate additional efforts to advance our fundamental knowledge of mechanisms involved in EC coupling and regulation of contractile function during cardiac maturation. Such studies will have important implications for the subsequent development of more rational and age-specific therapeutic strategies for infants and children with abnormal cardiac contractile function.

REFERENCES

1. Bers DM. 1991. Excitation-contraction coupling and cardiac contractile force. Kluwer Academic Publishers, The Netherlands.
2. Bers DM. 1996. Measurement of calcium transport in heart using modern approaches. New Horizons 4:36–44.
3. Fabiato A. 1985. Simulated calcium current can both cause calcium loading and trigger calcium release from the sarcoplasmic reticulum of a skinned canine cardiac Purkinje cell. J Gen Physiol 85:291–320.
4. Carl SL, Felix K, Caswell AH, Brandt NR, Ball WJ Jr., Vaghy PL, Meissner G, Ferguson DG. 1995. Immunolocalization of sarcolemmal dihydropyridine receptor and sarcoplasmic reticular triadin and ryanodine receptor in rabbit ventricle and atrium. J Cell Biol 129:672–682.
5. Sun X, Protasi F, Takahashi M, Takeshima H, Ferguson DG, Franzini-Armstrong C. 1995. Molecular architecture of membranes involved in excitation-contraction coupling of cardiac muscle. J Cell Biol 129:659–671.
6. Stern MD. 1998. Exploring local calcium feedback: trying to fool mother nature. J Gen Physiol 112:259–262.
7. Sham JSK, Cleemann L, Morad M. 1995. Functional coupling of Ca^{2+} channels and ryanodine receptors in cardiac myocytes. Proc Natl Acad Sci USA 92:121–125.
8. Shacklock PS, Wier WG, Balke CW. 1995. Local Ca^{2+} transients (Ca^{2+} sparks) originate at transverse tubules in rat heart cells. J Physiol (Lond) 487:601–608.
9. Wasserstrom JA, Vites AM. 1996. The role of Na^+-Ca^{2+} exchange in activation of excitation-contraction coupling in rat ventricular myocytes. J Physiol (Lond) 493:529–542.
10. Vornanen M, Shepherd N, Isenberg G. 1994. Tension-voltage relations of single myocytes reflect Ca release triggered by Na/Ca exchange at 35°C but not 23°C. Am J Physiol 267:C623–C632.
11. Sipido KR, Maes M, Van de Werf F. 1997. Low efficiency of Ca^{2+} entry through the Na^+-Ca^{2+} exchanger as trigger for Ca^{2+} release from the sarcoplasmic reticulum—A comparison between L-type Ca^{2+} current and reverse-mode Na^+-Ca^{2+} exchange. Circ Res 81:1034–1044.
12. Sipido KR, Callewaert G, Porciatti F, Vereecke J, Carmeliet E. 1995. $[Ca^{2+}]_i$-dependent membrane currents in guinea-pig ventricular cells in the absence of Na/Ca exchange. Pflugers Arch 430:871–878.

13. Sipido KR, Carmeliet E, Van der Werf F. 1998. T-type Ca^{2+} current as a trigger for Ca^{2+} release from the sarcoplasmic reticulum in guinea-pig ventricular myocytes. J Physiol (London) 508:439–451.

14. Ferrier GR, Redondo IM, Mason CA, Mapplebeck C, Howlett SE. 2000. Regulation of contraction and relaxation by membrane potential in cardiac ventricular myocytes. Am J Physiol 278:H1618–H1626.

15. Howlett SE, Zhu JQ, Ferrier GR. 1998. Contribution of a voltage-sensitive calcium release mechanism to contraction in cardiac ventricular myocytes. Am J Physiol 274:H155–H170.

16. Piacentino V, Dipla K, Gaughan JP, Houser SR. 2000. Voltage-dependent Ca^{2+} release from the SR of feline ventricular myocytes is explained by Ca^{2+}-induced Ca^{2+} release. Journal of Physiology-London 523:533–548.

17. Artman M. 1994. Developmental Changes in Myocardial Inotropic Responsiveness. R.G. Landes Company, Austin, TX.

18. Teitel DF. 1998. Physiologic development of the cardiovascular system in the fetus. In: Fetal and Neonatal Physiology. Polin RA, Fox WW, eds. W.B. Saunders Co., Philadelphia.

19. Anderson PAW. 1996. The heart and development. Semin Perinatol ••:482–509.

20. Pegg W, Michalak M. 1987. Differentiation of sarcoplasmic reticulum during cardiac myogenesis. Am J Physiol 252:H22–H31.

21. Nassar R, Reedy MC, Anderson PA. 1987. Developmental changes in the ultrastructure and sarcomere shortening of the isolated rabbit ventricular myocyte. Circ Res 61:465–483.

22. Nakanishi T, Seguchi M, Takao A. 1988. Development of the myocardial contractile system. Experientia 44:936–944.

23. Artman M, Graham TP, Boucek RJ. 1985. Effects of postnatal maturation on myocardial contractile responses to calcium antagonists and changes in contraction frequency. J Cardiovasc Pharmacol 7:850–855.

24. Fisher DJ, Tate CA, Phillips S. 1992. Developmental regulation of the sarcoplasmic reticulum calcium pump in the rabbit heart. Pediatr Res 31:474–479.

25. Kaufman TM, Horton JW, White DJ, Mahony L. 1990. Age-related changes in myocardial relaxation and sarcoplasmic reticulum function. Am J Physiol 259:H309–H316.

26. Huynh TV, Chen FH, Wetzel GT, Friedman WF, Klitzner TS. 1992. Developmental changes in membrane Ca^{2+} and K^+ currents in fetal, neonatal, and adult rabbit ventricular myocytes. Circ Res 70:508–515.

27. Wetzel GT, Chen FH, Klitzner TS. 1991. L- and T-type calcium channels in acutely isolated neonatal and adult cardiac myocytes. Pediatr Res 30:89–94.

28. Brillantes A-MB, Bezprozvannaya S, Marks AR. 1994. Developmental and tissue-specific regulation of rabbit skeletal and cardiac muscle calcium channels involved in excitation-contraction coupling. Circ Res 75:503–510.

29. Balaguru D, Haddock PS, Puglisi JL, Bers DM, Coetzee WA, Artman M. 1997. Role of the sarcoplasmic reticulum in contraction and relaxation of immature rabbit ventricular myocytes. J Mol Cell Cardiol 29:2747–2757.

30. Miller MS, Friedman WF, Wetzel GT. 1997. Caffeine-induced contractions in developing rabbit heart. Pediatr Res 42:287–292.

31. Varadi G, Mori Y, Mikala G, Schwartz A. 1995. Molecular determinants of Ca^{2+} channel function and drug action. Trends Pharmacol Sci 16:43–49.

32. Haase H. 2000. Expression of Ca^{2+} channel subunits during cardiac ontogeny in mice and rats: identification of fetal α_{1C} and β subunit isoforms. J Cell Biochem 76:695–703.

33. Kolossov E, Fleischmann BK, Liu Q, Bloch W, Viatchenko-Karpinski S, Manzke O, Ji GJ, Bohlen H, Addicks K, Hescheler J. 1998. Functional characteristics of ES cell-derived cardiac precursor cells identified by tissue-specific expression of the green fluorescent protein. J Cell Biol 143:2045–2056.

34. Wetzel GT, Chen FH, Klitzner TS. 1993. Ca^{2+} channel kinetics in acutely isolated fetal, neonatal, and adult rabbit cardiac myocytes. Circ Res 72:1065–1074.

35. Renaud JF, Fosset M, Kazazoglou T, Lazdunski M, Schmid A. 1989. Appearance and function of voltage-dependent Ca^{2+} channels during pre- and postnatal development of cardiac and skeletal muscles. Ann N Y Acad Sci 560:418–425.

36. Navaratnam S, Khatter JC. 1991. Increased [^{3}H]nitrendipine binding sites in rat heart during adult maturation and aging. Biochem Pharmacol 41:593–600.

37. Wibo M, Bravo G, Godfraind T. 1991. Postnatal maturation of excitation-contraction coupling in rat ventricle in relation to the subcellular localization and surface density of 1,4-dihydropyridine and ryanodine receptors. Circ Res 68:662–673.

38. An RH, Davies MP, Doevendans PA, Kubalak SW, Bangalore R, Chien KR, Kass RS. 1996. Developmental changes in β-adrenergic modulation of L-type Ca^{2+} channels in embryonic mouse heart. Circ Res 78:371–378.

39. Vornanen M. 1996. Contribution of sarcolemmal calcium current to total cellular calcium in postnatally developing rat heart. Cardiovasc Res 32:400–410.

40. Osaka T, Joyner RW. 1991. Developmental changes in calcium currents of rabbit ventricular cells. Circ Res 68:788–796.

41. Roca TP, Pigott JD, Clarkson CW, Crumb WJ. 1996. L-type calcium current in pediatric and adult human atrial myocytes: evidence for developmental changes in channel inactivation. Pediatr Res 40:462–468.

42. Hatem SN, Sweeten T, Vetter V, Morad M. 1995. Evidence for presence of Ca^{2+} channel-gated Ca^{2+} stores in neonatal human atrial myocytes. Am J Physiol 268:H1195–H1201.

43. Cohen NM, Lederer WJ. 1993. Calcium current in single human cardiac myocytes. J Cardiovasc Electrophysiol 4:422–437.

44. Rosemblit N, Moschella MC, Ondriasa E, Gutstein DE, Ondrias K, Marks AR. 1999. Intracellular calcium release channel expression during embryogenesis. Dev Biol 206:163–177.

45. Gorza L, Vettore S, Tessaro A, Sorrentino V, Vitadello M. 1997. Regional and age-related differences in mRNA composition of intracellular Ca^{2+}-release channels of rat cardiac myocytes. J Mol Cell Cardiol 29:1023–1036.

46. Ramesh V, Kresch MJ, Katz AM, Kim DH. 1995. Characterization of Ca^{2+}-release channels in fetal and adult rat hearts. Am J Physiol 269:H778–H782.

47. Seguchi M, Harding JA, Jarmakani JM. 1986. Developmental change in the function of sarcoplasmic reticulum. J Mol Cell Cardiol 18:189–195.

48. Haddock PS, Coetzee WA, Cho E, Porter L, Katoh H, Bers DM, Jafri MS, Artman M. 1999. Subcellular $[Ca^{2+}]_i$ gradients during excitation-contraction coupling in newborn rabbit ventricular myocytes. Circ Res 85:415–427.

49. Ostadalova I, Kolar F, Ostadal B, Rohlicek V, Rohlicek J, Prochazka J. 1993. Early postnatal development of contractile performance and responsiveness to Ca^{2+}, verapamil and ryanodine in the isolated rat heart. J Mol Cell Cardiol 25:733–740.

50. Brotto MAD, Creazzo TL. 1996. Ca^{2+} transients in embryonic chick heart: Contributions from Ca^{2+} channels and the sarcoplasmic reticulum. Am J Physiol 270:H518–H525.

51. Takeshima H, Komazaki S, Hirose K, Nishi M, Noda T, Iino M. 1998. Embryonic lethality and abnormal cardiac myocytes in mice lacking ryanodine receptor type 2. EMBO J 17:3309–3316.

52. Haddock PS, Coetzee WA, Artman M. 1997. Na^+/Ca^{2+} exchange current and contractions measured under Cl^--free conditions in developing rabbit hearts. Am J Physiol Heart Circ Physiol 273: H837–H846.

53. Kim H, Kim D, Lee I, Rah B, Sawa Y, Schaper J. 1992. Human fetal heart development after mid-term: morphometry and ultrastructural study. J Mol Cell Cardiol 24:949–965.

54. Hatem S, Bénardeau A, Rücker-Martin C, Marty I, de Chamnisso P, Villaz M, Mercadier J-J. 1997. Different compartments of sarcoplasmic reticulum participate in the excitation–contraction coupling process in human atrial myocytes. Circ Res 80:345–353.

55. Lipp P, Huser J, Pott L, Niggli E. 12-15-1996. Spatially non-uniform $Ca2^+$ signals induced by the reduction of transverse tubules in citrate-loaded guinea-pig ventricular myocytes in culture. J Physiol (Lond) 497:589–597.

56. Huser J, Lipsius SL, Blatter LA. 1996. Calcium gradients during excitation-contraction coupling in cat atrial myocytes. J Physiol 494:641–651.

57. Haddock PS, Artman M, Coetzee WA. 1998. Influence of postnatal changes in action potential duration on Na-Ca exchange in rabbit ventricular myocytes. Pflugers Arch-Eur J Physiol 435:789–795.

58. Klitzner TS, Chen F, Raven RR, Wetzel GT, Friedman WF. 1991. Calcium current and tension generation in immature mammalian myocardium: effects of diltiazem. J Mol Cell Cardiol 23:807–815.

59. Katsube Y, Yokoshiki H, Nguyen L, Yamamoto M, Sperelakis N. 1998. L-type Ca^{2+} currents in ventricular myocytes from neonatal and adult rats. Can J Physiol Pharmacol 76:873–881.

60. Barry WH, Bridge JHB. 1993. Intracellular calcium homeostasis in cardiac myocytes. Circulation 87:1806–1815.

61. Hryshko LV, Philipson KD. 1997. Sodium-calcium exchange: Recent advances. Basic Res Cardiol 92 Suppl. 1:45–51.

62. Levi AJ, Spitzer KW, Kohmoto O, Bridge JHB. 1994. Depolarization-induced Ca entry via Na-Ca exchange triggers SR release in guinea pig cardiac myocytes. Am J Physiol 266:H1422–H1433.

63. Leblanc N, Hume JR. 1990. Sodium current-induced release of calcium from cardiac sarcoplasmic reticulum. Science 248:372–376.
64. Koushik SV, Bundy J, Conway SJ. 1999. Sodium-calcium exchanger is initially expressed in a heart-restricted pattern within the early mouse embryo. Mech Dev 88:119–122.
65. Artman M. 1992. Sarcolemmal Na⁺-Ca²⁺ exchange activity and exchanger immunoreactivity in developing rabbit hearts. Am J Physiol 263:H1506–H1513.
66. Boerth SR, Zimmer DB, Artman M. 1994. Steady-state mRNA levels of the sarcolemmal Na⁺-Ca²⁺ exchanger peak near birth in developing rabbit and rat hearts. Circ Res 74:354–359.
67. Chen F, Mottino G, Klitzner TS, Philipson KD, Frank JS. 1995. Distribution of the Na⁺/Ca²⁺ exchange protein in developing rabbit myocytes. Am J Physiol 268:C1126–C1132.
68. Artman M, Ichikawa H, Avkiran M, Coetzee WA. 1995. Na⁺/Ca²⁺ exchange current density in cardiac myocytes from rabbits and guinea pigs during postnatal development. Am J Physiol 268: H1714–H1722.
69. Reed TD, Babu GJ, Ji Y, Zilberman A, Heyen MV, Wuytack F, Periasamy M. 2000. The expression of SR calcium transport ATPase and the Na⁺/Ca²⁺ exchanger are antithetically regulated during mouse cardiac development and in hypo/hyperthyroidism. J Mol Cell Cardiol 32:453–464.
70. Qu YX, Ghatpande A, El Sherif N, Boutjdir M. 2000. Gene expression of Na⁺/Ca²⁺ exchanger during development in human heart. Cardiovasc Res 45:866–873.
71. Vetter R, Studer R, Reinecke H, Kolár F, Ostádalová, I, Drexler H. 1995. Reciprocal changes in the postnatal expression of the sarcolemmal Na⁺-Ca²⁺-exchanger and SERCA2 in rat heart. J Mol Cell Cardiol 27:1689–1701.
72. Boerth SR, Artman M. 1996. Thyroid hormone regulates Na⁺-Ca²⁺ exchanger expression during postnatal maturation and in adult rabbit ventricular myocardium. Cardiovasc Res 31(S):E145–E152.
73. Matsuda T, Takuma K, Baba A. 1997. Na⁺-Ca²⁺ exchanger: Physiology and pharmacology. Jpn J Pharmacol 74:1–20.
74. Hilgemann DW, Ball R. 1996. Regulation of cardiac Na⁺, Ca²⁺ exchange and K_{ATP} potassium channels by PIP₂. Science 273:956–959.
75. Perchenet L, Hinde AK, Patel KCR, Hancox JC, Levi AJ. 2000. Stimulation of Na/Ca exchange by the β-adrenergic/protein kinase A pathway in guinea-pig ventricular myocytes at 37°C. Pflugers Arch 439:822–828.
76. Wahler GM, Dollinger SJ, Smith JM, Flemal KL. 1994. Time course of postnatal changes in rat heart action potential and in transient outward current is different. Am J Physiol 267:H1157–H1166.
77. Conforti L, Tohse N, Sperelakis N. 1993. Tetrodotoxin-sensitive sodium current in rat fetal ventricular myocytes—contribution to the plateau phase of action potential. J Mol Cell Cardiol 25:159–173.
78. Kato Y, Masumiya H, Agata N, Tanaka H, Shigenobu K. 1996. Developmental changes in action potential and membrane currents in fetal, neonatal and adult guinea pig ventricular myocytes. J Mol Cell Cardiol 28:1515–1522.
79. Agata N, Tanaka H, Shigenobu K. 1994. Effects of tetrodotoxin and low-sodium on action potential plateau of ventricular myocardium from neonatal and adult guinea-pigs. Comp Biochem Physiol [A] 107A:459–461.
80. Crumb WJ Jr, Pigott JD, Clarkson CW. 1995. Comparison of I_{to} in young and adult human atrial myocytes: Evidence for developmental changes. Am J Physiol 268:H1335–H1342.
81. Lucchesi PA, Sweadner KJ. 1991. Postnatal changes in Na, K-ATPase isoform expression in rat cardiac ventricle. J Biol Chem 299:9327–9331.
82. Hanson GL, Schilling WP, Michael LH. 1993. Sodium-potassium pump and sodium-calcium exchange in adult and neonatal canine sarcolemma. Am J Physiol 264:H320–H326.
83. Magyar CE, Wang JN, Azuma KK, McDonough AA. 1995. Reciprocal regulation of cardiac Na-K-ATPase and Na/Ca exchanger: Hypertension, thyroid hormone, development. Am J Physiol 269:C675–C682.
84. Kjeldsen K, Gron P. 1990. Age-dependent change in myocardial cardiac glycoside receptor (Na, K pump) concentration in children. J Cardiovasc Pharmacol 15:332–337.
85. Levesque PC, Clark CD, Zakarov SI, Rosenshtraukh LV, Hume JR. 1993. Anion and cation modulation of the guinea-pig ventricular action potential during β-adrenergic stimulation. Pflugers Archiv 424:54–62.
86. Díaz ME, Cook SJ, Chamunorwa JP, Trafford AW, Lancaster MK, O'Neill SC, Eisner DA. 1996. Variability of spontaneous Ca²⁺ release between different rat ventricular myocytes is correlated with Na⁺-Ca²⁺ exchange and [Na⁺]ᵢ. Circ Res 78:857–862.

87. Artman M, Henry G, Coetzee WA. 2000. Cellular basis for age-related differences in cardiac excitation-contraction coupling. Prog Pediatr Cardiol 11:185–194.
88. Berlin JR, Bassani JWM, Bers DM. 1994. Intrinsic cytosolic calcium buffering properties of single rat cardiac myocytes. Biophys J 67:1775–1787.
89. Delbridge LMD, Bassani JWM, Bers DM. 1996. Steady-state twitch Ca^{2+} fluxes and cytosolic Ca^{2+} buffering in rabbit ventricular myocytes. Am J Physiol 270:C192–C199.
90. Bassani RA, Shannon TR, Bers DM. 1998. Passive Ca^{2+} binding in ventricular myocardium of neonatal and adult rats. Cell Calcium 23:433–442.
91. Fan J, Shuba YM, Morad M. 1996. Regulation of cardiac sodium-calcium exchanger by β-adrenergic agonists. Proc Natl Acad Sci USA 93:5527–5532.
92. Rakotonirina A, Soustre H. 1989. Effects of isoprenaline on tonic tension and Na-Ca exchange in frog atrial fibres. Gen Physiol Biophys 8:313–326.
93. He SW, Ruknudin A, Bambrick LL, Lederer WJ, Schulze DH. 1998. Isoform-specific regulation of the Na^+/Ca^{2+} exchanger in rat astrocytes and neurons by PKA. J Neurosci 18:4833–4841.
94. Nicoll DA, Longoni S, Philipson KD. 1990. Molecular cloning and functional expression of the cardiac Na^+-Ca^{2+} exchanger. Science 250:562–565.
95. Maltsev VA, Ji GJ, Wobus AM, Fleischmann BK, Hescheler J. 1999. Establishment of β-adrenergic modulation of L-type Ca^{2+} current in the early stages of cardiomyocyte development. Circ Res 84:136–145.
96. Kuznetsov V, Pak E, Robinson RB, Steinberg SF. 1995. $β_2$-adrenergic receptor actions in neonatal and adult rat ventricular myocytes. Circ Res 76:40–52.
97. Pavoine C, Magne S, Sauvadet A, Pecker F. 2000. Evidence for a $β_2$-adrenergic/arachidonic acid pathway in ventricular cardiomyocytes. J Biol Chem 274:628–637.
98. Zeiders JL, Seidler FJ, Iaccarino G, Koch WJ, Slotkin TA. 2000. Ontogeny of cardiac β-adrenoceptor desensitization mechanisms: agonist treatment enhances receptor/G protein transduction rather than eliciting uncoupling. J Mol Cell Cardiol 31:413–423.

B. Ostadal, M. Nagano and N.S. Dhalla (eds.).
CARDIAC DEVELOPMENT. Copyright © 2002.
Kluwer Academic Publishers. Boston.
All rights reserved.

DEVELOPMENTAL CHANGES OF SARCOPLASMIC RETICULAR CALCIUM ION TRANSPORT AND PHOSPHOLAMBAN IN RAT HEART

ROLAND VETTER, UWE REHFELD, CHRISTOPH REISSFELDER, WOLFGANG WEIß, FRANTIŠEK KOLÁŘ,[1] and MARTIN PAUL

Institute of Clinical Pharmacology and Toxicology, Benjamin Franklin Medical Center, Freie Universität Berlin, Germany; [1] Institute of Physiology, Academy of Sciences of the Czech Republic, Prague, Czech Republic

Summary. This comparative study investigates the relationship between sarcoplasmic reticulum (SR) calcium (Ca^{2+}) ATPase transport activity and phospholamban (PLB) phosphorylation in whole cardiac homogenates around birth and during postnatal development until weaning. At fetal day 20, the rate of homogenate oxalate-supported Ca^{2+} uptake was 23% of that at postnatal day 6 (0.34 ± 0.08 vs 1.46 ± 0.37 nmoles Ca^{2+}/mg wet ventricular weight/min, respectively; $P < 0.05$). This was accompanied by a 2-fold gain in heart mass. Between postnatal days 6 and 21, there occurred a further 4-fold increase in heart mass which was accompanied by only a 1.3-fold increase in SR Ca^{2+} transport activity. Levels of phosphorylated PLB formed *in vitro* in the presence of radiolabelled ATP and catalytic subunit of protein kinase A increased approx. 4-fold between fetal day 20 and postnatal day 21. In this early developmental period, SR Ca^{2+}-transport values were linearly related to the respective ^{32}P-PLB levels suggesting coordinated developmental changes of SR Ca^{2+} ATPase and PLB. Developmental changes in SR Ca^{2+} transport and ^{32}P-PLB levels were thyroid hormone(TH)-dependent as revealed from analysis of these parameters in 21-day-old rats with experimentally induced eu-, hypo- and hyperthyroid states. It appears that TH-dependent changes in the phosphorylation of PLB play a major role for the increase in SR Ca^{2+} transport activity between birth and weaning.

Key words: Sarcoplasmic Reticulum, Calcium ATPase, Phospholamban, Development, Thyroid hormones

Addresses for mailing proofs: Roland Vetter, MD, Institute of Clinical Pharmacology and Toxicology, Benjamin Franklin Medical Center, Freie Universität Berlin, Garystrasse 5, D-14195 Berlin (Dahlem), Germany. Phone: +49-30-8445 1721; Fax: +49-30-8445 1762; e-mail: rvetter@zedat.fu-berlin.de

INTRODUCTION

Postnatal maturation of the rat heart is characterized by a rapid increase in its mass and contractile performance that matches the increased functional demands during postnatal growth. Cardiac growth in the perinatal period is mainly due to hyperplasia whereas cellular hypertrophy of cardiomyocytes appears to be the sole growth mechanism at later stages [1]. The increase in cardiomyocyte size is associated with an accumulation of many different types of cellular proteins due to an accelerated protein synthesis [2]. This appears to be particularly true for proteins of the sarcoplasmic reticulum (SR). The SR in cardiac muscle regulates the relaxation of the muscle and acts as a source of Ca^{2+} for myofilament activation during the excitation-contraction coupling process [3]. Several previous studies have shown that this process undergoes developmental changes during fetal and postnatal heart growth. For example, a progressive postnatal increase in the rate of cardiac relaxation in rodents such as rabbit and rat [4,5] is paralleled by an increased Ca^{2+} transporting activity of the cardiac SR [5–10]. Recent evidence points to a developmentally regulated elevation in the expression of the SR Ca^{2+} ATPase isoform SERCA2a in the myocardium as an important contributing mechanism to these changes [6–8,11,12]. In addition, alterations in membrane lipids [13,14] as well as levels and state of phosphorylation of the Ca^{2+}-ATPase modulatory protein phospholamban (PLB) could be other contributing factors [15–18]. Phospholamban, a homopentameric SR protein has been shown to regulate the rate of SR Ca^{2+} transport through changes in the affinity of the Ca^{2+}-ATPase for Ca^{2+}. The Ca^{2+} transporting activity of this enzyme is suppressed while PLB is dephosphorylated. This inhibition is relieved upon phosphorylation of this protein by cyclic AMP(cAMP)-dependent protein kinase (at serine 16) which in intact tissue occurs in response to β-adrenergic stimulation [15–17]. Phospholamban can also become phosphorylated at a distinct amino acid residue (at threonine 17) by Ca^{2+}-dependent calmodulin (CaM) kinase II [16,18]. As the SR plays a central role in cardiac excitation-contraction coupling, we initiated a comparative study on the Ca^{2+} transport function and PLB of this intracellular organelle in the late fetal/early postnatal period in rats. Since thyroid hormone (TH) levels increase in postnatal life and are essential for maturation of myocardial Ca^{2+} handling, the question was addressed as to whether developmental changes in SR Ca^{2+} transport and PLB are TH-dependent.

MATERIALS AND METHODS

Animals

Hearts of Wistar rats ranging in age from fetal day 15 to day 21 after birth were used. Litters of newborn Wistar rats were evened to eight pups per dam and maintained throughout experiment. Some of them were made hypothyroid by the administration of 0.05% 6-n-propyl-2-thiouracil (PTU) in drinking water given to nursing mothers from postnatal day 2 to day 12 and to 21. Hyperthyroidism was induced by daily subcutaneous injections of L-triiodothyronine (T$_3$; 10 μg/100 g body weight) in the same period of time. Euthyroid control rats received no treatment. In another group of animals, the PTU-induced hypothyroidism was simultaneously treated with $2.5\,\mu g\,T_3/100\,g$ body weight. This lower dose of T_3 was selected because $10\,\mu g\,T_3/100\,g$ B.W./d caused high mortality in PTU-treated animals. After sacrifying the animals by cervical dislocation, the heart was rapidly removed and immersed in ice-cold solution containing 130 mM NaCl, 30 mM KCl and 10 mM histidine (pH 7.4). The isolated ventricles were blotted, immediately frozen in liquid nitrogen and stored at $-80°C$ until used for biochemical analysis. Animal care and experimental procedure were in accordance with institutional guidelines.

Preparation of tissue homogenates

Tissue homogenates were prepared from ventricular tissue of single hearts or several pooled hearts under stringent phosphoprotein protection conditions as described elsewhere [19]. The final homogenate was filtered through polyamide gauze (90 μm mesh; NeoLab, Heidelberg, Germany) and kept in a tube on ice. A sample of this homogenate was used within 10 min for the measurement of oxalate-supported Ca^{2+} uptake. Other samples were immediately frozen in liquid nitrogen and stored at $-80°C$ until use for the quantitation of PLB, SR Ca^{2+} ATPase and protein. For ELISA of PLB, tissue homogenates were treated with 0.6 M KCl in order to remove contractile proteins as described elswhere [19].

Biochemical and immunochemical assays

The assay of protein [12], oxalate-supported Ca^{2+} uptake into SR vesicles at 37°C and 0.21 μM free Ca^{2+} concentration [19], SDS-polyacrylamide gel electrophoresis [12], protein kinase A-catalyzed phosphorylation of PLB [12,19], Western blotting [12], ELISA for PLB [12] have all been described in previous papers.

Statistical analysis

Values are presented as mean ± SD unless stated otherwise. Statistical analysis was performed by Student's t-test for unpaired observations or one way analysis of variance followed by Bonferroni group-to-group comparisons. Statistical significance was assumed at $P < 0.05$.

RESULTS

Postnatal changes in ventricular weight and protein

Figure 1 shows the postnatal changes in ventricular weight and ventricular proteins in the early postnatal growth period between day 1 and day 21 in Wistar rats. Initial experiments showed no differences in either body or heart weight of male and female rats, thus all the data were combined. The results show a more than 6-fold increase in ventricular weight between postnatal days 1 and 21. These changes were paralleled by an approx. 3-fold increase in total ventricular protein content indicating that the synthesis of cardiac proteins is extremely high in this period. It is particularly noteworthy that gain in ventricular weight and protein was highest in the first 6 day after birth.

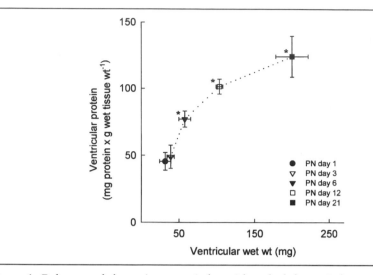

Figure 1. Early postnatal changes in rat ventricular weight and whole ventricular protein content between postnatal (PN) day 1 and 21. Ventricular weight is the sum of left and right ventricular weight. Values are mean ± SD for 5 to 6 hearts in each age group. *P < 0.05 vs. day 1 and day 3.

Developmental changes in SR Ca²⁺ uptake and phospholamban phosphorylation

Figure 2 shows the relationship between rate values of oxalate-supported SR Ca^{2+} uptake in whole ventricular homogenates and ventricular weight between fetal day 20 and postnatal day 21. There occurred an almost linear 4-fold increase in the rate of SR Ca^{2+} uptake between fetal day 20 and postnatal day 6. The SR Ca^{2+} transport activity was further increased by 32% between postnatal days 6 and 21. Addition of catalytic (C) subunit of protein kinase A (PKA) resulted in an increased Ca^{2+} uptake rate at all developmental stages studied. By contrast, inhibition of endogenous PKA by 10 μM of the PKA inhibitor peptide [PKI(6–22)amide] caused a marked reduction in Ca^{2+} uptake at all developmental stages studied (Fig. 3). These results indicate that the cardiac SR Ca^{2+} pump activity of fetal and newborn rats can be modulated by PKA-catalyzed phosphorylation of PLB. Figure 3 also shows the developmental changes between fetal day 15 and postnatal day 21 in the content of radiolabelled ^{32}P-PLB that was formed after incubation of cardiac homogenates in the presence of saturating [γ-^{32}P]ATP concentration and an excess of exogenous C subunit of PKA. The results show that the in vitro ^{32}P incorporation into PLB increased from low values at fetal day 15 to maximal values obtained at day 21. There occurred an approx. 4-fold increase in the content of radiolabelled ^{32}P-PLB between fetal day 20 and postnatal day 6. The amount of formed ^{32}P-PLB was only 1.2-fold increased between postnatal days 6 and 21.

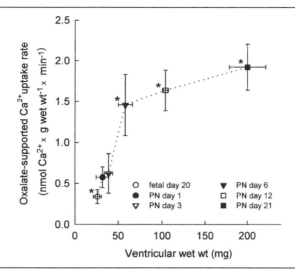

Figure 2. Relationship between ventricular mass and homogenate oxalate-supported sarcoplasmic reticular Ca^{2+} transport during perinatal and postnatal (PN) development. Ventricular weight is the sum of left and right ventricular weight. For Ca^{2+} uptake homogenates (60 μg wet tissue wt) were incubated in 250 μl medium containing (in mM) 40 imidazol (pH 7.0), 100 KCl, 10 $MgCl_2$, 5 Tris-ATP, 6 phosphocreatine, 10 K-oxalate, 10 NaN_3, 0.2 EGTA, and 0.1 $^{45}CaCl_2$ at 37°C. Values are mean ± SD for 5 to 6 hearts in each age group. *$P < 0.05$ vs. day 1.

Relationship between oxalate-supported Ca^{2+} uptake and phospholamban phosphorylation

In order to examine whether the postnatal changes in SR Ca^{2+} pump activity and PLB phosphorylation occur in a coordinated manner, Ca^{2+} uptake rates were plotted against the amount of ^{32}P-PLB formed *in vitro* in the presence of C subunit of PKA. Figure 3 shows the relationship between SR Ca^{2+} uptake rate and PLB phosphorylation from fetal day 15 to day 21 post partum. The results show a linear relationship between SR Ca^{2+} uptake and PLB phosphorylation for the data of 15 and 20 day-old fetal hearts and 1, 3, 6, 12 and 21 day old animals. This linear relationship was observed for the protein kinase-stimulated Ca^{2+} uptake (Fig. 3A) as well as for the respective Ca^{2+} uptake values determined after complete suppression of PKA-catalyzed *in vitro* phosphorylation of PLB in the Ca^{2+} uptake assay using a highly potent peptide inhibitor of PKA (Fig. 3B). Thus, the developmental increase in SR Ca^{2+} uptake is matched by a proportional increase in the fraction of cardiac PLB that can be phosphorylated *in vitro* by PKA. The level of the nonphosphorylated PLB fraction is low at birth and is increasing steadily with further postnatal development.

Thyroid status, Ca^{2+} uptake and in vitro phosphorylation of phospholamban

As TH levels increase in the postnatal life and are essential for maturation of SR Ca^{2+} handling the influence of thyroid status on the postnatal increase of both SR

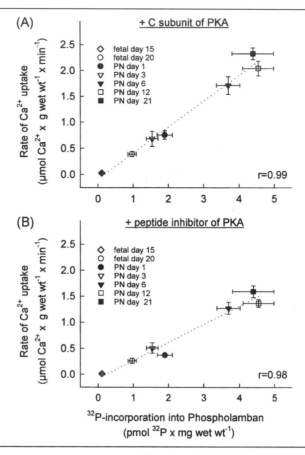

Figure 3. Relationship between the amount of ^{32}P-phospholamban formed *in vitro* and the rate of oxalate-supported Ca^{2+} uptake in ventricular homogenates of fetal and postnatal (PN) rat heart. Ca^{2+} uptake was measured in the presence of either (A) 2 μM exogeneous catalytic (C) subunit of protein kinase A (PKA) or (B) 10 μM synthethic peptide inhibitor of PKA. Values are mean ± SD for 5 to 6 different hearts in each group. For fetal day 15, several hearts were pooled to obtain a sufficient amount of tissue. See also Materials and Methods.

Ca^{2+} pump activity and *in vitro* phosphorylation of PLB were examined. For this purpose, SR oxalate-supported Ca^{2+} uptake and PKA-catalyzed *in vitro* phosphorylation of PLB was analyzed in ventricular homogenates of 21-day old euthyroid, hypothyroid and hyperthyroid animals (Fig. 4). In hypothyroid hearts, the Ca^{2+} uptake rate was 41% of euthyroid controls. A similar decline was observed if SR Ca^{2+} uptake was assayed in the presence of the Ca^{2+} release channel inhibitor ruthenium red (data not shown). In the same homogenates of hypothyroid animals, *in vitro* incorporation of ^{32}P into PLB was elevated by 44% compared to euthyroid controls. These changes in hypothyroidism were reversed by simultaneous treatment

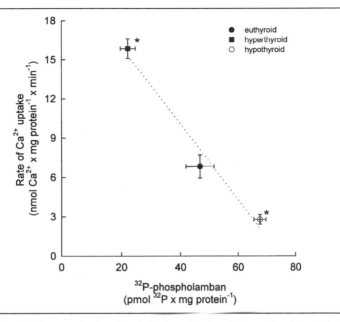

Figure 4. Relationship between *in vitro* phospholamban phosphorylation catalyzed by added catalytic (C) subunit of protein kinase A and rate of oxalate-supported sarcoplasmic reticular Ca^{2+} uptake in ventricular homogenates of 21-day-old rats with different thyroid status. Hyperthyroidism was produced by injection of $10\,\mu g/d/100\,g$ BW of 3,3',5-triiodothyronine (T_3) from day 2 to 21 post partum. Pups were made hypothyroid by giving to nursing mothers drinking water containing 0.05% 6-*n*-propyl-2-thiouracil for the same period. Values are means ± SEM for 6 euthyroid, hyperthyroid and hypothyroid rats in each group. *$P < 0.05$ vs. values of euthyroid animals. For conditions of Ca^{2+} uptake and phosphorylation experiments see Materials and Methods.

with PTU and T_3 (data not shown). As shown in Fig. 4, hyperthyroid rats exhibited opposite changes. An increase in the rate of Ca^{2+} uptake by 132% was accompanied by a decrease (−52% vs. euthyroid control) in the amount of ^{32}P-PLB formed *in vitro* in the presence of C subunit of PKA.

As the values for SR Ca^{2+} uptake in Fig. 4 do not reflect maximum uptake rates, additional measurements were made in membrane preparations over a wide range of free Ca^{2+} ion concentrations to determine V_{max} and EC_{50} values for Ca^{2+} (for details see [12]). Compared to euthyroid controls, the maximum rate value was found to be reduced by 73% in PTU-treated animals. In hyperthyroidism, the V_{max} value was not significantly different from controls. By contrast, the EC_{50} value for Ca^{2+} was significantly increased in postnatal hypothyroidism and decreased in hyperthyroid myocardium. In line with this finding, a 1.6-, 1.9- and 1.1-fold stimulation of SR Ca^{2+} uptake (at $0.21\,\mu M$ free Ca^{2+}) was observed in eu-, hypo- and hyperthyroidism, respectively, after phosphorylation with C subunit of PKA (data not shown).

To examine whether the TH-dependent alterations in SR Ca^{2+} uptake and PLB phosphorylation are accompanied by changes at the level of the two respective pro-

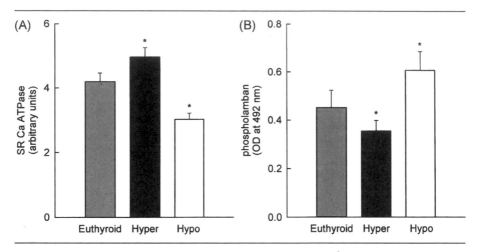

Figure 5. Immunoreactive protein levels of the sarcoplasmic reticular Ca^{2+} ATPase SERCA2 (A) and phospholamban (B) in cardiac homogenates of euthyroid, hyperthyroid (Hyper), and hypothyroid (Hypo) 21-day-old rats. Values are means ± SD for 8 animals in each group. *P < 0.05 vs. euthyroid controls. The amount of tissue protein per lane and well was 5 and 2.5 μg for determination of SERCA2a (Western blot) and phospholamban (ELISA) levels, respectively. For detailed experimental conditions see Materials and Methods.

teins, semi-quantitative Western blot analysis (for SR Ca^{2+} ATPase) and an ELISA for PLB [12] were performed. The immunoreactive band of the cardiac SR Ca^{2+} ATPase was found at 100 kD (data not shown). As shown in Fig. 5, hypothyroidism elevated the protein level of PLB by 35% compared with the euthyroid state, while SR Ca^{2+} ATPase protein level decreased by 21%. Both changes were reversed by T_3 treatment of hypothyroid animals (data not shown). By contrast, hyperthyroidism elevated the protein level of the SR Ca^{2+} ATPase by 18% but decreased PLB level by 28% compared to euthyroid controls (Fig. 5). Taken together the TH-dependent changes in the levels of the two proteins were rather small compared to the above described marked changes in SR Ca^{2+} uptake and *in vitro* PLB phosphorylation. It thus appears that TH-dependent changes in phosphorylation of PLB rather than altered SR Ca^{2+}-ATPase/PLB expression play a major role in the T_3-dependent control of SR Ca^{2+} transport activity in the postnatal development of rat heart with different thyroid states.

DISCUSSION

The aim of the present study was to define late fetal and early postnatal changes of the cardiac SR Ca^{2+} uptake activity and PLB phosphorylation in rats and to investigate whether an altered thyroid status is capable to modulate these parameters in the early postnatal period. During developmental heart growth, both the transcription of genes encoding SR proteins and Ca^{2+} transport catalyzed by the SR Ca^{2+} pump are increased in a characteristic manner. The steady state mRNA levels of the

SR Ca^{2+} pump and SR Ca^{2+} release channel increase steadily [7,8,20,21], whereas PLB mRNA levels appear not to change significantly [21]. Although an altered mRNA level is an important determinant of SR protein synthesis, it is not the sole factor regulating net Ca^{2+} pump activity.

Ca^{2+} uptake and phospholamban phosphorylation during rat heart development

In the present study, the SR Ca^{2+} transport activity was measured as oxalate-supported Ca^{2+} uptake in whole tissue homogenates which excludes the risk of purifying non-representative SR populations and other uncertainties associated with the use of purified membrane preparations [22,23]. For Ca^{2+} uptake experiments, a submicromolar free Ca^{2+} concentration was chosen which reveals the inhibitory influences of nonphosphorylated PLB on the Ca^{2+} pump. Phosphorylation of PLB increases the rate-limiting decomposition rate of the intermediate phosphoenzyme of the Ca^{2+} pump that forms during each Ca^{2+} translocation cycle [17]. Phosphorylation of this protein also increases the Ca^{2+} sensitivity of the Ca^{2+} pump [17]. However, the techniques for determining the effect of PLB phosphorylation on Ca^{2+} transport rate cannot resolve all individual influences. The main problem resides in the fact that the absolute *in vivo* status of PLB phosphorylation at the cAMP- and the calmodulin-dependent sites is difficult to evaluate although an indirect phosphorylation technique (so-called "back phosphorylation") has been successfully applied in previous canine and rat studies [24,25]. To obtain additional information of the influence of thyroid hormones on the postnatal changes in SR Ca^{2+} handling and PLB, the oxalate-supported SR Ca^{2+} uptake, the *in vitro* phosphorylation of PLB catalyzed by C subunit of PKA and the respective immunoreactive protein levels were determined at different thyroid states. We show that the Ca^{2+} uptake activity of the cardiac SR increases steadily between fetal day 15 and postnatal day 21. This gain in Ca^{2+} uptake activity could be observed after maximal phosphorylation of PLB in the presence of C subunit of PKA, after inhibition of endogenous cAMP-dependent protein kinase by a specific inhibitory peptide, and in the presence of the SR Ca^{2+} release channel inhibitor ruthenium red (data not shown). Thus, the developmental increase of net oxalate-supported Ca^{2+} uptake appears not to be due to developmental differences in the ratio of phosphorylated-to-nonphosphorylated PLB or changes in Ca^{2+} flux through SR Ca^{2+} release channels. It is an interesting finding of this work that the developmental changes in SR Ca^{2+} uptake and *in vitro* phosphorylation of PLB by C subunit of PKA were found to be linearly related between fetal day 15 and postnatal day 21. In contrast to matured hearts, sympathetic innervation is poorly developed in the late fetal and early postnatal period [26] and phosphorylation of PLB in the intact heart is expected to be low [24,25]. Under conditions of low *in vivo* phosphorylation, changes in the amount of ^{32}P-PLB formed *in vitro* can be considered as a measure of relative changes of the tissue level of PLB. Therefore, the observed correlation between the increase in homogenate SR Ca^{2+} uptake and the increase in ^{32}P-PLB between fetal day 15 and postnatal day 21 suggests that the late fetal/early postnatal SR Ca^{2+} handling and PLB biosynthesis occur in a coordinated manner. In this context, it should be noted that tissue handling, Ca^{2+} uptake and phosphorylation experiments were performed under conditions which protect phosphoproteins pre-existing *in vivo* from dephosphorylation after removal of the hearts [12,19].

A possible alternative mechanism for developmental increase in SR Ca^{2+} transport activity is an elevated expression of the Ca^{2+} pump gene. In fact, an elevated expression of the slow skeletal/cardiac SR Ca^{2+} ATPase isoform SERCA2a is, at least partially, responsible for the developmental increase in the SR Ca^{2+} transport activity during postnatal heart growth of rodents such as rat and rabbit [7,8,10,20]. This mechanism may also contribute to the observed developmental increase in SR Ca^{2+} pumping. Moreover, other influences arising from possible differences in membrane lipids [13,14] or Ca^{2+} pump modulation by Ca^{2+}/calmodulin-dependent phosphorylation/dephosphorylation processes should not dismissed [18,27,28].

Thyroid status, Ca^{2+} uptake and in vitro phosphorylation of phospholamban

Thyroid hormone levels increase postnatally [29] and the results of the present study demonstrate that abolishing this neonatal thyroid surge in rats prevented the normal postnatal increase in SR Ca^{2+} sequestering activity [20]. The marked depression of the SR Ca^{2+} pump activity observed after administration of PTU is entirely consistent with previous studies in developing [30,31] and adult rat hearts [32,33]. We found that the expression of the cardiac SR Ca^{2+} pump protein was downregulated in hypothyroid 21-day-old animals. Recently, similar results have been reported in hypothyroid rabbits of the same age; however, Ca^{2+}-pump expression remained constant in this model, probably due to insufficient reduction of TH level in the blood [34].

Our finding that the level of immunoreactive PLB was enhanced in hypothyroid hearts is concordant with previous studies in adult rats [35] and postnatal rat heart membranes [12]. By contrast, either no change [36] or a decrease in PLB expression [37] have been observed in hypothyroid rabbits. This suggests species-dependent differences in responsiveness of PLB gene to thyroid hormones. The results of phosphorylation experiments show that *in vitro* ^{32}P incorporation into PLB was significantly increased in hypothyroidism. This elevation was higher than could be expected from the increase in tissue level of PLB. Although we did not determine the absolute basal phosphorylation in the tissue, our data suggest that the *in vivo* phosphorylation of PLB is lower in hypothyroid hearts compared to euthyroid and hyperthyroid ones, that is most probably due to a lower adrenergic responsiveness [38]. Taken together these data indicate that in developing hypothyroid ventricles, the alteration of SR Ca^{2+} transport rates is accomplished in part by decreasing the number of Ca^{2+} pump molecules. In addition, higher PLB expression and most likely reduced *in vivo* phosphorylation of this protein result in a marked increase in levels of nonphosphorylated PLB. As nonphosphorylated PLB suppresses the SR Ca^{2+} pump, a marked decrease in the SR Ca^{2+} uptake rate occurs. Hyperthyroidism was associated with opposite changes in the SR Ca^{2+} uptake activity. Elevated rate of SR Ca^{2+} uptake in ventricular homogenates that was observed after T_3 treatment confirms earlier data obtained with the same model in whole tissue homogenates [30] or isolated membranes [12]. Similar results have been also described in TH-treated adult rat hearts [39] and neonatal rat cardiomyocytes [40]. By contrast, Wibo et al. did not observe an anticipated increase in the thapsigargin-sensitive SR Ca^{2+}-ATPase activity in cardiac homogenates in 21-day-old hyperthyroid rats [41].

In contrast to Ca^{2+} uptake, the level of Ca^{2+} pump protein was only moderately elevated in hyperthyroid hearts as compared to euthyroid controls. This suggests that normal postnatal level of thyroid hormones in the blood which is known to reach peak values during the third postnatal week [29], might be sufficient for maximal stimulation of SR Ca^{2+} pump expression in the rat heart. In line with this view, T_3 administration accelerated the normal postnatal increase in densities of ryanodine receptors and β-adrenoceptors, and the redistribution of L-type Ca^{2+} channels from nonjunctional to junctional domains of the sarcolemma and T-tubules in 7- and 14-day-old rats [41] but not in 21-day-old rats [31]. In contrast to our results, earlier reports have shown that adult hyperthyroid animals exhibited a marked higher expression of cardiac SR Ca^{2+} pump [34,36,37,42] than age-matched euthyroid controls. This may be related to the fact that the level of thyroid hormones in the blood of adult rats is only about half of that in 3-week-old animals [29]. However, other regulatory mechanisms than altered expression of the respective genes seem to be responsible for elevated SR Ca^{2+} uptake in 21-day-old hyperthyroid rats. Our data together with previous reports [12,36,37,40] indicate that the expression of cardiac PLB is significantly depressed in hyperthyroidism. Moreover, *in vitro* ^{32}P incorporation into this protein was also markedly decreased suggesting that the ratio of phosphorylated to nonphosphorylated PLB was increased by T_3 treatment. We assume that the reduction in inhibitory nonphosphorylated PLB due to its decreased expression and enhanced *in vivo* phosphorylation of PLB, rather than enhanced SR Ca^{2+} pump expression, account primarily for elevated SR Ca^{2+} transport activity in postnatal hyperthyroidism. Hypothyroidism prevented the changes particularly due to altered expression of the SR Ca^{2+} pump. In addition, increased levels of PLB and reduced PKA-catalyzed *in vivo* phosphorylation of this protein contribute to suppression of the cardiac SR Ca^{2+} transport activity in this state. By contrast, a moderate decline in expression of PLB and a strong enhancement of *in vivo* phosphorylation of this regulatory protein are most likely the major contributing mechanisms for an elevated SR Ca^{2+} transport activity in postnatal hyperthyroidism rather than an alteration in Ca^{2+} pump level. Thus, thyroid hormones are important candidate hormones determining the postnatal development of myocardial SR Ca^{2+} handling.

ACKNOWLEDGEMENTS

This work was supported by a grant of the FSP "Herz-Kreislauf-Erkrankungen" of the Benjamin Franklin Medical Center. We wish to thank Ursula Jacob-Müller and Norbert Hinz for excellent technical assistance.

REFERENCES

1. Clubb FJ, Jr, Bell PD, Kriseman JD, Bishop SP. 1987. Myocardial cell growth and blood pressure development in neonatal spontaneously hypertensive rats. Lab Invest 56:189–197.
2. Morgan HE, Gordon EE, Kira Y, Chua HL, Russo LA, Peterson CJ, McDermott PJ, Watson PA. 1987. Biochemical mechanisms of cardiac hypertrophy. Annu Rev Physiol 49:533–543.
3. Fozzard H. 1977. Heart: Excitation-contraction coupling. Annu Rev Physiol 41:201–220.
4. Maylie JG. 1982. Excitation-contraction coupling in neonatal and adult myocardium of cat. Am J Physiol 242:H834–H843.
5. Nakanishi T, Seguchi M, Takao A. 1988. Development of the myocardial contractile system. Experientia 44:936–944.
6. Chemla D, Lecarpentier Y, Martin JL, Clergue M, Antonetti A, Hatt PY. 1986. Relationship between inotropy and relaxation in rat myocardium. Am J Physiol 250:H1008–1016.
7. Komuro I, Kurabayashi M, Shibazaki Y, Takaku F, Yazaki Y. 1989. Molecular cloning and characterization of a Ca^{2+} + Mg^{2+}-dependent adenosine triphosphatase from rat cardiac sarcoplasmic reticulum. Regulation of its expression by pressure overload and developmental stage. J Clin Invest 83: 1102–1108.
8. Lompre AM, Lambert F, Lakatta EG, Schwartz K. 1991. Expression of sarcoplasmic reticulum Ca^{2+}-ATPase and calsequestrin genes in rat heart during ontogenic development and aging. Circ Res 69:1380–1388.
9. Nayler WG, Fassold E. 1977. Calcium accumulating and ATPase activity of cardiac sarcoplasmic reticulum before and after birth. Cardiovasc Res 11:231–237.
10. Vetter R, Kemsies C, Schulze W. 1987. Sarcolemmal Na^+-Ca^{2+} exchange and sarcoplasmic reticulum Ca^{2+} uptake in several cardiac preparations. Biomed Biochim Acta 46:S375–S381.
11. Fisher DJ, Tate CA, Phillips S. 1992. Developmental regulation of the sarcoplasmic reticulum calcium pump in the rabbit heart. Pediatr Res 31:474–479.
12. Cernohorský J, Kolář F, Pelouch V, Korecky B, Vetter R. 1998. Thyroid control of sarcolemmal Na^+/Ca^{2+} exchanger and SR Ca^{2+}-ATPase in developing rat heart. Am J Physiol 275:H264–H273.
13. Katz AM, Nash-Adler P, Watras J, Messineo FC, Takenaka H, Louis CF. 1982. Fatty acid effects on calcium influx and efflux in sarcoplasmic reticulum vesicles from rabbit skeletal muscle. Biochim Biophys Acta 687:17–26.
14. Martonosi A, Donley J, Halpin RA. 1968. Sarcoplasmic reticulum. 3. The role of phospholipids in the adenosine triphosphatase activity and Ca^{++} transport. J Biol Chem 243:61–70.
15. Colyer J. 1993. Control of the calcium pump of cardiac sarcoplasmic reticulum. A specific role for the pentameric structure of phospholamban? Cardiovasc Res 27:1766–1771.
16. Wegener AD, Simmerman HK, Lindemann JP, Jones LR. 1989. Phospholamban phosphorylation in intact ventricles. Phosphorylation of serine 16 and threonine 17 in response to beta-adrenergic stimulation. J Biol Chem 264:11468–11474.
17. Tada M, Katz AM. 1982. Phosphorylation of the sarcoplasmic reticulum and sarcolemma. Annu Rev Physiol 44:401–423.
18. Lindemann JP, Watanabe AM. 1985. Phosphorylation of phospholamban in intact myocardium. Role of Ca^{2+}-calmodulin-dependent mechanisms. J Biol Chem 260:4516–4525.
19. Freestone N, Singh J, Krause E-G, Vetter R. 1996. Early postnatal changes in sarcoplasmic reticulum calcium transport function in spontaneously hypertensive rats. Mol Cell Biochem 163/164:57–66.
20. Vetter R, Studer R, Reinecke H, Kolář F, Ostadalova I, Drexler H. 1995. Reciprocal changes in the postnatal expression of the sarcolemmal Na^+-Ca^{2+}-exchanger and SERCA2 in rat heart. J Mol Cell Cardiol 27:1689–1701.
21. Arai M, Otsu K, MacLennan DH, Periasamy M. 1992. Regulation of sarcoplasmic reticulum gene expression during cardiac and skeletal muscle development. Am J Physiol 262:C614–C620.
22. Feher JJ, Briggs FN, Hess ML. 1980. Characterization of cardiac sarcoplasmic reticulum from ischemic myocardium: comparison of isolated sarcoplasmic reticulum with unfractionated homogenates. J Mol Cell Cardiol 12:427–432.
23. Solaro RJ, Briggs FN. 1974. Estimating the functional capabilities of sarcoplasmic reticulum in cardiac muscle. Calcium binding. Circ Res 34:531–540.
24. Karczewski P, Vetter R, Holtzhauer M, Krause EG. 1986. Indirect technique for the estimation of cAMP-dependent and Ca^{2+}/calmodulin-dependent phospholamban phosphorylation state in canine heart in vivo. Biomed Biochim Acta 45:S227–S231.
25. Karczewski P, Bartel S, Krause EG. 1990. Differential sensitivity to isoprenaline of troponin I and phospholamban phosphorylation in isolated rat hearts. Biochem J 266:115–122.

26. Kirby ML. 1988. Role of extracardiac factors in heart development. Experientia 44:944–951.
27. Napolitano R, Vittone L, Mundina C, Chiappe de Cingolani G, Mattiazzi A. 1992. Phosphorylation of phospholamban in the intact heart. A study on the physiological role of the Ca^{2+}-calmodulin-dependent protein kinase system. J Mol Cell Cardiol 24:387–396.
28. Hawkins C, Xu A, Narayanan N. 1994. Sarcoplasmic reticulum calcium pump in cardiac and slow twitch skeletal muscle but not fast twitch skeletal muscle undergoes phosphorylation by endogenous and exogenous Ca^{2+}/calmodulin-dependent protein kinase. Characterization of optimal conditions for calcium pump phosphorylation. J Biol Chem 269:31198–31206.
29. Vigouroux E. 1976. Dynamic study of postnatal thyroid function in the rat. Acta Endocrinol (Copenh) 83:752–762.
30. Kolář F, Seppet EK, Vetter R, Procházka J, Grünermel J, Zilmer K, Oštádal B. 1992. Thyroid control of contractile function and calcium handling in neonatal rat heart. Pflugers Arch 21:26–31.
31. Wibo M, Kolář F, Zheng L, Godfraind T. 1995. Influence of thyroid status on postnatal maturation of calcium channels, β-adrenoreceptors and cation transport ATPases in rat ventricular tissue. J Mol Cell Cardiol 27:1731–1743.
32. Beekman RE, van Hardeveld C, Simonides WS. 1989. On the mechanism of the reduction by thyroid hormone of β-adrenergic relaxation rate stimulation in rat heart. Biochem J 259:229–236.
33. Black SC, McNeill JH, Katz S. 1993. Cardiac sarcoplasmic reticulum calcium transport activity of thyroidectomized rats: the role of endogenous myocardial acylcarnitines and calcium pump protein. Pharmacology 46:130–141.
34. Boerth SR, Artman M. 1996. Thyroid hormone regulates Na^+-Ca^{2+} exchanger expression during postnatal maturation and in adult rabbit ventricular myocardium. Cardiovasc Res 31:E145–E152.
35. Kiss E, Jakab G, Kranias EG, Edes I. 1994. Thyroid hormone-induced alterations in phospholamban protein expression. Circ Res 75:245–251.
36. Nagai R, Zarain-Herzberg A, Brandl CJ, Fujii J, Tada M, MacLennan DH, Alpert NR, Periasamy M. 1989. Regulation of myocardial Ca^{2+}-ATPase and phospholamban mRNA expression in response to pressure overload and thyroid hormone. Proc Natl Acad Sci USA 86:2966–2970.
37. Arai M, Otsu K, MacLennan DH, Alpert NR, Periasamy M. 1991. Effect of thyroid hormone on the expression of messenger RNA encoding sarcoplasmic reticulum proteins. Circ Res 69:266–276.
38. Williams LT, Lefkowitz RJ, Watanabe AM, Hathaway DR, Besch HR. 1977. Thyroid hormone regulation of β adrenergic receptor number. J Biol Chem 252:2787–2789.
39. Limas CJ. 1978. Enhanced phosphorylation of myocardial sarcoplasmic reticulum in experimental hyperthyroidism. Am J Physiol 234:H426–H431.
40. Kimura Y, Otsu K, Nishida K, Kuzuya T, Tada M. 1994. Thyroid hormone enhances Ca^{2+} pumping activity of the cardiac sarcoplasmic reticulum by increasing Ca^{2+}-ATPase and decreasing phospholamban expression. J Mol Cell Cardiol 26:1145–1154.
41. Wibo M, Feron O, Zheng L, Maleki M, Kolář F, Godfraind T. 1998. Thyroid status and postnatal changes in subsarcolemmal distribution and isoform expression of rat cardiac dihydropyridine receptors. Cardiovasc Res 37:151–159.
42. Rohrer D, Dillmann WH. 1988. Thyroid hormone markedly increases the mRNA coding for sarcoplasmic reticulum Ca^{2+}-ATPase in the rat heart. J Biol Chem 63:6941–6944.

B. Ostadal, M. Nagano and N.S. Dhalla (eds.).
CARDIAC DEVELOPMENT. Copyright © 2002.
Kluwer Academic Publishers. Boston.
All rights reserved.

SARCOPLASMIC RETICULUM FUNCTION IN THE DEVELOPING HEART

RANA M. TEMSAH, THOMAS NETTICADAN,
and NARANJAN S. DHALLA

Institute of Cardiovascular Sciences, St. Boniface General Hospital Research Centre and
Department of Physiology, Faculty of Medicine, University of Manitoba, Winnipeg, Canada

Summary. In view of the critical role of sarcoplasmic reticulum (SR) in regulating Ca^{2+}-movements and thereby modulating cardiac contractility in the adult hearts, several studies have been carried out to understand its contribution in cardiac contraction and relaxation processes at early stages of myocardial development. The contractile characteristics of the neonatal heart are weak in comparison to the adult heart. Sparse sympathetic innervation and an immature SR were suggested to be factors contributing to reduced contractility of the neonatal heart. SR Ca^{2+}-uptake and release activities as well as expression of the SR Ca^{2+}-cycling proteins have been reported to increase after birth. The presence of protein kinases and phosphatases in early stages of development indicate a role for the regulatory mechanisms in maintaining SR Ca^{2+}-transport. However, increased expression of phosphatases in the early stages suggest enhanced dephosphorylation of SR proteins. There is a lack of effects of Ca^{2+}-channel inhibitors on neonatal hearts and increased Na^{+}-Ca^{2+}-exchanger function in the fetal and neonatal in comparison to the adult heart. Thus, in view of the reduced SR function at early stages of development, the SR does not appear to play a major role in the regulation of cardiac contractility during the fetal and neonatal stages.

Key words: Sarcoplasmic reticulum, Cardiac development, Fetal heart, Neonatal heart

Address correspondence to: Dr. Naranjan S. Dhalla, Institute of Cardiovascular Sciences, St. Boniface General Hospital Research Centre, 351 Taché Avenue, Winnipeg, Manitoba R2H 2A6, Canada. Tel: (204) 235-3417; Fax: (204) 233-6723; e-mail: cvso@sbrc.ca

INTRODUCTION

It is now well established that calcium is an essential cation for the maintenance of cellular integrity, regulation of metabolism, cell growth and cell proliferation [1]. This cation also plays an important role in regulating cardiomyocyte function on a beat-to-beat basis. A large gradient of Ca^{2+} (about 10,000 fold) across the cardiomyocyte membrane is maintained by coordinated functioning of different cellular organelles such as sarcolemma (SL) and sarcoplasmic reticulum (SR). The concentration of ionized Ca^{2+} in the extracellular space is about 1.25 mM whereas the intracellular Ca^{2+} concentration ranges between 10^{-7} M and 10^{-5} M during diastole and systole, respectively. In view of the critical role of SR in the regulation of intracellular Ca^{2+} in cardiomyocytes and the progressive increase in the ability of myocardium to generate contractile force during development, this article is focused on the ontogenic development of cardiac SR function.

PHYSIOLOGICAL AND BIOCHEMICAL ASPECTS OF SR SYSTEM

In adult cardiomyocytes, both SL and SR are considered to be the major organelles involved in the regulation of intracellular Ca^{2+} concentration ($[Ca^{2+}]_i$) on a beat-to-beat basis [2] (Fig. 1A). Depolarization of the SL membrane permits entry of a relatively small amount of Ca^{2+} from the extracellular space (primary source of Ca^{2+}) via L-type Ca^{2+}-channels [3]. This small amount of $[Ca^{2+}]_i$ triggers the release of a large amount of Ca^{2+} from the SR store through Ca^{2+}-release channels; a phenomenon known as Ca^{2+}-induced-Ca^{2+}-release [3,4]. The Ca^{2+} released from the SR activates the contractile filaments resulting in cardiac contraction. For the occurrence of cardiac relaxation, the level of $[Ca^{2+}]_i$ is restored to the resting level by the reuptake of Ca^{2+} by the SR Ca^{2+}-pump ATPase [5,6], and extrusion of Ca^{2+} out of the cell by the Na^+-Ca^{2+}-exchanger [7,8] as well as the SL Ca^{2+}-pump ATPase. At this point, it is important to mention that the contribution of these systems is species dependent. Bers et al [7,9] have shown that SR Ca^{2+}-pump ATPase is responsible for 92% of Ca^{2+} uptake while 7% of Ca^{2+} is removed by the Na^+-Ca^{2+}-exchanger in rat ventricular myocardium. On the other hand, the SR Ca^{2+}-pump ATPase removes 70–75% of Ca^{2+} whereas 25–30% is removed by Na^+-Ca^{2+}-exchanger in human, rabbit, cat, ferret and guinea pig hearts. The SL Ca^{2+}-pump ATPase has been considered to be of minor importance in the regulation of intracellular Ca^{2+}. Although nuclei and mitochondria are also known to accumulate a large amount of Ca^{2+}, they do not play a role in regulating the intracellular Ca^{2+} on a beat-to-beat basis.

Ultrastructural studies of ventricular myocardial cells have revealed that the SR is composed of at least three distinct structures [10]: a) network SR which represents the major region of the SR surrounding the myofibrils [11], b) peripheral SR and interior-junctional SR represent regions closely apposed to the SL and T-tubules, respectively; these are composed of cisternae and longitudinal regions where the former is connected by junctional processes called "feet" [11,12], and c) corbular SR that is confined to the I-band of the sarcomere. Both the junctional SR and

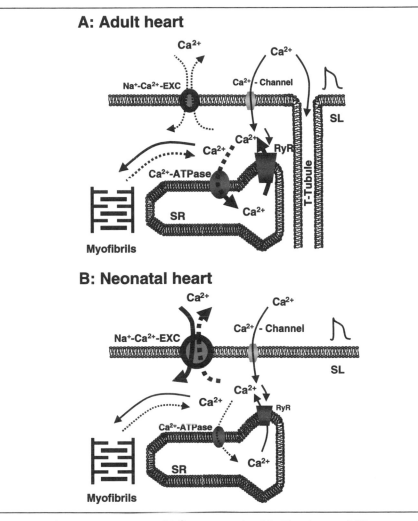

Figure 1. Schematic representation of Ca^{2+}-movement in adult (A) and neonatal (B) myocytes. SL, sarcolemma; SR, sarcoplasmic reticulum; T-tubule, transverse tubule; Na^+-Ca^{2+}-EXC, Na^+-Ca^{2+}-exchanger; Ca^{2+}-ATPase, Ca^{2+}-pump ATPase; RyR, ryanodine receptor. The thickness of the arrows indicates the relative contribution of the Ca^{2+}-handling mechanisms in regulating Ca^{2+}-movements.

corbular SR are extensions of the network SR. The SR membranes are composed of several proteins that are of functional significance among which are; Ca^{2+}-release channels or ryanodine receptors (RyR), SR Ca^{2+}-pump ATPase (SERCA), phospholamban (PLB) and calsequestrin (CQS).

Cardiac contraction is triggered by the release of Ca^{2+} from the SR during the open state of Ca^{2+}-release channels or RyR. The channel acquired this nomenclature from its capability to bind to ryanodine which is a highly toxic plant alkaloid and induces different effects depending on the concentrations applied [13]. Nanomolar concentrations are known to keep the channel in an open state, whereas concentrations higher than $10\,\mu M$ can completely close the channel. In cardiomyocytes, two different Ca^{2+}-release channels have been identified: RyR which is most abundant and relevant to excitation-contraction coupling; and the inositol 3, 4, 5-triphosphate receptor which is of low density in the SR [14]. Using molecular cloning analysis, RyR was detected in three different isoforms (RyR1, RyR2 and RyR3) encoded by three different genes. RyR2 is the only isoform expressed in cardiac tissue [15–17] and is considered the largest protein identified in the SR (565 kDa) [17]. It consists of over 5,000 amino acids [18,19] and is composed of four monomers that form a tetrameric structure. RyR forms a functional complex due to its association with several other proteins: CQS, junctin, triadin and FK506 binding protein (FKBP) [20]. Stoke and Wagenknecht [21] have suggested that the unusual high molecular mass of RyR may be due to numerous endogenous modulatory ligands including calmodulin and FKBP [14]. RyR is also known to be phosphorylated by Ca^{2+}/calmodulin dependent protein kinase (CaMK) and by cAMP-dependent protein kinase (PKA) [17,22,23] resulting in enhanced Ca^{2+}-release. Anatomically, the proximity between the L-type Ca^{2+}-channels on the T-tubules and RyR at the cisternae of the SR allows what is known by Ca^{2+}-induced-Ca^{2+}-release phenomenon [3].

SERCA is encoded by three highly homologous genes: SERCA1, SERCA2, and SERCA3 [24]. SERCA1a and 1b isoforms are expressed in adult and neonatal fast-twitch skeletal muscles, respectively [25]. SERCA2a is the cardiac and slow-twitch skeletal isoform [26], whereas SERCA2b is expressed in smooth muscle and non-muscle tissues [27]. SERCA3 is a non-muscle isoform and it is mainly expressed in epithelial and endothelial cells [28]. It is now well established that SERCA2a is the only isoform expressed in normal or diseased myocardium [29–31]. SERCA2a protein (105 kDa) exhibits Ca^{2+}-stimulated and Mg^{2+}-dependent ATPase activity and thus serves as a Ca^{2+}-pump [32,33]. It is localized mainly in the longitudinal portion of the SR [34] and constitutes 35–40% of the SR proteins [35,36]. By the hydrolysis of one molecule of ATP, the Ca^{2+}-pump transports two Ca^{2+}-ions against a high ionic gradient ranging between $100\,nM - 10\,\mu M$ in the cytosol and $1\,mM$ in the SR [9]. SERCA2a activity determines the amount of Ca^{2+} sequestered in the SR as well as the amount of Ca^{2+} available for release in the next wave of excitation and is responsible for the restoration of Ca^{2+} gradient between intracellular and SR lumen side. This protein is therefore essential for the determination of the rate and extent of relaxation and the rate and amplitude of contraction. SERCA2a is also known to undergo direct phosphorylation by CaMK at Ser-38 [37] resulting in enhanced Ca^{2+}-uptake in the SR.

PLB is a regulatory phosphoprotein in the SR membrane that is remarkably conserved since it is encoded by one gene in all species and is expressed in the cardiac and slow skeletal muscle [38]. Cardiac PLB exists in two forms, the pentameric form and the monomeric form [39–41]. The pentameric form (27 kDa) is composed of 5 identical subunits which upon boiling in sodium dodecyl sulphate buffer dissociates into identical monomers (6 kDa) having 52 amino acids [42–44]. Since the pentameric and monomeric forms of PLB are under dynamic equilibrium, it has been suggested that the pentameric form may be an inactive reservoir for the active monomeric form [45]. Immunohistochemical studies have shown that PLB is localized in the SR with the highest distribution in the longitudinal region of the SR and co-localized with SERCA2a. This anatomical proximity indicates the functional correlation between both proteins. PLB has been identified as the principal substrate phosphorylated by PKA at Ser-16, CaMK at Thr-17, protein kinase C at Ser-10 and by cGMP-dependent protein kinase [23,43,46–48]. PLB phosphorylation *in vivo* has been postulated to play a key role in mediating a lusitropic effect (cardiac relaxation) and the inotropic effect (rate of contraction) of the β-adrenergic system [46].

CQS is a high-capacity moderate affinity Ca^{2+}-binding protein which stores Ca^{2+} in the SR lumen [49–51]. Among the two isoforms of CQS only one isoform is expressed in the developing, adult and aging cardiac tissue [52–54]. CQS (55 kDa) is composed of 396 amino acid residues and is anchored to the cisternae part of the SR in close proximity with RyR [55]. CQS, RyR and other SR proteins (FKBP, junctin and triadin) are hypothesized to form a functional complex for the coordination of Ca^{2+}-release [20]. Although, CQS is known to be a preferred substrate for phosphorylation by casein kinase II at Ser-378 both *in vivo* and *in vitro* [56], the functional consequence of this phosphorylation is not yet understood.

SARCOPLASMIC RETICULUM IN THE DEVELOPING HEART

There is a growing body of evidence in literature suggesting structural and functional differences between the fetal, neonatal and adult SR. These studies started three decades ago and were triggered by the differences observed in cardiac performance by some investigators [57,58]. Fetal and neonatal cardiac muscles developed less peak tension and its velocity of shortening was reduced when compared to the adult cardiac muscle. These differences were accounted for by the relatively less sympathetic innervation of the fetal and neonatal muscle resulting in lower levels of endogenous catecholamines [57,59]. Further studies in this area revealed another possible explanation i.e. the developmental changes in the SR structure and consequently its function. The content of the SR was reported to be less in the 1-day old neonatal heart in comparison to that in the adult cat [60]. The evidence for SR maturation immediately after birth was supported by several observations detailed below.

First, the phenomenon of Ca^{2+}-induced-Ca^{2+}-release was shown to occur in neonatal rat heart after birth [61] and progressed subsequently with development [62]. A major reason for the absence of Ca^{2+}-induced-Ca^{2+}-release before birth could be the absence of T-tubules in the fetal stage; T-tubules have been reported to develop in cardiomyocytes after 8–10 days of birth [63]. Second, Ryanodine binding and the expression of RyR protein have been reported to be low in fetal and neonatal heart in comparison to adult hearts [64,65]. In fact, the RyR protein content has been reported to increase with age [66] and these observations are consistent with lower SR Ca^{2+}-release activity in the neonatal hearts. Using electron microscopy RyR protein has been detected as early as day 4 of fetal life [67]. Reduced Ca^{2+}-ATPase activity and SR Ca^{2+}-uptake have also been reported in the fetal and neonatal hearts in comparison to adult hearts [68–71]. Some studies [66,69,70,72] have shown that fetal and neonatal hearts expressed lower levels of SERCA2a protein and PLB in comparison to adult hearts. The immunofluoresence labeling technique made it possible to identify the presence of SERCA2a at an early stage of the development of chick myocardium (9–10 days fetal) [73]. It appeared in the single tubular heart concurrent with the time the first heart beat occurred [73]. Interestingly, later studies using in situ hybridization technique confirmed that SERCA2a is expressed at a significantly low level in the myocardium at day 9 fetal, while PLB appeared at 12 days fetal [74]. These observations suggest that the SR function increases with development (Fig. 1A and 1B). In comparison to adult hearts both higher and lower levels of CQS protein have been reported in fetal hearts [69,70]. CQS mRNA is expressed at a high level (50% of the maximum) in all age groups although it peaked at day 4 of neonatal life [75]. Third, Pegg and Michalak [70] reported that PLB in the fetal SR membranes was phosphorylated by PKA but not by endogenous CaMK. On the other hand Narayanan et al. [66] have reported that RyR, SERCA2a and PLB were phosphorylated by the endogenous CaMK as early as day 21 of fetal life. The rabbit myocardium expressed CaMK (δ-isoform) at day 21 of fetal life and reached its maximal level just before birth and then declined to lower levels immediately after birth. The levels of the endogenous CaMK in adults was the same as that after birth but significantly lower than that prior to birth. The protein contents of protein phosphatase types 1 and 2A in adult ventricular preparations were lower in comparison to neonatal preparations. These results were consistent with reduced PLB phosphorylation in adult ventricular preparations in comparison to neonatal [71]. Furthermore, these observations suggest that enhanced dephosphorylation may be a contributory factor for reduced SR function of the neonatal hearts.

Finally, Na^+-dependent Ca^{2+}-uptake was reported to be significantly higher in the fetal and neonatal hearts when compared to adult hearts [76]. Increased Na^+-Ca^{2+}-exchange function was consistent with the markedly higher content of the exchanger protein in fetal and neonatal hearts [76]. These observations suggested an abundant and highly developed exchanger and an important role for the exchanger in relaxation of the fetal and neonatal hearts. On the other hand, the maximal contraction amplitude of adult myocytes was almost completely suppressed but the contraction in neonatal myocytes was unaffected upon blocking the L-type Ca^{2+}-current [77]. Furthermore, voltage gated Ca^{2+}-current amplitude has been reported to increase with maturation [78]. These results suggest that the Ca^{2+} required for contraction in neonatal myocytes may be via Ca^{2+} influx by reverse Na^+-Ca^{2+} exchange (Fig. 1A and 1B). All the above observations point out to a dominant role for the Na^+-Ca^{2+}-exchanger in the immature heart that appeared to decline with the maturation of the SR during the course of development.

In conclusion the SR appears to be immature in the fetal and newborn hearts and therefore plays a less prominent role in cardiac contractility in the early stages of development. On the other hand the Na^+-Ca^{2+}-exchanger plays a dominant role during the early stages. A reversal of the roles of the Na^+-Ca^{2+}-exchanger and SR takes place with age. A decline in the dominance of the exchanger occurs with subsequent maturation of the SR with age.

ACKNOWLEDGEMENTS

The work reported in this study was supported by a grant from the Canadian Institutes of Health Research (CIHR Group in Experimental Cardiology). NSD holds the CIHR/Pharmaceutical Research and Development Chair in Cardiovascular Research supported by Merck Frosst Canada. RMT is a pre-doctoral fellow of the Heart and Stroke Foundation of Canada.

REFERENCES

1. Dhalla NS, Pierce GN, Panagia V, Singal PK, Beamish RE. 1982. Calcium movements in relation to heart function. Basic Res Cardiol 77:117–139.
2. Dhalla NS, Temsah RM. 2001. Sarcoplasmic reticulum and cardiac oxidative stress: an emerging target for heart disease. Emerging Therapeutic Targets 5:205–217.
3. Fabiato A. 1983. Calcium-induced release of calcium from the cardiac sarcoplasmic reticulum. Am J Physiol 245:C1–14.
4. Wier WG. 1990. Cytoplasmic [Ca^{2+}] in mammalian ventricle: dynamic control by cellular processes. Annu Rev Physiol 52:467–485.
5. Lewartowski B, Wolska B. 1993. The effect of thapsigargin on sarcoplasmic reticulum Ca^{2+} content and contractions of single myocytes of rat ventricular myocardium. J Physiol Pharmacol 44:243–250.
6. Lipp P, Pott L, Callewaert G, Carmeliet E. 1992. Calcium transients caused by calcium entry are influenced by the sarcoplasmic reticulum in guinea-pig atrial myocytes. J Physiol (Lond) 454:321–338.
7. Bassani JW, Bassani RA, Bers DM. 1994. Relaxation in rabbit and rat cardiac cells: species-dependent differences in cellular mechanisms. J Physiol (Lond) 476:279–293.
8. Negretti N, O'Neill SC, Eisner DA. 1993. The relative contributions of different intracellular and sarcolemmal systems to relaxation in rat ventricular myocytes. Cardiovasc Res 27:1826–1830.
9. Bers, DM. Ca transport during contraction and relaxation in mammalian ventricular muscle. In Hasenfuss G and Just H, eds. Alterations of excitation-contraction coupling in the failing human heart. New York, Springer-Verlag. 1998, 1–16.
10. Jewett PH, Leonard SD, Sommer JR. 1973. Chicken cardiac muscle: its elusive extended junctional sarcoplasmic reticulum and sarcoplasmic reticulum fenestrations. J Cell Biol 56:595–600.
11. Forbes MS, Sperelakis N. 1983. The membrane systems and cytoskeletal elements of mammalian myocardial cells. Cell Muscle Motil 3:89–155.
12. Sommer JR, Waugh RA. 1976. The ultrastructure of the mammalian cardiac muscle cell-with special emphasis on the tubular membrane systems. A review. Am J Pathol 82:192–232.
13. Rousseau E, Smith JS, Meissner G. 1987. Ryanodine modifies conductance and gating behavior of single Ca^{2+} release channel. Am J Physiol 253:C364–C368.
14. Marks AR. 1997. Intracellular calcium-release channels: regulators of cell life and death. Am J Physiol 272:H597–H605.
15. Marks AR, Tempst P, Hwang KS, Taubman MB, Inui M, Chadwick C, Fleischer S, Nadal-Ginard B. 1989. Molecular cloning and characterization of the ryanodine receptor/junctional channel complex cDNA from skeletal muscle sarcoplasmic reticulum. Proc Natl Acad Sci USA 86:8683–8687.
16. Otsu K, Willard HF, Khanna VK, Zorzato F, Green NM, MacLennan DH. 1990. Molecular cloning of cDNA encoding the Ca^{2+} release channel (ryanodine receptor) of rabbit cardiac muscle sarcoplasmic reticulum. J Biol Chem 265:13472–13483.

17. Takeshima H, Yamazawa T, Ikemoto T, Takekura H, Nishi M, Noda T, Iino M. 1995. Ca²⁺-induced Ca²⁺ release in myocytes from dyspedic mice lacking the type-1 ryanodine receptor. EMBO J 14: 2999–3006.

18. Inui M, Saito A, Fleischer S. 1987. Isolation of the ryanodine receptor from cardiac sarcoplasmic reticulum and identity with the feet structures. J Biol Chem 262:15637–15642.

19. Takeshima H, Nishimura S, Matsumoto T, Ishida H, Kangawa K, Minamino N, Matsuo H, Ueda M, Hanaoka M, Hirose T. 1989. Primary structure and expression from complementary DNA of skeletal muscle ryanodine receptor. Nature 339:439–445.

20. Zhang L, Kelley J, Schmeisser G, Kobayashi YM, Jones LR. 1997. Complex formation between junctin, triadin, calsequestrin, and the ryanodine receptor. Proteins of the cardiac junctional sarcoplasmic reticulum membrane. J Biol Chem 272:23389–23397.

21. Stokes DL, Wagenknecht T. 2000. Calcium transport across the sarcoplasmic reticulum: structure and function of Ca²⁺-ATPase and the ryanodine receptor. Eur J Biochem 267:5274–5279.

22. Witcher DR, Kovacs RJ, Schulman H, Cefali DC, Jones LR. 1991. Unique phosphorylation site on the cardiac ryanodine receptor regulates calcium channel activity. J Biol Chem 266:11144–11152.

23. Takasago T, Imagawa T, Furukawa K, Ogurusu T, Shigekawa M. 1991. Regulation of the cardiac ryanodine receptor by protein kinase-dependent phosphorylation. J Biochem (Tokyo) 109:163–170.

24. Arai M, Matsui H, Periasamy M. 1994. Sarcoplasmic reticulum gene expression in cardiac hypertrophy and heart failure. Circ Res 74:555–564.

25. Brandl CJ, Green NM, Korczak B, MacLennan DH. 1986. Two Ca²⁺ ATPase genes: homologies and mechanistic implications of deduced amino acid sequences. Cell 44:597–607.

26. Zarain-Herzberg A, MacLennan DH, Periasamy M. 1990. Characterization of rabbit cardiac sarco(endo)plasmic reticulum Ca²⁺-ATPase gene. J Biol Chem 265:4670–4677.

27. Lytton J, Zarain-Herzberg A, Periasamy M, MacLennan DH. 1989. Molecular cloning of the mammalian smooth muscle sarco(endo)plasmic reticulum Ca²⁺-ATPase. J Biol Chem 264:7059–7065.

28. Anger M, Samuel JL, Marotte F, Wuytack F, Rappaport L, Lompre AM. 1994. In situ mRNA distribution of sarco(endo)plasmic reticulum Ca²⁺-ATPase isoforms during ontogeny in the rat. J Mol Cell Cardiol 26:539–550.

29. Lompre AM, Anger M, Levitsky D. 1994. Sarco(endo)plasmic reticulum calcium pumps in the cardiovascular system: function and gene expression. J Mol Cell Cardiol 26:1109–1121.

30. Nagai R, Zarain-Herzberg A, Brandl CJ, Fujii J, Tada M, MacLennan DH, Alpert NR, Periasamy M. 1989. Regulation of myocardial Ca²⁺-ATPase and phospholamban mRNA expression in response to pressure overload and thyroid hormone. Proc Natl Acad Sci USA 86:2966–2970.

31. de la BD, Levitsky D, Rappaport L, Mercadier JJ, Marotte F, Wisnewsky C, Brovkovich V, Schwartz K, Lompre AM. 1990. Function of the sarcoplasmic reticulum and expression of its Ca²⁺-ATPase gene in pressure overload-induced cardiac hypertrophy in the rat. Circ Res 66:554–564.

32. Komuro I, Kurabayashi M, Shibazaki Y, Takaku F, Yazaki Y. 1989. Molecular cloning and characterization of a Ca²⁺ + Mg²⁺-dependent adenosine triphosphatase from rat cardiac sarcoplasmic reticulum. Regulation of its expression by pressure overload and developmental stage. J Clin Invest 83:1102–1108.

33. Brandl CJ, deLeon S, Martin DR, MacLennan DH. 1987. Adult forms of the Ca²⁺-ATPase of sarcoplasmic reticulum. Expression in developing skeletal muscle. J Biol Chem 262:3768–3774.

34. Jorgensen AO, Shen AC, MacLennan DH, Tokuyasu KT. 1982. Ultrastructural localization of the Ca²⁺ + Mg²⁺-dependent ATPase of sarcoplasmic reticulum in rat skeletal muscle by immunoferritin labeling of ultrathin frozen sections. J Cell Biol 92:409–416.

35. Fabiato A, Fabiato F. 1979. Calcium and cardiac excitation-contraction coupling. Annu Rev Physiol 41:473–484.

36. Tada M, Yamamoto T, Tonomura Y. 1978. Molecular mechanism of active calcium transport by sarcoplasmic reticulum. Physiol Rev 58:1–79.

37. Toyofuku T, Curotto Kurzydlowski K, Narayanan N, MacLennan DH. 1994. Identification of Ser38 as the site in cardiac sarcoplasmic reticulum Ca²⁺-ATPase that is phosphorylated by Ca²⁺/calmodulin-dependent protein kinase. J Biol Chem 269:26492–26496.

38. Simmerman HK, Jones LR. 1998. Phospholamban: protein structure, mechanism of action, and role in cardiac function. Physiol Rev 78:921–947.

39. Bidlack JM, Shamoo AE. 1980. Adenosine 3′,5′-monophosphate-dependent phosphorylation of a 6000 and a 22,000 dalton protein from cardiac sarcoplasmic reticulum. Biochim Biophys Acta 632:310–325.

40. Jones LR, Besch HR, Jr., Fleming JW, McConnaughey MM, Watanabe AM. 1979. Separation of vesicles of cardiac sarcolemma from vesicles of cardiac sarcoplasmic reticulum. Comparative biochemical analysis of component activities. J Biol Chem 254:530–539.
41. Will H, Levchenko TS, Levitsky DO, Smirnov VN, Wollenberger A. 1978. Partial characterization of protein kinase-catalyzed phosphorylation of low molecular weight proteins in purified preparations of pigeon heart sarcolemma and sarcoplasmic reticulum. Biochim Biophys Acta 543:175–193.
42. Wegener AD, Jones LR. 1984. Phosphorylation-induced mobility shift in phospholamban in sodium dodecyl sulfate-polyacrylamide gels. Evidence for a protein structure consisting of multiple identical phosphorylatable subunits. J Biol Chem 259:1834–1841.
43. Wegener AD, Simmerman HK, Liepnieks J, Jones LR. 1986. Proteolytic cleavage of phospholamban purified from canine cardiac sarcoplasmic reticulum vesicles. Generation of a low resolution model of phospholamban structure. J Biol Chem 261:5154–5159.
44. Jones LR, Simmerman HK, Wilson WW, Gurd FR, Wegener AD. 1985. Purification and characterization of phospholamban from canine cardiac sarcoplasmic reticulum. J Biol Chem 260:7721–7730.
45. Kimura Y, Kurzydlowski K, Tada M, MacLennan DH. 1997. Phospholamban inhibitory function is activated by depolymerization. J Biol Chem 272:15061–15064.
46. Le Peuch CJ, Haiech J, Demaille JG. 1979. Concerted regulation of cardiac sarcoplasmic reticulum calcium transport by cyclic adenosine monophosphate dependent and calcium-calmodulin-dependent phosphorylations. Biochemistry 18:5150–5157.
47. Simmerman HK, Collins JH, Theibert JL, Wegener AD, Jones LR. 1986. Sequence analysis of phospholamban. Identification of phosphorylation sites and two major structural domains. J Biol Chem 261:13333–13341.
48. Tada M, Kirchberger MA. 1975. Regulation of calcium transport by cyclic AMP. A proposed mechanism for the beta-adrenergic control of myocardial contractility. Acta Cardiol 30:231–237.
49. Mitchell RD, Simmerman HK, Jones LR. 1988. Ca^{2+} binding effects on protein conformation and protein interactions of canine cardiac calsequestrin. J Biol Chem 263:1376–1381.
50. Jorgensen AO, Campbell KP. 1984. Evidence for the presence of calsequestrin in two structurally different regions of myocardial sarcoplasmic reticulum. J Cell Biol 98:1597–1602.
51. Jorgensen AO, Shen AC, Campbell KP. 1985. Ultrastructural localization of calsequestrin in adult rat atrial and ventricular muscle cells. J Cell Biol 101:257–268.
52. Yano K, Zarain-Herzberg A. 1994. Sarcoplasmic reticulum calsequestrin: structural and functional properties. Mol Cell Biochem 135:61–70.
53. Arai M, Alpert NR, Periasamy M. 1991. Cloning and characterization of the gene encoding rabbit cardiac calsequestrin. Gene 109:275–279.
54. Fliegel L, Ohnishi M, Carpenter MR, Khanna VK, Reithmeier RA, MacLennan DH. 1987. Amino acid sequence of rabbit fast-twitch skeletal muscle calsequestrin deduced from cDNA and peptide sequencing. Proc Natl Acad Sci USA 84:1167–1171.
55. MacLennan DH, Wong PT. 1971. Isolation of a calcium-sequestering protein from sarcoplasmic reticulum. Proc Natl Acad Sci USA 68:1231–1235.
56. Cala SE, Jones LR. 1991. Phosphorylation of cardiac and skeletal muscle calsequestrin isoforms by casein kinase II. Demonstration of a cluster of unique rapidly phosphorylated sites in cardiac calsequestrin. J Biol Chem 266:391–398.
57. Friedman WF. 1972. The intrinsic physiologic properties of the developing heart. Prog Cardiovasc Disease 15:87–111.
58. Davies P, Dewar J, Tynan M, Ward R. 1975. Post-natal developmental changes in the length-tension relationship of cat papillary muscles. J Physiol 253:95–102.
59. Friedman WF, Pool PE, Jacobowitz D, Seagren SC, Braunwald E. 1968. Sympathetic innervation of the developing rabbit heart. Biochemical and histochemical comparisons of fetal, neonatal, and adult myocardium. Circ Res 23:25–32.
60. Maylie JG. 1982. Excitation-contraction coupling in neonatal and adult myocardium of cat. Am J Physiol 242:H834–H843.
61. Fabiato A, Fabiato F. 1978. Calcium-induced release of calcium from the sarcoplasmic reticulum of skinned cells from adult human, dog, cat, rabbit, rat, and frog hearts and from fetal and new-born rat ventricles. Ann N Y Acad Sci 307:491–522.
62. Fabiato A. 1982. Calcium release in skinned cardiac cells: variations with species, tissues, and development. Fed Proc 41:2238–2244.
63. Hoerter J, Mazet F, Vassort G. 1981. Perinatal growth of the rabbit cardiac cell: possible implications for the mechanism of relaxation. J Mol Cell Cardiol 13:725–740.

64. Fitzgerald M, Neylon CB, Marks AR, Woodcock EA. 1994. Reduced ryanodine receptor content in isolated neonatal cardiomyocytes compared with the intact tissue. J Mol Cell Cardiol 26:1261–1265.
65. Ramesh V, Kresch MJ, Katz AM, Kim DH. 1995. Characterization of Ca^{2+}-release channels in fetal and adult rat hearts. Am J Physiol 269:H778–H782.
66. Xu A, Hawkins C, Narayanan N. 1997. Ontogeny of sarcoplasmic reticulum protein phosphorylation by Ca^{2+}-calmodulin-dependent protein kinase. J Mol Cell Cardiol 29:405–418.
67. Protasi F, Sun XH, Franzini-Armstrong C. 1996. Formation and maturation of the calcium release apparatus in developing and adult avian myocardium. Dev Biol 173:265–278.
68. Nayler WG, Fassold E. 1977. Calcium accumulating and ATPase activity of cardiac sarcoplasmic reticulum before and after birth. Cardiovasc Res 11:231–237.
69. Mahony L, Jones LR. 1986. Developmental changes in cardiac sarcoplasmic reticulum in sheep. J Biol Chem 261:15257–15265.
70. Pegg W, Michalak M. 1987. Differentiation of sarcoplasmic reticulum during cardiac myogenesis. Am J Physiol 252:H22–H31.
71. Gombosova I, Boknik P, Kirchhefer U, Knapp J, Luss H, Muller FU, Muller T, Vahlensieck U, Schmitz W, Bodor GS, Neumann J. 1998. Postnatal changes in contractile time parameters, calcium regulatory proteins, and phosphatases. Am J Physiol 274:H2123–H2132.
72. Szymanska G, Grupp IL, Slack JP, Harrer JM, Kranias EG. 1995. Alterations in sarcoplasmic reticulum calcium uptake, relaxation parameters and their responses to beta-adrenergic agonists in the developing rabbit heart. J Mol Cell Cardiol 27:1819–1829.
73. Jorgensen AO, Bashir R. 1984. Temporal appearance and distribution of the $Ca^{2+} + Mg^{2+}$ ATPase of the sarcoplasmic reticulum in developing chick myocardium as determined by immunofluorescence labeling. Dev Biol 106:156–165.
74. Moorman AF, Vermeulen JL, Koban MU, Schwartz K, Lamers WH, Boheler KR. 1995. Patterns of expression of sarcoplasmic reticulum Ca^{2+}-ATPase and phospholamban mRNAs during rat heart development. Circ Res 76:616–625.
75. Lompre AM, Lambert F, Lakatta EG, Schwartz K. 1991. Expression of sarcoplasmic reticulum Ca^{2+}-ATPase and calsequestrin genes in rat heart during ontogenic development and aging. Circ Res 69:1380–1388.
76. Artman M. 1992. Sarcolemmal Na^+-Ca^{2+} exchange activity and exchanger immunoreactivity in developing rabbit hearts. Am J Physiol 263:H1506–H1513.
77. Wetzel GT, Chen F, Klitzner TS. 1995. Na^+/Ca^{2+} exchange and cell contraction in isolated neonatal and adult rabbit cardiac myocytes. Am J Physiol 268:H1723–H1733.
78. Wetzel GT, Chen F, Klitzner TS. 1991. L- and T-type calcium channels in acutely isolated neonatal and adult cardiac myocytes. Pediatr Res 30:89–94.

B. Ostadal, M. Nagano and N.S. Dhalla (eds.).
CARDIAC DEVELOPMENT. Copyright © 2002.
Kluwer Academic Publishers. Boston.

DIFFERENCES IN CALCIUM HANDLING AND REGULATORY MECHANISMS BETWEEN NEONATAL AND ADULT HEARTS

NARANJAN S. DHALLA, IVANA OSTADALOVA,[1]
BOHUSLAV OSTADAL,[1] SUSHMA A. MENGI, VIJAYAN ELIMBAN,
and MOHINDER S. NIJJAR

Institute of Cardiovascular Sciences, St. Boniface General Hospital Research Centre &
Department of Physiology, Faculty of Medicine University of Manitoba, Winnipeg, Canada and
[1] Institute of Physiology, Czech Academy of Sciences Prague, Czech Republic

Summary. Although the neonatal heart develops less contractile force in comparison to the adult heart, it is much more tolerant with respect to ischemia-reperfusion injury, occurrence of Ca^{2+}-paradox and catecholamine-induced cardiotoxicity. By employing 5 day old neonatal and 250 day old adult rats, we have shown that the density of L-type Ca^{2+}-channels as well as the activities of sarcolemmal Na^{+}-Ca^{2+} exchanger and Ca^{2+}-pump were higher in the neonatal heart. On the other hand, basal and isoproterenol-stimulated adenylyl cyclase activities as well as sarcolemmal Na^{+}-K^{+} ATPase and ^{3}H-ouabain binding activities in the neonatal hearts were lower in comparison to the adult hearts. The immaturity of sarcoplasmic reticulum in the neonatal heart was evident from the low Ca^{2+}-pump, Ca^{2+}-release and ^{3}H-ryanodine binding activities in comparison to the adult heart. While Ca^{2+}-uptake activity in neonatal heart mitochondria was higher, mitochondrial ATPase activity was lower when compared to those in the adult heart. These data provide evidence that the Ca^{2+}-handling abilities and regulatory mechanisms in neonatal and adult hearts are different from each other and these differences may explain the weakness of cardiac function as well as increased tolerance of the neonatal heart to different pathophysiological interventions.

Key words: Cardiomyocyte calcium-handling, Sarcolemmal Ca^{2+}-pump, Sarcoplasmic reticular Ca^{2+}-pump, Na^{+}-Ca^{2+} exchanger, Na^{+}-K^{+} ATPase, Ca^{2+}-release channels, L-type Ca^{2+}-channels, β-adrenoceptor-adenylyl cyclase

Address for Correspondence: Dr. Naranjan S. Dhalla, Institute of Cardiovascular Sciences, St. Boniface General Hospital Research Centre, 351 Tache Avenue, Winnipeg, MB, R2H 2A6, Canada. Tel: (204) 235-3417; Fax: (204) 233-6723; e-mail: cvso@sbrc.ca

INTRODUCTION

In view of the critical role of Ca^{2+} in the processes of cardiac contraction and relaxation, extensive studies have been carried out over the past 40 years to understand the basic mechanisms, which determine Ca^{2+} movements in cardiomyocytes [1–11]. It has become clear that different subcellular organelles such as sarcolemma (SL), sarcoplasmic reticulum (SR), mitochondria and nucleus, by virtue of their ability to bind and accumulate Ca^{2+}, are intimately involved in controlling the intracellular Ca^{2+} in the cardiac muscle. Although mitochondria are capable of accumulating a large amount of Ca^{2+}, their participation in regulating the intracellular Ca^{2+} in the heart on a beat-to-beat basis is not fully understood. On the other hand, both SL and SR have been shown to contain some high affinity sites for Ca^{2+} and are thus considered to maintain a large concentration gradient between the intracellular and extracellular compartments. It should be noted that the extracellular concentration of Ca^{2+} is about $1.25\,mM$ whereas the intracellular concentration of Ca^{2+} varies between 0.1 to $10\,\mu M$ during contraction and relaxation phases of the myocardium. Depolarization of cardiomyocytes has been shown to open Ca^{2+}-channels present in the SL membrane and permit the entry of a small amount of Ca^{2+} into cardiomyocytes. This influx of Ca^{2+} then releases Ca^{2+} from the SR stores through the activation and opening of Ca^{2+}-release channels or ryanodine receptors in the SR membrane. The increase in intracellular Ca^{2+} promotes the binding of Ca^{2+} with troponin and thus suppresses the inhibitory effect of troponin on actin and myosin; this allows the thick and thin filaments to slide for the occurrence of cardiac contraction. The energy of cardiac contraction is provided by the hydrolysis of ATP due to the activation of myofibrillar ATPase by Ca^{2+}. On the other hand, relaxation of the cardiac muscle occurs as a consequence of removal of Ca^{2+} from troponin due to a decrease in the intracellular concentration of Ca^{2+} mainly upon the activation of SR Ca^{2+}-pump ATPase and sequestering of Ca^{2+} in the SR tubules. A small amount of Ca^{2+} is also extruded from the cytoplasm by the activation of Ca^{2+}-pump ATPase and Na^{+}-Ca^{2+} exchanger, which are present in the SL membrane. The energy for the processes of both contraction and relaxation is provided in the form of ATP by mitochondria through the Ca^{2+}-regulated mechanisms. In view of these events, it is evident that both SR and SR membranes mainly and mitochondria to some extent are known to regulate the intracellular concentration of Ca^{2+} in adult cardiomyocytes. Although nucleus is also considered to accumulate Ca^{2+}, its role in the regulation of Ca^{2+} in cardiomyocytes remains to be explored. In this article, it is intended to discuss the contribution of SR, mitochondria and SL in handling the intracellular Ca^{2+} in neonatal and adult cardiomyocytes. In addition, it is planned to examine the role of β-adrenoceptor-adenylyl cyclase system as well as Na^{+}-K^{+} ATPase in regulating the intracellular Ca^{2+} in neonatal and adult cardiomyocytes.

Cardiac function in neonatal heart

The cardiac muscle from neonatal hearts is known to generate less contractile force in comparison to that from the adult hearts [12–14]. Such a difference in cardiac

Table 1. Cardiac performance and
pathologic responses of neonatal and adult hearts

A. Heart function:	Weak contractile force development
B. Pathologic responses:	
Ischemia-reperfusion injury	Increased tolerance
Ca^{2+}-paradoxic injury	Increased tolerance
Catecholamine-induced toxicity	Increased tolerance

function between neonatal and adult hearts may be due to difference in the abilities of cardiomyocytes to handle Ca^{2+} with respect to the interaction and regulation of Ca^{2+} by SL, SR, mitochondria and myofibrils [15,16]. This concept is consistent with the observations that the neonatal heart function is more dependent upon Ca^{2+} influx from the extracellular source whereas the adult heart function depends upon the release of Ca^{2+} from the intracellular stores [17,18]. Furthermore, low contents of myofibrillar proteins as well as difference in the composition of myofibrils for myosin isozymes have been considered to explain the ability of neonatal heart to develop less contractile force in comparison to the adult heart. In fact, it appears that the behaviour of cardiomyocytes and subcellular organelles in the neonatal heart is different from that of the adult heart. This view is substantiated by the observations that the neonatal heart not only generates less contractile force, but its responses to various pathological interventions are also different from those for the adult heart (Table 1). It should be pointed out, however, that these developmental changes in functional, metabolic and molecular behaviour of the heart are species, sex and age dependent [15,19,20] and thus some caution should be exercised while interpreting the data at different stages of development. In addition, the translation of some ex vivo data on cardiac responses to inotropic agents and vasopressors to in vivo situations should be done with great care because the pharmacokinetics of cardiovascular drugs in neonatal animals have been reported to be different from those in the adult animals [21]. Accordingly, no effort was made to discuss differences between the responses of neonatal and adult hearts to various pharmacologic agents.

Mechanisms of Ca^{2+}-movements in neonatal heart

Although a great deal of work has been carried out to identify the role of SL, SR and mitochondria in controlling calcium movements in the adult heart, the information on these aspects in the neonatal heart is limited [15,16]. In this regard, SL Na^+-K^+ ATPase and ^3H-ouabain binding were lower whereas Na^+-Ca^{2+} exchange, Ca^{2+}-flux and passive Ca^{2+}-binding activities in the neonatal rabbit heart were comparable to those in the adult heart [22,23]. Some investigators have reported no change in the SR Ca^{2+} load but neonatal cells were found to exhibit smaller Ca^{2+}-release from the SR during contraction and greater Ca^{2+}-removal by SL Na^+-Ca^{2+} exchange during relaxation in comparison to the adult heart [24,25]. On the other

Table 2. ^{3}H-nitrendipine binding to crude membranes from neonatal and adult rat hearts

	Adult	Neonatal
B_{max} (fmol/mg)	180 ± 14	342 ± 21*
Kd (nM Ca^{2+})	0.44 ± 0.05	0.52 ± 0.07
Non-specific binding (fmol/mg)	19.4 ± 1.7	23.0 ± 3.1

Each value is a mean ± S.E. of 4 preparations. Methods for the isolation of crude membranes and determination of ^{3}H-nitrendipine binding were same as described earlier (32). * $P < 0.05$ compared to adult.

hand, both SR Ca^{2+}-uptake and mRNA for Ca^{2+}-pump protein (SERCA2a) in neonatal heart have been reported to be less than those in the adult rat heart [16,26]. It was interesting to note that in contrast to the adult heart, infusion of angiotensin in neonatal animals resulted in depression of the SR SERCA2a and Ca^{2+}-release channel genes as well as SL Na^+-Ca^{2+} exchange gene [27]. It is also pointed out that the L-type Ca^{2+}-channels in the neonatal rat ventricle were observed to be predominantly present in the SL membrane whereas these were more abundant in T-tubules in the adult heart [28]. No difference in SL Na^+-Ca^{2+} exchange between neonatal and adult hearts was observed while both SL Na^+-K^+ ATPase activity and ouabain binding in the neonatal heart were less than those in the adult heart [29]. These differences in the Na^+-K^+ ATPase were found to be due to differences in the amounts of the isozymes subunits in the neonatal and adult hearts [30]. Furthermore, increased mitochondrial Ca^{2+}-uptake in the neonatal rat heart in comparison to the adult heart [16] was related to the mitochondrial uniporter rather than to the modification of the driving force of Ca^{2+}-transport [31].

In order to gain indepth information and appreciate the significance of differences in the mechanisms of Ca^{2+}-handling by neonatal and adult cardiomyocytes, we employed ventricular tissue from 5 day old (neonatal) and 250 day old (adult) rats. Crude membranes as well as SL, SR and mitochondrial preparations were isolated from left ventricles according to the methods described elsewhere [32–37]. ^{3}H-nitrendipine binding (marker for SL L-type Ca^{2+} channels), SL ATP-dependent Ca^{2+}-uptake and Ca^{2+}-stimulated ATPase (index for SL Ca^{2+}-pump), SL Na^+-dependent Ca^{2+}-uptake (marker for Na^+-Ca^{2+} exchange), ^{3}H-ryanodine-sensitive Ca^{2+}-release and ryanodine binding (index for SR Ca^{2+}-release channels), SR Ca^+-uptake and Ca^{2+}-stimulated ATPase (index for SR Ca^{2+}-pump) as well as mitochondrial Ca^{2+}-uptake and ATPase (marker for mitochondrial uniporter activity) were determined by techniques used previously in our laboratory [32–37]. The data in Table 2 indicate that maximal ^{3}H-nitrendipine binding in the neonatal heart was higher than that in the adult heart without any changes in the ligand affinity ($1/K_d$). Likewise, the SL Ca^{2+}-pump and Na^+-dependent Ca^{2+}-uptake activities in the neonatal hearts were higher than those in the adult hearts (Tables 3 and 4). These results can be interpreted to suggest that both Ca^{2+}-influx and Ca^{2+}-efflux activities in the neonatal hearts may play a predominant role in contraction and relaxation processes

Table 3. Sarcolemmal Ca^{2+}-pump
activity in neonatal and adult rat hearts

	Adult	Neonatal
ATP-dependent Ca^{2+}-uptake (nmol/mg/min)	14.2 ± 1.7	26.4 ± 1.5*
Ca^{2+}-stimulated ATPase (μmol Pi/mg/hr)	12.6 ± 0.9	24.1 ± 0.8*
Mg^{2+} ATPase (μmol Pi/mg/hr)	81.0 ± 3.8	78.9 ± 4.2

Each value is a mean ± S.E. of 4 experiments. Sarcolemmal vesicles were isolated and both Ca^{2+}-uptake and ATPase activities were determined according to the procedures described elsewhere (33, 34). * $P < 0.05$ compared to adult.

Table 4. Sarcolemmal Na^+-dependent
Ca^{2+}-uptake in neonatal and adult rat hearts

	Adult	Neonatal
V_{max} (nmol/mg/2 sec)	13.5 ± 0.6	34.1 ± 2.5*
K_m (μM Ca^{2+})	22.4 ± 1.2	23.5 ± 1.8
Non-specific Ca^{2+}-binding (nmol/mg/2 sec)	3.2 ± 0.5	3.4 ± 0.4

Each value is a mean ± S.E. of 5 preparations. Sarcolemmal vesicles were isolated and Na^+-dependent Ca^{2+}-uptake parameters (V_{max} and K_m) were measured according to the procedures described elsewhere (33, 34). * $P < 0.05$ compared to adult.

Table 5. Sarcoplasmic reticular Ca^{2+}-
release activities in neonatal and adult rat hearts

	Adult	Neonatal
Ryanodine-sensitive Ca^{2+}-release (nmol/mg/15 sec)	9.4 ± 1.5	2.3 ± 0.3*
B_{max} for ^3H-ryanodine binding (fmol/mg)	1625 ± 138	500 ± 40*

Each value is a mean ± S.E. of 5 preparations. Sarcoplasmic reticular vesicles were isolated and Ca^{2+}-release activity and ryanodine binding were determined by procedures described elsewhere (35, 36). * $P < 0.05$ compared with adult.

in comparison to the adult heart. On the other hand, the SR ryanodine-sensitive Ca^{2+}-release activity and ^3H-ryanodine binding as well as SR Ca^{2+}-uptake and Ca^{2+}-stimulated ATPase activities in the neonatal hearts were lower than those in the adult hearts (Tables 5 and 6). These results indicate that both SR Ca^{2+}-release channels and Ca^{2+}-pump mechanisms in the neonatal hearts may not play any major role in contraction and relaxation processes in comparison to the adult hearts. In contrast to SR, mitochondrial Ca^{2+}-uptake was higher whereas Mg^{2+} ATPase activity was lower in the neonatal heart in comparison to those in the adult heart (Table 7). This seems to suggest that mitochondria may play a greater role in controlling

Table 6. Sarcoplasmic reticular Ca^{2+}-pump activities in neonatal and adult rat hearts

	Adult	Neonatal
Ca^{2+}-uptake (nmol/mg/min)	65 ± 4.1	23 ± 2.3*
Ca^{2+}-stimulated ATPase (nmol/mg/min)	204 ± 17.2	68 ± 4.9*

Each value is a mean ± S.E. of 6 preparations. Sarcoplasmic reticular vesicles were isolated and Ca^{2+}-pump and ATPase activities were determined by procedures described elsewhere (35). * $P < 0.05$ compared with adult.

Table 7. Mitochondrial Ca^{2+}-uptake in neonatal and adult rat hearts

	Adult	Neonatal
Ca^{2+}-uptake (nmol/mg/5 min)	25 ± 1.4	42 ± 3.9*
Mg^{2+} ATPase (μmol Pi/mg/5 min)	8.4 ± 0.9	5.2 ± 0.6*

Each value is a mean ± S.E. of 6 preparations. Mitochondria were isolated and Ca^{2+}-uptake as well as ATPase activities were determined by procedures described elsewhere (37). * $P < 0.05$ compared with adult.

the intracellular Ca^{2+} in comparison to SR in the neonatal hearts. These data provide evidence that the mechanisms involved in Ca^{2+}-handling in neonatal hearts are different from those in the adult hearts.

Regulation of intracellular Ca^{2+} in neonatal heart

Although Na^+-K^+ ATPase, adenylyl cyclase and β-adrenoceptors present in the SL membrane are not Ca^{2+}-cycling proteins per se, these proteins are known to regulate both Ca^{2+}-influx and Ca^{2+}-efflux activities across the SL membrane [1,5,9]. Stimulation of β-adrenoceptor-adenylyl cyclase system promotes Ca^{2+}-influx across SL and Ca^{2+}-accumulation in the SR tubules by phosphorylation of L-type Ca^{2+}-channels as well as Ca^{2+}-pump and Ca^{2+}-release proteins, respectively. Accordingly, SL membranes were isolated from neonatal (5 days old) and adult (250 days old) rat hearts for the determination of Na^+-K^+ ATPase and ^3H-ouabain binding [33] whereas crude membranes were isolated for the determination of adenylyl cyclase and $β_1$-adrenoceptors as well as $β_2$-adrenoceptors [38,39]. The data in Table 8 indicate that both Na^+-K^+ ATPase and ^3H-ouabain binding were lower in the neonatal SL in comparison to those in the SL preparation from the adult heart. This observation would mean that the reduced Na^+-pump activity in neonatal heart would result in elevated levels of Na^+ which would then produce higher levels of intracellular Ca^{2+} by affecting the Na^+-Ca^{2+} exchanger. Likewise, both the basal and isoproterenol-stimulated adenylyl cyclase activities were lower in the neonatal hearts without any difference in the NaF-stimulated and forskolin-stimulated adenylyl cyclase activities in the adult hearts (Table 9). However, no difference between neonatal and adult hearts was seen with respect to the characteristics of $β_1$-adrenoceptor or $β_2$-adrenoceptors (Table 10).

Table 8. Sarcolemmal Na$^+$-K$^+$ ATPase activity
and ouabain-binding in neonatal and adult rat hearts

	Adult	Neonatal
Na$^+$-K$^+$ ATPase (μmol Pi/mg/hr)	23.6 ± 1.7	6.1 ± 0.8★
Ouabain-sensitive Na$^+$-K$^+$ ATPase (μmol Pi/mg/hr)	5.0 ± 0.8	1.2 ± 0.3★
B$_{max}$ for ^{3}H-ouabain binding (pmol/mg)	19.8 ± 0.2	4.1 ± 0.4★

Each value is a mean ± S.E. of 6 preparations. Sarcolemmal preparation was isolated and ATPase activity as well as ouabain binding were determined by procedures described elsewhere (33). ★ P < 0.05 compared to adult.

Table 9. Adenylyl cyclase activities of
crude membranes from neonatal and adult hearts

	Adult	Neonatal
	(pmol cAMP/mg/min)	
Basal	60 ± 4.1	41 ± 3.2★
NaF-stimulated	146 ± 13	135 ± 11
Forskolin-stimulated	526 ± 48	504 ± 37
Isoproterenol-stimulated	72 ± 4.5	56 ± 3.2★

Each value is mean ± S.E. of 4 preparations. Crude membranes were isolated and adenylyl cyclase activities in the absence or presence of different stimulators were determined according to the procedures described elsewhere (38). ★ P < 0.05 compared to adult.

Table 10. Binding characteristics of ^{125}I-cyanopindolol
to crude membranes from neonatal and adult rat hearts

	Adult	Neonatal
A. β$_1$-adrenergic receptor		
B$_{max}$ (fmol/mg)	80 ± 5.6	95 ± 7.2
K$_d$ (pmol)	35 ± 2.6	34 ± 3.7
B. β$_2$-adrenergic receptor		
B$_{max}$ (fmol/mg)	21 ± 1.9	23 ± 1.6
K$_d$ (pmol)	16 ± 0.7	18 ± 1.3

Each value is a mean ± S.E. of 5 preparations. Crude membranes were isolated and the characteristics β$_1$-adrenergic and β$_2$-adrenergic receptors were determined by procedures described elsewhere (39). ★ P < 0.05 compared to adult.

The lower isoproterenol-stimulated adenylyl cyclase activity in the neonatal heart may not be due to β$_1$-adrenoceptors but instead may be a consequence of reduced protein content of adenylyl cyclase. Furthermore, these results indicate that the β-adrenoceptor-adenylyl cyclase system may be associated with less entry of Ca^{2+} from the extracellular source in the neonatal hearts. Nonetheless, the observed differences in both Na$^+$-K$^+$ ATPase and basal as well as isoproterenol-stimulated adenylyl cyclase can be seen to reflect some differences in the regulatory mechanisms for Ca^{2+}-handling by the neonatal and adult hearts.

Reponses of neonatal hearts to pathophysiological interventions

The ischemic adult heart, when not reperfused after a certain period of ischemia, exhibits poor recovery with respect to cardiac performance as well as SL and SR functions [40–42]. However, the neonatal heart has been observed to be less sensitive to the ischemia-reperfusion injury [43–46]. Such a difference between the neonatal and adult heart has been considered to be due to immaturity of key enzymes such as SR Ca^{2+}-stimulated ATPase and 5'-nucleotidease [47,48], differences in myocardial metabolism [49] and better endothelial responses as well as improved coronary flow [50]. Since the neonatal heart is also more resistant to injury due to Ca^{2+}-paradoxic phenomenon [51,52], which is known to be associated with the occurrence of intracellular Ca^{2+}-overload [53], it is possible that greater resistance of neonatal heart to ischemia-reperfusion injury may be a consequence of attenuated development of the intracellular Ca^{2+}-overload. It is pointed out that reperfusion of hearts with Ca^{2+}-free medium followed by reperfusion with medium containing Ca^{2+} (Ca^{2+} paradox) has been shown to produce changes similar to those seen in the ischemia-reperfused hearts [53–56]. In view of the role of oxidative stress in the genesis of ischemia-reperfusion injury [55–57], it is likely that larger amounts of antioxidants and other antioxidative factors may be present in the neonatal heart in comparison to the adult hearts. It should be noted that neonatal hearts were less sensitive to catecholamines with respect to producing inotropic effect as well as apoptosis in comparison to the adult hearts [58,59]. Since the high levels of circulating catecholamines are also known to produce cardiotoxicity due to oxidative stress and subsequent occurrence of intracellular Ca^{2+}-overload [60], it is evident that the increased tolerance of neonatal hearts for exhibiting cardiotoxic effects [19] may be related to the higher level of antioxidative reserve in comparison to the adult hearts. Thus it seems likely that in comparison to the adult heart, higher tolerance of the neonatal heart may be due to its resistance for the development of intracellular Ca^{2+}-overload.

CONCLUSIONS

From the foregoing discussion, it is apparent that the weaker ability of neonatal heart to develop contractile force in comparison to the adult heart may not only be due to the sparse contractile machinery but may also depend upon the immaturity of SR for Ca^{2+}-release and Ca^{2+}-uptake. The increased dependence of neonatal heart on extracellular Ca^{2+} for contraction may be a consequence of increased Ca^{2+}-influx due to increased density of L-type Ca^{2+}-channels in the SL membranes as well as high modulatory effect of low levels of Na^+-K^+ ATPase on the Na^+-Ca^{2+} exchanger. On the other hand, increased SL Na^+-Ca^{2+} exchange and Ca^{2+}-pump activities in the neonatal heart may play a dominant role in cardiac relaxation and this is in contrast to the adult heart where SR Ca^{2+}-pump is known to be a major player in this regard. The increased tolerance of the neonatal heart for ischemia-reperfusion injury, occurrence of Ca^{2+}-paradox and catecholamine-induced cardiotoxicity may be related to its resistance for the development of intracellular Ca^{2+}-overload as a consequence of higher activities of SL Na^{+}-Ca^{2+} exchange and Ca^{2+}-pump for the removal of Ca^{2+} from cardiomyocytes as well as higher ability of mitochondria to accumulate Ca^{2+}.

ACKNOWLEDGEMENTS

The work reported in this article was supported by a grant from the Canadian Institutes of Health Research (CIHR) Group in Experimental Cardiology. NSD holds CIHR/Research & Development Chair in Cardiovascular Research supported by Merck Frosst, Canada. SAM was a visiting scientist from S.N.D.T. Women's University, Mumbai, India.

REFERENCES

1. Dhalla NS, Ziegelhoffer A, Harrow JAC. 1977. Regulatory role of membrane systems in heart function. Can J Physiol Pharmacol 55:1211–1234.
2. Dhalla NS, Das PK, Sharma GP. 1978. Subcellular basis of contractile failure. J Mol Cell Cardiol 10:363–385.
3. Chapman RA. 1979. Excitation-contraction coupling in cardiac muscles. Prog Biophys Mol Biol 35:1–52.
4. Lullman H, Peters T. 1979. Plasmalemmal calcium in cardiac excitation-contraction coupling in heart muscle. Prog Pharmacol 2:1–57.
5. Dhalla NS, Pierce GN, Panagia V, Singal PK, Beamish RE. 1982. Calcium movements in relation to heart function. Basic Res Cardiol 77:117–139.
6. Tsien RW. 1983. Calcium channels in excitable cell membranes. Annu Rev Physiol 45:341–358.
7. Reuter H. 1985. Calcium movements through cardiac cell membranes. Med Res Rev 5:427–440.
8. Carafoli E. 1987. Intracellular calcium homeostasis. Annu Rev Biochem 56:395–433.
9. Dhalla NS, Dixon IMC, Beamish RE. 1991. Biochemical basis of heart function and contractile failure. J Appl Cardiol 6:7–30.
10. Carafoli E, Chiesi M. 1992. Calcium pumps in the plasma and intracellular membranes. Curr Top Cell Regul 32:209–241.
11. Dhalla NS, Wang X, Beamish RE. 1996. Intracellular calcium handling in normal and failing hearts. Exptl Clin Cardiol 1:7–20.
12. Jarmakani JM, Nakanishi T, George BL, Bers DM. 1982. The effect of extracellular calcium on myocardial mechanical function in the neonatal rabbit. Dev Pharmacol Ther 5:1–52.
13. Katz AM. 1991. Maturational changes in excitation-contraction coupling in mammalian myocardium. J Am Cell Cardiol 17:218–225.
14. Ostadalova I, Kolar F, Ostadal B, Rohlicek J, Prochazka J. 1993. Early postnatal development on contractile performance and responsiveness to calcium, verapamil and ryanodine in the isolated rat heart. J Mol Cell Cardiol 25:733–740.
15. Nijjar MS, Dhalla NS. 1997. Biochemical basis of calcium-handling in developing myocardium. In B Ostadal, M Nagano and NS Dhalla (eds), The Developing Heart. Philadelphia: Lippincott-Raven Publishers, pp. 189–217.
16. Sulakhe PV, Dhalla NS. 1970. Excitation-contraction coupling in heart. IV. Energy-dependent calcium transport in the myocardium. Life Sci 9.1363–1370.
17. Seguchi M, Harding JA, Jarmakani JM. 1986. Developmental change in the function of sarcoplasmic reticulum. J Mol Cell Cardiol 18:189–195.
18. Bers DM, Philipson KD, Langer GA. 1981. Cardiac contractility and sarcolemmal calcium binding in several cardiac muscle preparation. Am J Physiol 240:H576–583.
19. Ostadal B, Beamish RE, Barwinsky J, Dhalla NS. 1989. Ontogenetic development of cardiac sensitivity to catecholamines. J Appl Cardiol 4:467–486.

20. Ostadal B, Ostadalova I, Dhalla NS. 1999. Development of cardiac sensitivity to oxygen deficiency: Comparative and ontogenetic aspects. Physiol Rev 79:635–659.
21. Steinberg C, Notterman DA. 1994. Pharmacokinetics of cardiovascular drugs in children. Inotropes and vasopressors. Clin Pharmacokinet 27:345–367.
22. Hanson GL, Schilling WP, Michael LH. 1993. Sodium-potassium pump and sodium-calcium exchange in adult and neonatal canine cardiac sarcolemmal. Am J Physiol 264:H320–H326.
23. Meno H, Jarmakani JM, Philipson KD. 1988. Sarcolemmal calcium kinetics in the neonatal heart. J Mol Cell Cardiol 20:585–591.
24. Balaguru D, Haddock PS, Puglisi JL, Bers DM, Coetzee WA, Artman M. 1997. Role of the sarcoplasmic reticulum in contraction and relaxation of immature rabbit ventricular myocytes. J Mol Cell Cardiol 29:2747–2757.
25. Chen F, Ding S, Lee BS, Wetzel GT. 2000. Sarcoplasmic reticulum Ca(2+) ATPase and cell contraction in developing rabbit heart. J Mol Cell Cardiol 32:745–755.
26. Ribadeau-Dumas A, Brady M, Boateng SY, Schwartz K, Boheler KR. 1999. Sarco(endo)plasmic reticulum Ca(2+)-ATPase (SERCA2) gene products are regulated post-transcriptionally during rat cardiac development.
27. Ju H, Scammel-La Fleur T, Dixon IMC. 1996. Altered mRNA abundance of calcium transport genes in cardiac myocytes induced by angiotensin II. J Mol Cell Cardiol 28:1119–1128.
28. Wibo M, Bravo G, Godfraind T. 1991. Postnatal maturation of excitation-contraction coupling in rat ventricle in relation to the subcellular localization and surface density of 1,4-dihyropyridine and ryanodine receptors. Circ Res 68:662–673.
29. Hanson GL, Schilling WP, Michael LH. 1993. Sodium-potassium pump and sodium-calcium exchange in adult and neonatal canine cardiac sarcolemmal. Am J Physiol 264:H320–H326.
30. Lucchesi PA, Sweadner KJ. 1991. Postnatal changes in Na,K-ATPase isoform expression in rat cardiac ventricle. Conservation of biphasic ouabain affinity. J Biol Chem 266:9327–9331.
31. Bassani RA, Fagian MM, Bassani JW, Vercesi AE. 1998. Changes in calcium uptake rate by rat cardiac mitochondria during postnatal development. J Mol Cell Cardiol 30:2013–2023.
32. Dixon IMC, Lee SL, Dhalla NS. 1990. Nitrendipine binding in congestive heart failure due to myocardial infarction. Circ Res 66:782–788.
33. Dixon IMC, Hata T, Dhalla NS. 1992. Sarcolemmal Na⁺-K⁺ ATPase activity in congestive heart failure due to myocardial infarction. Am J Physiol 262:C664–C671.
34. Dixon IMC, Hata T, Dhalla NS. 1992. Sarcolemmal Ca²⁺-transport in congestive heart failure due to myocardial infarction in rats. Am J Physiol 262:H1387–H1394.
35. Ganguly PK, Pierce GN, Dhalla KS, Dhalla NS. 1983. Defective sarcoplasmic reticular calcium transport in diabetic cardiomyopathy. Am J Physiol 244:E528–E535.
36. Osada M, Netticadan T, Tamura K, Dhalla NS. 1998. Modification of ischemia-reperfusion-induced changes in cardiac sarcoplasmic reticulum by preconditioning. Am J Physiol 247:H2025–H2034.
37. Pierce GN, Dhalla NS. 1985. Heart mitochondrial function in chronic experimental diabetes in rats. Can J Cardiol 1:48–54.
38. Sethi R, Dhalla KS, Beamish RE, Dhalla NS. 1997. Differential changes in left and right ventricular adenylyl cyclase activities in congestive heart failure. Am J Physiol 272:H884–H893.
39. Persad S, Elimban V, Siddiqui F, Dhalla NS. 1999. Alterations in cardiac membrane β-adrenoceptor and adenylyl cyclase due to hypochlorous acid. J Mol Cell Cardiol 31:101–111.
40. Temsah RM, Netticadan T, Chapman D, Takeda S, Mochizuki S, Dhalla NS. 1999. Alterations in sarcoplasmic reticulum function and gene expression in ischemia-reperfused rat heart. Am J Physiol 277:H584–H594.
41. Dhalla NS, Panagia V, Singal PK, Makino N, Dixon IMC, Eyolfson DA. 1988. Alterations in heart membrane calcium transport during the development of ischemia-reperfusion injury. J Mol Cell Cardiol 20 (Suppl. II):3–13.
42. Temsah RM, Dyck C, Netticadan T, Chapman D, Elimban V, Dhalla NS. 2000. Effect of β-adrenoceptor blockers on sarcoplasmic reticular function and gene expression in the ischemic-reperfused heart. J Pharmacol Exp Therap 293:15–23.
43. Riva E, Hearse DJ. 1993. Age-dependent changes in myocardial susceptibility to ischemic injury. Cardioscience 4:85–92.
44. Kohman LJ, Veit LJ. 1991. Neonatal myocardium resists reperfusion injury. J Surg Res 51:133–137.
45. Pridjian AK, Levitsky S, Krukenkamp I, Silverman NA, Feinberg H. 1987. Developmental changes in reperfusion injury. A comparison of intracellular cation accumulation in the newborn, neonatal and adult heart. J Thorac Cardiovasc Surg 93:428–433.

46. Murashita T, Borgers M, Hearse DJ. 1992. Developmental changes in tolerance to ischaemia in the rabbit heart: disparity between interpretations of structural, enzymatic and functional indices of injury. J Mol Cell Cardiol 24:1143–1154.
47. Quantz M, Tchervenkov C, Chiu RC. 1992. Unique responses of immature hearts to ischemia. Functional recovery versus initiation of contracture. J Thorac Cardiovasc Surg 103:927–935.
48. Grosso MA, Banerjee A, St Cyr JA, Rogers KB, Brown JM, Clarke DR, Campbell DN, Harken AH. 1992. Cardiac 5'-nucleotidase activity increases with age and inversely relates to recovery from ischemia. J Thorac Cardiovasc Surg 103:206–209.
49. Wittnich C. 1992. Age-related differences in myocardial metabolism affects response to ischemia. Age in heart tolerance to ischemia. Am J Cardiovasc Pathol 4:175–180.
50. Hiramatsu T, Zund G, Schermerhorn ML, Shinoka T, Miura T, Mayer JE Jr. 1995. Age differences in effects of hypothermic ischemia on endothelial and ventricular function. Ann Thorac Surg 60 (Suppl 6):S501–S504.
51. Ucmura S, Young H, Matsuoka S, Nakanishi T, Jarmakani JM. 1985. Calcium paradox in the neonatal heart. Can J Cardiol 1:114–120.
52. Elz JS, Nayler WG. 1987. Quantification of calcium paradox in neonatal rat hearts. Am J Physiol 253:H1358–H1364.
53. Alto LE, Dhalla NS. 1979. Myocardial cation contents during induction of the calcium paradox. Am J Physiol 237:H713–H719.
54. Yates JC, Dhalla NS. 1975. Structural and functional changes associated with failure and recovery of hearts after perfusion with Ca^{++}-free medium. J Mol Cell Cardiol 7:91–103.
55. Dhalla NS, Elmoselhi AB, Hata T, Makino N. 2000. Status of myocardial antioxidants in ischemia-reperfusion injury. Cardiovasc Res 47:446–456.
56. Dhalla NS, Temsah RM, Netticadan T. 2000. Role of oxidative stress in cardiovascular diseases. J Hypertension 18:655–673.
57. Dhalla NS, Golfman L, Takeda S, Takeda N, Nagano M. 1999. Evidence for the role of oxidative stress in acute ischemic heart disease: A brief review. Can J Cardiol 15:587–593.
58. Sun LS. 1999. Regulation of myocardial beta-adrenergic receptor function in adult and neonatal rabbits. Biol Neonate 76:181–192.
59. Shyu KG, Kuan P, Chang ML, Wang BW, Huang FY. 2000. Effects of norepinephrine on apoptosis in rat neonatal cardiomyocytes. J Formos Med Assoc 99:412–418.
60. Dhalla KS, Rupp H, Beamish RE, Dhalla NS. 1996. Mechanisms of alterations in cardiac membrane Ca^{2+} transport due to excess catecholamines. Cardiovasc Drugs Therapy 10:231–238.

B. Ostadal, M. Nagano and N.S. Dhalla (eds.).
CARDIAC DEVELOPMENT. Copyright © 2002.
Kluwer Academic Publishers. Boston.
All rights reserved.

METABOLIC DIFFERENCES BETWEEN PEDIATRIC AND ADULT HEARTS: IMPLICATIONS FOR CARDIAC SURGERY

M.-S. SULEIMAN PHD,[1] H. IMURA MD,[1] M. CAPUTO MD,[1]
G.D. ANGELINI FRCS,[1] P. MODI FRCS,[1] R. ASCIONE MD,[1]
A. LOTTO MD,[1] A. PARRY FRCS,[2] and A. PAWADE FRCS[2]

Bristol Heart Institute[1], University of Bristol, Bristol Royal Infirmary, and The Royal Hospital for Sick Children[2], Bristol BS2 8HW, UK

Summary. Recent evidence suggests that during open heart surgery, pediatric hearts are more vulnerable to reperfusion injury compared to adult hearts. Metabolic differences between pediatric and adult myocardium may, in part, be responsible for the reported increased vulnerability of pediatric hearts. The aim of this work was to compare the metabolic state of both pediatric and adult hearts prior to open heart surgery. Ventricular biopsies were collected at the beginning of crossclamp time from hearts of 42 pediatric and 41 adult patients. Adenine nucleotides (ATP, ADP, AMP), purines (inosine, adenosine), amino acids (glutamate and alanine) and lactate were determined in all biopsies. There were no differences in the myocardial concentration of ATP, ADP, AMP, inosine and adenosine between pediatric and adult hearts. However, pediatric hearts had significantly higher lactate levels and lower levels of amino acids compared to adult hearts. These metabolic differences may offer an explanation for why pediatric hearts show more reperfusion injury than adult hearts during open heart surgery.

Key words: pediatric, myocardium, metabolism.

INTRODUCTION

Major advances have been made in the preservation of myocardial function during open heart surgery, since the introduction of cardioplegic arrest [1]. Although myocar-

Author for correspondence: M-S Suleiman, Bristol Heart Institute, University of Bristol, Bristol Royal Infirmary, Bristol BS2 8HW. Tel: 0117-9283519; Fax: 0117-9299737; e-mail: M.S.Suleiman@bristol.ac.uk

dial protection strategies have been originally designed to protect adult hearts, they have been adopted uncritically for pediatric cardiac surgery [2]. Available laboratory data has been inconclusive in explaining the vulnerability of the immature myocardium to cardiac surgery [3,4]. The majority of experimental reports suggest that developing mammalian hearts are more resistant to the damaging effects of cardiac insults than adult hearts [2–9]. This improved tolerance has been attributed to differences in vascular resistance, calcium mobilization and metabolism [6,10–13]. Others, however, have reported that the immature myocardium is more vulnerable to injury than the adult heart [14–17]. Experimental laboratory research investigating the cardioprotective action of cardioplegic solutions have also been inconclusive, not least because of species-dependent and age-related differences [16,18–22].

Significant reperfusion injury, as measured by postoperative release of myocardial markers of injury, occurs during pediatric open heart surgery [23,24]. The extent of this injury was significantly more than what was seen in adult hearts following open heart surgery using similar or different techniques of myocardial protection and similar ischemic times [23,25–28]. The mechanisms responsible for the increased susceptibility of pediatric hearts to ischemia/reperfusion injury during surgery are not presently known. In this study we investigated whether there are metabolic differences between pediatric and adult hearts which may offer an explanation for the increased vulnerability of pediatric hearts to reperfusion injury. In order to achieve this we measured the resting myocardial concentration of important metabolites in ventricular biopsies collected from hearts of pediatric and adult patients undergoing open heart surgery.

MATERIALS AND METHODS

Eighty three patients (42 pediatric and 41 adult) were recruited in this study. Pediatric patients were undergoing a variety of corrective surgery for congenital heart disease. Adult patients were undergoing surgery for either aortic valve disease (n = 25) or coronary artery disease (n = 16).

Pre-operative characteristics are summarized in Tables 1 and 2. All surgery was elective with no emergency operations. Ethical approval from the local authority and informed consent were obtained for all patients.

Collection of ventricular biopsies and extraction of metabolites

Myocardial biopsies were collected immediately after institution of cardiopulmonary bypass and before cross clamping the aorta. In pediatric patients, myocardial biopsies were collected from the right ventricle (free wall of the trabecular portion) through the tricuspid valve by direct resection with surgical scissors. Myocardial biopsies were collected from adult hearts using a "Trucut" needle. In patients with ischemic heart disease, the biopsies were collected from the apex of the left ventricle. However, in the cases of patient with aortic valve disease, biopsies were collected from both left and right ventricles. Each biopsy specimen (3–10 mg) was immediately frozen in liquid nitrogen until processing for the analysis of cellular metabolites.

Table 1. Pediatric patients characteristics

		n = 42
Age		
	Mean	24 ± 5 months
	Range	(1–120)
Body Weight (kg)		10.0 ± 1.3
		(3–40)
Sex (male/female)		28/14
Pathology†		
	VSD	12
	TOF	9
	AVSD	3
	PA or PS	3
	TAPVD and TGA	5
	ASD or P-AVSD	1
	Mitral or Aortic valve	3
	Others	6

†VSD, Ventricular Septal Defect; TOF, Tetralogy Of Fallott, AVSD, Atrio-Ventricular Septal Defect; PA, Pulmonary Atresia; PS, Pulmonary Stenosis; TAPVD, Total Anomalus Pulmonary Vein Drainage; TGA, Transposition of Great Arteries; ASD, Atrial Septal Defect; P-AVSD, Partial AVSD.

Table 2. Adult patients characteristics

	Pathology	
	Aortic Valve (n = 25)	Coronary (n = 16)
Male/Female	19/6	14/2
Age (years)	66 ± 2	63 ± 2
BMI	30.9 ± 1.4	26.2 ± 1.0
Hypertension	11	6
Hypercholesterolemia	5	11
Diabetes mellitus	1	2
Smoking	7	14
Ejection fraction		
Good (<49%)	21	12
Fair (30–49%)	4	4
Trans-valvular peak gradient (mmHg)	76.1 ± 2.6	
Canadian class:		
I	7	0
II	6	2
III	5	8
IV	7	6
NYHA class:		
I	7	6
II	10	0
III	7	10
IV	1	0

Data are presented as mean ± Standard error or number. BMI = Body Mass Index; NYHA = New York Heart Association.

Table 3. The myocardial concentration of intracellular
metabolites (nmol/mg protein) in hearts of pediatric and adult patients

	Pediatric (n = 42)	Ischemic (n = 16)	Hypertrophic (n = 25)	Normal (n = 25)
ATP	43.8 ± 2.0	41.2 ± 3.3	40.6 ± 2.0	40.6 ± 2.5
ADP	22.6 ± 1.7	20.8 ± 1.7	20.8 ± 1.3	19.6 ± 1.4
AMP	5.6 ± 0.7	5.0 ± 0.5	5.1 ± 0.6	4.5 ± 0.5
ATP/ADP	2.30 ± 0.16	2.06 ± 0.12	2.04 ± 0.11	2.21 ± 0.15
ATP + ADP + AMP	72 ± 3	67 ± 5	66 ± 3	65 ± 4
Inosine	1.21 ± 0.15	1.15 ± 0.14	1.71 ± 0.25	1.46 ± 0.23
Adenosine	0.66 ± 0.08	0.46 ± 0.06	0.70 ± 0.10	0.70 ± 0.13

Determination of metabolites in biopsy specimen

Adenine nucleotides (ATP, ADP and AMP), purines (adenosine and inosine), lactate
and the free amino acids glutamate and alanine were measured in all biopsies
collected.

Adenine nucleotides and purines in the neutralized extract were separated and
quantified using an HPLC method based on previous reports [25,29]. Lactate was
determined using a diagnostic kit from Sigma. Amino acids were determined according to the Water's Pico-Tag method and similar to that reported earlier [25,27].

Data collection and analysis

All clinical and biochemical data were expressed as mean ± standard error of mean
(SEM). Statistical intergroup analysis was carried out using ANOVA. Correlation
matrix and coefficients were calculated and the significance determined using
Fisher's r to z. The statistical analyses were carried out using a statview package.

RESULTS

There were no significant differences in the myocardial concentration of energy rich
phosphates ATP, ADP, AMP between pediatric hearts and different types of adult
hearts (Table 3). Furthertmore, the myocardial concentration of purines (inosine and
adenosine) was similar for both pediatric and adult hearts. In contrast, the concentration of lactate in pediatric hearts was more than three fold higher than in adult
hearts (Fig. 1). There were no differences in the concentration of lactate between
ischemically diseased (45 ± 15 nmol/mg protein), hypertrophic left ventricle (69 ±
20 nmol/mg protein) or normal right ventricle (60 ± 12 nmol/mg protein) of adult
hearts. The myocardial concentration of the amino acid glutamate in pediatric hearts
was significantly lower than in ischemic and in hypertrophic adult myocardium (Fig.
2A). Although the concentration of glutamate tended to be lower in pediatric compared to normal adult myocardium, this difference did not reach statistical significance (p = 0.09). The amino acid alanine, a byproduct of glutamate metabolism
in the heart, was found at significantly lower concentration in pediatric hearts
compared to adult hearts (Fig. 2B).

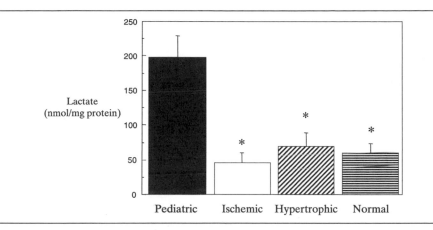

Figure 1. The myocardial concentration of lactate measured in biopsy specimen collected from pediatric hearts and from adult hearts (ischemic, hypertrophic and normal ventricles). *P < 0.05 versus pediatric.

In order to establish whether the concentration of different metabolites in individual patients correlated (increased or decreased) with each other, the correlation matrix for each group of patients, was constructed (Table 4). ADP versus AMP and ATP versus glutamate showed a strong positive correlation in all groups (p < 0.001). As the correlation between ATP and glutamate is likely to have implications for the utilization of glutamate for energy production, detailed information about the extent of this relationship is shown as scattergrams (Fig. 3).

DISCUSSION

Recent evidence suggests that during open heart surgery, pediatric hearts are more vulnerable to reperfusion injury than adult hearts (see Introduction). The underlying mechanisms responsible for the increased susceptibility of pediatric hearts to ischemia/reperfusion injury are not presently known. These may include differences in myocardial calcium handling and in metabolic properties. Calcium handling properties have been used to explain differences between adult and immature animal heart [30]. Whether these properties also change during development of human heart is presently unknown.

Although the preoperative metabolic state of pediatric and adult hearts was similar for most metabolites (Table 3) biopsies of pediatric hearts had significantly and markedly higher concentrations of lactate compared to adults. The heart is an omnivore and can utilize lactate for energy production [31]. Our finding that pediatric hearts contain relatively elevated levels of lactate suggests that their ability to utilize lactate as a substrate for energy production is not fully developed like in adult hearts. During cardioplegic ischemic arrest, adult human hearts accumulate lactate [25,27], which can then be used as a source of energy during reperfusion. This may not be

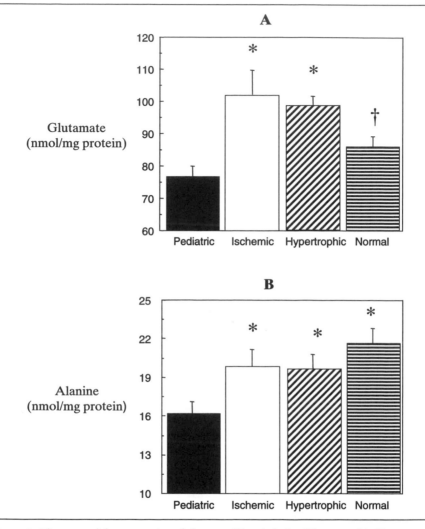

Figure 2. The myocardial concentration of glutamate (A) and alanine (B) measured in biopsy specimen collected from pediatric and adult hearts. For the sake of clarity, y-axis does not start at 0.0. *P < 0.05 versus pediatric; †P < 0.05 versus ischemic.

the case in pediatric hearts as they have markedly higher levels of lactate. In fact we have recently found that pediatric hearts do not tend to accumulate lactate during ischaemia [Imura et al., unpublished observations]. Such differences may explain the significantly higher reperfusion damage of pediatric hearts during surgery compared to adult hearts. Lactate has also been implicated in the regulation of K_{ATP} channel activity [32]. Whether this effect is age-dependent requires further investigation.

Table 4. Correlation Coefficients for myocardial metabolites in pediatric and adult hearts

Pediatric

	ATP	ADP	AMP	Inosine	Adenosine	Lactate	Glutamate	Alanine
ATP	1.00	0.37	−0.06	0.01	−0.10	−0.20	**0.80**	0.14
ADP	0.37	1.00	**0.78**	0.45	0.32	0.09	0.37	0.32
AMP	−0.06	**0.78**	1.00	0.65	0.39	0.01	0.02	0.15
Inosine	0.01	0.45	0.65	1.00	0.68	−0.10	0.09	0.32
Adenosine	−0.10	0.32	0.39	0.68	1.00	−0.04	0.02	0.10
Lactate	−0.20	0.09	0.01	−0.10	−0.04	1.00	−0.20	0.20
Glutamate	**0.80**	0.37	0.02	0.09	0.02	−0.20	1.00	−0.03
Alanine	0.14	0.32	0.15	0.32	0.10	0.20	−0.03	1.00

Ischemic

	ATP	ADP	AMP	Inosine	Adenosine	Lactate	Glutamate	Alanine
ATP	1.00	0.72	0.40	0.33	−0.19	−0.09	**0.87**	0.47
ADP	0.72	1.00	**0.89**	0.62	0.06	0.20	0.75	0.46
AMP	0.40	**0.89**	1.00	0.65	0.20	0.26	0.53	0.40
Inosine	0.30	0.62	0.65	1.00	0.47	0.41	0.58	0.63
Adenosine	−0.19	0.06	0.20	0.47	1.00	−0.07	0.02	0.15
Lactate	−0.09	0.20	0.26	0.41	−0.07	1.00	0.11	0.34
Glutamate	**0.87**	0.75	0.53	0.58	0.02	0.11	1.00	0.71
Alanine	0.47	0.46	0.40	0.63	0.15	0.34	0.71	1.00

Hypertrophic

	ATP	ADP	AMP	Inosine	Adenosine	Lactate	Glutamate	Alanine
ATP	1.00	0.59	0.22	0.25	0.00	0.12	**0.71**	0.35
ADP	0.59	1.00	**0.85**	0.37	0.43	0.63	0.62	0.17
AMP	0.22	**0.85**	1.00	0.25	0.61	0.70	0.39	−0.09
Inosine	0.25	0.37	0.25	1.00	0.38	−0.01	0.40	0.14
Adenosine	0.00	0.43	0.61	0.38	1.00	0.15	0.19	−0.02
Lactate	0.12	0.63	0.70	−0.01	0.15	1.00	0.31	0.15
Glutamate	**0.71**	0.62	0.39	0.40	0.19	0.31	1.00	0.26
Alanine	0.35	0.17	−0.09	0.14	−0.02	0.15	0.26	1.00

Normal

	ATP	ADP	AMP	Inosine	Adenosine	Lactate	Glutamate	Alanine
ATP	1.00	0.08	−0.04	−0.09	0.08	−0.19	**0.71**	0.30
ADP	0.08	1.00	**0.89**	0.38	0.53	−0.20	0.07	0.15
AMP	−0.04	**0.89**	1.00	0.43	0.68	−0.04	−0.15	0.18
Inosine	−0.09	0.38	0.43	1.00	0.57	−0.24	−0.16	0.12
Adenosine	0.08	0.53	0.68	0.57	1.00	−0.14	0.03	0.26
Lactate	−0.19	−0.20	−0.40	−0.24	−0.10	1.00	0.04	0.27
Glutamate	**0.71**	0.07	−0.15	−0.16	0.03	0.04	1.00	0.45
Alanine	0.30	0.15	0.18	0.12	0.26	0.27	0.45	1.00

Coefficients in bold are for metabolites with strong and highly significant ($P < 0.001$) positive correlation in all groups.

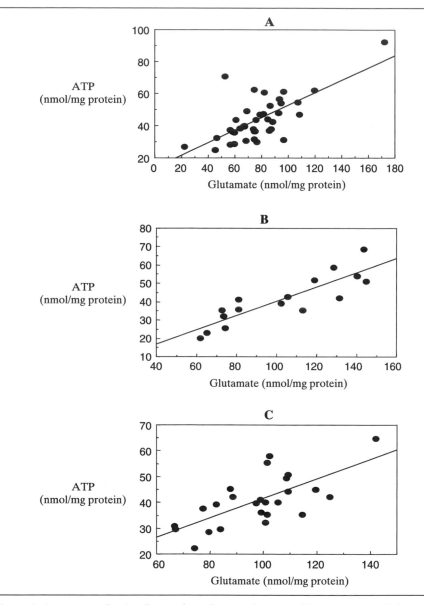

Figure 3. Scattergarms showing the correlation between the myocardial concentration of glutamate and ATP in pediatric (A), adult ischemic (B) and hypertrophic (C) hearts. Simple linear regression is used to fit the data.

In addition to lactate, both glutamate and alanine tended to be different between pediatric and adult hearts. Glutamate is used to enrich cardioplegia to protect the heart against ischemia/reperfusion damage [33]. It provides metabolic support at the substrate level phosphorylation where glutamate and pyruvate are converted to alanine and α-ketoglutarate [34,35]. In fact we have shown that the human myocardium utilizes glutamate during ischemia and early after reperfusion [25,27,28]. Therefore the lower concentration of glutamate in pediatric hearts compared to adult hearts may render the pediatric hearts having less substrates available for energy production during cardiac insults. The strong correlation between the concentrations of ATP and glutamate adds weight to the suggestion that the metabolism of glutamate has strong energy implications. The lower levels of alanine are consistent with pediatric heart cells having less glutamate than adult hearts, as alanine is a byproduct of glutamate.

In this study we present novel data showing that the metabolic state of pediatric hearts is different to that of adult hearts, irrespective of pathology. In particular, this work suggests that the metabolism of lactate is poor in pediatric hearts and along with lower levels of glutamate, may render the pediatric hearts more susceptible to ischemia and reperfusion injury. This finding will help in formulating strategies aimed at protecting the pediatric myocardium during open heart surgery.

ACKNOWLEDGEMENTS

We acknowledge the help of members of staff in pediatric cardiac surgery at the Children Hospital in Bristol and Anne Moffat for her excellent technical assistance. This study was supported by grants from the British Heart Foundation (GDA is a BHF Professor of Cardiac Surgery), the Garefield Western Trust, and the National Heart Research Fund.

REFERENCES

1. Melrose DG, Dreyer B, Bentall HH, et al. 1955. Elective cardiac arrest. J Thorac Cardiovasc Surg 2:21–22.
2. Hammon JW. 1995. Myocardial protection in the immature heart. Ann Thorac Surg 60:839–842.
3. Ostadal B, Ostadalova I, Dhalla NS. 1999. Development of cardiac sensitivity to oxygen deficiency: comparative and ontogenetic aspects. Physiol Rev 79(3):635–659.
4. Ostadal B, Kolar F, Parratt JR, et al. 1998. Tolerance to ischemia and ischemic preconditioning in neonatal rat heart. J Mol Cell Cardiol 30:857–865.
5. Linakis JG, Raymond RM. 1999. Effect of amiloride on age-dependent cardiac dysfunction after ischemia/reperfusion in the isolated, perfused rat heart. Shock 11:218–223.
6. Southworth R, Shattock MJ, Hearse DJ, et al. 1998. Developmental differences in superoxide production in isolated guinea-pig hearts during reperfusion. J Mol Cell Cardiol 30:1391–1399.
7. Starnes JW, Bowles DK, Seiler KS. 1997. Myocardial injury after hypoxia in immature adult and aged rats. Aging-Clin Experimental Res 9:268–276.
8. Murashita T, Borgers M, Hearse DJ. 1992. Developmental changes in tolerance to ischemia in the rabbit heart: Disparity between interpretations of structural, enzymatic and functional indices of injury. J Mol Cell Cardiol 24:1143–1154.
9. Murphy CE, Salter DR, Morris JJ, et al. 1986. Age-related differences in adenine nucleotide metabolism during in vivo global ischemia. Surg Forum 37:288–290.

10. Jonas RA. 1998. Myocardial protection for neonates and infants. Thorac Cardiovasc Surg 46:288–291.
11. Itoi T, Lopaschuk GD. 1996. Calcium improves mechanical function and carbohydrate metabolism following ischemia in isolated bi-ventricular working hearts from immature rabbits. J Mol Cell Cardiol 28:1501–1514.
12. Matherne GP, Berr SS, Headrick JP. 1996. Integration of vascular, contractile, and metabolic responses to hypoxia: Effects of maturation and adenosine. Am J Physiol 39:R895–R905.
13. Lopaschuk GD, Spafford MA. 1992. Differences in myocardial ischemic tolerance between 1-day-old and 7-day-old rabbits. Can J Physiol Pharmacol 70:1315–1323.
14. Pearl JM, Laks H, Drinkwater DC, et al. 1993. Normocalcemic blood or crystalloid cardioplegia provides better neonatal myocardial protection than does low-calcium cardioplegia. J Thorac Cardiovasc Surg 105:201–206.
15. Carr LJ, Vanderwerf QM, Anderson SE, et al. 1992. Age-related response of rabbit heart to normothermic ischemia: A 31P-MRS study. Am J Physiol 262:H391–H398.
16. Kempsford RD, Hearse DJ. 1990. Protection of the immature heart Temperature-dependent beneficial or detrimental effects of multidose crystalloid cardioplegia in the neonatal rabbit heart. J Thorac Cardiovasc Surg 99:269–279.
17. Watanabe H, Yokosawa T, Eguchi S, et al. 1989. Functional and metabolic protection of the neonatal myocardium from ischemia. Insufficient protection by cardioplegia. J Thorac Cardiovasc Surg 97:50–58.
18. Bolling K, Kronon M, Allen BS, et al. 1997. Myocardial protection in normal and hypoxically stressed neonatal hearts: The superiority of blood versus crystalloid cardioplegia. J Thorac Cardiovasc Surg 113:994–1003.
19. Karck M, Ziemer G, Haverich A. 1996. Myocardial protection in chronic volume overload hypertrophy of immature rat hearts. Eur J Cardiothorac Surg 10:690–698.
20. Corno AF, Bethencourt DM, Laks H, et al. 1987. Myocardial protection in the neonatal heart. A comparison of topical hypothermia and crystalloid and blood cardioplegic solutions. J Thorac Cardiovasc Surg 93:163–172.
21. Baker JE, Boerboom LE, Olinger GN. 1990. Is protection of ischemic neonatal myocardium by cardioplegia species dependent? J Thorac Cardiovasc Surg 99:280–287.
22. Baker EJ, Boerboom LE, Olinger GN, Baker JE. 1995. Tolerance of the developing heart to ischemia: impact of hypoximia from birth. Am J Physiol 268:H1165–H1173.
23. Taggart DP, Hadjinikolas L, Wong K, et al. 1996. Vulnerability of pediatric myocardium to cardiac surgery. Heart 76:214–217.
24. Imura H, Caputo M, Ascione R, Pawade A, Suleiman M-S, Angelini GD. Cardiac troponin I is a predictor of early clinical outcome in arterial switch operation. Presented at the 14th Annual Meeting of the European Association for Cardio-Thoracic Surgery. Frankfurt 7–11 October 2000; Abstract Book: P140.
25. Suleiman M-S, Dihmis WC, Caputo M, et al. 1997. Changes in myocardial concentration of glutamate and aspartate during coronary artery surgery. Am J Physiol 272:H1063–H1069.
26. Caputo M, Ascione R, Angelini GD, et al. 1998. The end of the cold era: from intermittent cold to intermittent warm blood cardioplegia. Eur J Cardiothorac Surg 14:467–475.
27. Caputo M, Dihmis WC, Bryan AJ, et al. 1998. Warm blood hyperkalaemic reperfusion (hot shot) prevents myocardial substrate derangement in patients undergoing coronary artery bypass surgery. Eur J Cardiothorac Surg 13:559–564.
28. Caputo M, Bryan AJ, Calafiore AM, et al. 1998. Intermittent antegrade hyperkalemic warm blood cardioplegia supplemented with magnesium prevents myocardial substrate derangement in patients undergoing coronary artery bypass surgery. Eur J Cardiothoracic Surg 14:596–601.
29. Smolensky RT, Lachno DR, Ledingham SJM, et al. 1996. Determination of sixteen nucleotides, nucleosides and bases using high-performance liquid chromatography and its application to the study of purine metabolism in hearts for transplantation. J Chromatography 527:414–420.
30. Cyran SE, Phillips J, Ditty S, et al. 1993. Developmental differences in cardiac myocyte calcium homeostasis after steady-state potassium depolarization-mechanisms and implications for cardioplegia. J Pediat 122:77–83.
31. Goodwin GW, Taegtmeyer. 2000. Improved energy homeostasis of the heart in the metabolic state of exercise. Am J Physiol (in press).
32. Baker JE, Curry BD, Olinger GN, et al. 1997. Increased tolerance of the chronically hypoxic immature heart to ischemia Contribution of the KATP channel. Circulation 95:1278–1285.

33. Buckberg GD. 1995. Update on current techniques of myocardial protection. Ann Thorac Surg 60:805–814.
34. Mudge GH, Mills RM, Taegtmeyer H, et al. 1976. Alterations of myocardial aminoacid metabolism in chronic ischaemic heart disease. J Clin Invest 58:1185–1192.
35. Pisarenko OI. 1996. Mechanisms of myocardial protection by amino acids: facts and hypothesis. Clin Exp Pharm Physiol 23:627–633.

B. Ostadal, M. Nagano and N.S. Dhalla (eds.).
CARDIAC DEVELOPMENT. Copyright © 2002.
Kluwer Academic Publishers. Boston.
All rights reserved.

MOLECULAR PHENOTYPE OF THE DEVELOPING HEART WITH A CONGENITAL ANOMALY

THEODORUS H.F. PETERS,[1,2] LENNART KLOMPE,[1,2] AD J.J.C. BOGERS,[2] and HARI S. SHARMA[1]

Departments of [1] Pharmacology and [2] Cardio-thoracic Surgery, Erasmus University Medical Center Rotterdam, Rotterdam, The Netherlands

Summary. A high prevalence of congenital heart malformations accounts for defects in the outflow tract accompanied with right ventricular hypertrophy (RVH), such as in case of tetralogy of Fallot (ToF) and in pulmonary atresia (PA) with a ventricular septal defect (VSD). The etiology and contributing molecular events in cardiovascular malformations are poorly understood. These patients require primary corrective surgical repair at young age, which is now a treatment of choice where closing of the VSD and removing the right ventricular outflow tract obstruction are performed. In the past years, we have been investigating the myocardial molecular phenotype at various stages of RVH in ToF and PA/VSD. In the study, summarised in this chapter, we assessed the surface area of cells in right ventricular biopsies and examined the myocardial fibrosis by measuring total collagen and fibronectin expression both at mRNA and protein level. Assessment of myocardial cell hypertrophy revealed significantly enlarged (p < 0.01) cells in adult (>25 yr.) patients with ToF as compared to age matched controls. Immunohistochemical staining of biopsies for collagen followed by video image analysis showed significantly enhanced interstitial collagen levels in adult ToF as compared to young (<2 yr.) controls (p < 0.05) and young ToF patients (p < 0.01). In PA/VSD patients however, interstitial collagen levels did not change as compared to respective age matched controls. Interestingly, peri-vascular collagen deposition increased in young ToF patients as compared to young and adult controls. In contrast, the staining levels of both collagens and fibronectin were lower in the PA/VSD patients as compared to respective controls. Interstitial expression of fibronectin in ToF patents remained unchanged. RT-PCR

Address for correspondence: Hari S. Sharma, M.Phil., Ph.D., Institute of Pharmacology, Erasmus University Medical Center, Dr. Molewaterplein 50, 3015 GE Rotterdam, The Netherlands. Tel: + 31 10 4087963; Fax: + 31 10 408 9458; e-mail: SHARMA@FARMA.FGG.EUR.NL

analysis for collagen Iα, collagen III and fibronectin expression levels in PA/VSD patients showed only higher collagen III mRNA expression in PA/VSD patients as compared to respective age matched controls. We conclude that the enhanced myocyte size and increased extracellular matrix deposition and disarray of collagen and fibronectin are signs of fibrosis during RVH that contribute to diminished right ventricular function in patients with ToF and PA/VSD.

Key words: tetralogy of Fallot, right ventricle, hypertrophy, pulmonary atresia, and fibrosis

INTRODUCTION

The high mortality rate in children with congenital heart disease (CHD), a most common human birth defect, remains a major challenge in paediatric care world wide. Tetralogy of Fallot (ToF) is a common form of cyanotic congenital heart disease. One of the main features of ToF is right ventricular hypertrophy (RVH) due to pressure overload caused by (sub) pulmonary stenosis and/or due to volume overload caused by a ventricular septal defect [1]. ToF can be characterised by a subaortic ventricular septum defect (VSD), dextroposition of the aorta orifice (overriding the VSD), (sub)valvular pulmonary stenosis, resulting in hypoxemia due to diminished pulmonary flow [1]. The infundibular pulmonary stenosis can be more or less severe depending on the degree of malformation, the prominence of the outlet septum and the extent of RVH. Complete obstruction of the right ventricular outflow tract in ToF is known as pulmonary atresia with ventricular septal defect (PA/VSD). This complicated form of ToF with PA/VSD has been found to be associated with the presence of multiple systemic aorto-pulmonary collateral arteries (SPCAs). The VSD and right ventricular outflow tract obstruction lead to an equal systolic pressure in both ventricles and aorta, causing a varying degree of right to left shunting with central cyanosis and hypoxemia.

Without appropriate treatment, ToF ultimately results in cyanotic complications and cardiac failure. For these reasons, nearly 70% of patients with ToF require an operation during the first year of life [2]. Primary corrective surgical repair at young age is the treatment of choice and consists of closing the VSD and removing the right ventricular outflow tract obstruction. The aim of this strategy is to relieve the hypoxemia, to eliminate the stimulus for the adaptive RVH as well as preserving right ventricular function and electrical stability of the myocardium [3] and to encourage the normal development of the pulmonary vasculature [4]. If the pulmonary arterial system is incomplete or small, palliative surgery may improve the clinical situation and prepare for later correction. Due to improved peri-operative care, the results of primary repair have increased dramatically in the past decades. On long-term follow up some patients however, show pulmonary regurgitation after primary correction, causing right ventricular failure due to volume-overload. For these patients further secondary corrective surgery later in life is performed by implanting a pulmonary allograft heart valve between the right ventricle and the pulmonary artery. Despite adequate surgical procedures, it is not yet established that the RVH will completely regress and normal cardiac performance takes place. Therefore, it is our working hypothesis that molecular and cellular characteristics of the right ventricular myocardium at corrective and redo surgery will correlate with the clinical condition of the patient and with cardiac prognosis. However, no data are available on myocardial phenotype in human ToF.

Right ventricular hypertrophy

Right ventricular hypertrophy with expansion of cardio-myocytes in human ToF, is a response to the increased pressure overload caused by (sub) pulmonary stenosis or atresia in combination with the ventricular septal defect. Those responses lead to remodelling of the myocardium and to the development of fibrosis [5,3,6]. Changes in cardiac extracellular matrix proteins have been observed in association with cardiac hypertrophy [6,7]. Recently, a histopathological study on ToF myocardial tissue biopsies reported that the myocardial cell diameter was reduced in postoperative patients as compared to preoperative patients with ToF, but postoperative cellular diameter was still larger than that in the age matched normal subjects [8,9]. These findings suggest that RVH after corrective surgery of ToF can regress to some extent provided that residual pulmonary stenosis can be avoided. Until now, no data on molecular markers or their dynamics in RVH in human ToF are available. Several animal models of ventricular hypertrophy have been described [10–13], but none can approximate the ToF situation in humans.

Experimental animal studies however have provided some insight into the morphological and cellular changes in the hypertrophic myocardium in response to volume or pressure overload. A battery of genes including immediate early genes (like proto-oncogenes, c-fos, c-jun and c-myc), genes from the fetal period (like ANF, β-MHC and α-skeletal actin) and several other extracellular matrix regulating genes have been implicated in the cellular alterations leading to ventricular hypertrophy [10–12]. It is believed that alterations in gene expression reflect a shift towards a more embryonic program [14] that might play an important role in the myocardial adaptation in response to increased work load [15]. Furthermore, it is known from animal studies that inhibitors of angiotensin-converting enzyme can reverse the accumulation of fibrotic material [16] and provide further support for the suggestion that the trigger for extracellular matrix production during cardiac hypertrophy is induced by circulating substances [17].

Beside the morphological changes of the cardio-myocytes during hypertrophy, the myocardium require proportionate increase of coronary flow or growth of the coronary vasculature (angiogenesis) to compensate for the increased workload. It has been suggested that mechanical factors like stretch, shear stress, and wall tension may provide an initial stimulus for capillary angiogenesis during cardiac hypertrophy [13]. A number of peptide growth factors, like VEGF and TGF-β_1, are believed to play a role in modulating the angiogenesis during cardiac hypertrophy. However, it is still not clarified whether those altered expression patterns are general markers of cardiac hypertrophy or markers of a specific parallel pathogenic process such as in case of ToF. The information on the complex cascade of molecular mechanisms contributing to RVH in human cases of ToF is very limited and warrants further investigations.

Myocardial fibrosis

RVH leads to remodelling of the myocardium and to the accumulation of fibrotic material [5,18,3]. Under normal physiological conditions, collagenous cardiac proteins or extracellular matrix proteins, like collagen, fibronectin, glycoproteins, proteoglycans and elastin, serve for organisation and support of myocytes and the capillary network [19]. They direct among other things contractile force generated by cardiac myocytes, contribute to the passive stretch characteristics of the ventricle and serve to restore the ventricular myocytes to precontraction length. The increased accumulation of extracellular matrix proteins during myocardial fibrosis results in an increase of myocardial muscle stiffness and declining contractile performance [17,5]. Fibronectin and collagen type I and III are major components of the interstitial fibrillar network and it is assumed that the encoding genes are regulated by fibroblasts [5,6,17]. Animal studies showed increased level of mRNA of those markers during cardiac hypertrophy. Also the expression of TGF-β_1 is upregulated during pressure overload cardiac hypertrophy, which is believed to be one of the mechanisms by which fibrosis is activated in the heart. Active TGF-β_1 increases fibronectin and collagen expression in a variety of cell types and stimulates their incorporation in the extracellular matrix [5,6,20].

Collagens: One of the major contributing factors to myocardial fibrosis is a disproportionate accumulation, either reactive or reparative, of collagens [21–24]. Collagen fibers are organised in the collagen network found in the extracellular space of the myocardium [21,24]. The collagen concentration of the right ventricle is about 30% greater than the left ventricle, because its myocytes are smaller [25] and the highest depositions have been observed in the outflow tract and subendocardium [26]. The myocytes represent only one-third of the number of cells, but their volume accounts for over two-third of the myocardium, whereas the number of fibroblasts may represent as much as two-third of the cells [27]. There are five collagen subtypes present in the myocardium, type I, III, IV, V and VI. Most collagen subtypes in the heart are exclusively produced by cardiac fibroblasts [21]. The I and III collagen subtypes are the most abundant forms. Collagen type I represents 80% of the total cardiac collagen content and is the major collagenous product of cardiac fibroblasts [21], which is important for the cardiac strength and stiffness [24]. Collagen type III represents about 12% of total cardiac collagen content and participate in tissue elasticity [21,28]. The collagen fibres have several supporting and structural functions to provide myocardial stiffness and tensile strenghth [23,29,30]. When the collagen network is damaged, the myocyte support is compromised and allows tissue expansion [31]. Experimental [32] and clinical data [33] show that a rise in the collagen and fibronectin content increases the myocardial stiffness and promotes abnormalities of cardiac function during hypertrophy. Studying the expression and localization of genes encoding for fibronectin, collagens and collagenases at all stages of RVH in ToF may further elucidate the dynamics of the collagen network and myocardial fibrosis.

Fibronectin: Fibronectin is a glycoprotein located in the extracellular matrix and serves as a bridge between cardiac myocytes and interstitial collagen mesh network [19]. In the myocardium, fibronectin is homogeneously localised throughout the extracellular space. During the development of cardiac hypertrophy due to pressure overload, fetal fibronectin has been shown to accumulate in rats [32]. Fibronectin binds collagen and modulates the collagen fibrillogenesis, resulting in higher collagen type I concentration and a lower collagen type III concentration [34]. Fibronectin has been found to influence diverse processes including cell growth, adhesion, migration, and wound repair. Both fibronectin and collagen (subtype I and III) were found to be up regulated during RVH in humans [5].

MATERIALS AND METHODS

Right ventricular biopsies

The study was approved by the Medical Ethical Committee of the University Hospital Rotterdam (MEC153.268/1996/119). The group of patients operated upon for correction of ToF (ToF-1) consisted of 16 patients. The younger patients are grouped in the ToF-1a group (12 patients) with a mean age of 0.8 years (range 0.4–1.8 years) at the time of operation. The older patients are grouped in the ToF-1b group (4 patients), their mean age at the time of operation was 31.6 years (range 30.6–34.0 years). The group of patients operated upon for pulmonary allograft implantation late after correction of ToF (ToF-2) consisted of 9 patients, with a mean age of 30.0 years (range 19.3–38.8 years). The group of patients operated for the correction of PA/VSD consisted of 14 patients with a mean age of 2.54 years (range 0.76–5.51 years). The control group consisted of 11 heart donors who died due to non-cardiac complications and was further sub-divided in to young control group (C-1, n = 5) with a mean age of 4.9 years (range 0.0–13.3 years) and adult control group (C-2, n = 6) with a mean age of 29.8 (range 21.6–44.6 years). ToF-1 group consisted of removed endomyocardial tissue from the right ventricular outflow tract of patients with preserved pulmonary valve function or a transmural sample from the incision level of anterior right ventricular wall of patients with a transannular patch. In late secondary surgery after correction of ToF (ToF-2) pulmonary allografts were implanted as previously described [35,36] and biopsies consisted of tissue from the anterior free wall of the right ventricle. At clinical analysis all ToF-1 patients showed RVH and all ToF-2 patients showed RVH as well as right ventricular dilatation. There was no operative or other early mortality. There were no complications that could be attributed to taking the biopsies. Part of the myocardial tissue biopsies were fixed in 4% paraformaldehyde in PBS for 24 hours at room temperature and further processed for dehydration and embedding in paraffin for histological and immunohistochemical studies. Another part was immediately frozen in liquid nitrogen for mRNA expression studies.

Gomori reticuline staining

For determining the myocyte surface area, the cell (membrane) reticuline fibres were stained by routine Gomori's reticuline staining technique [37] in 5 μm thick sections. After the silver staining was developed, slides were mounted and visualised under light microscope.

Collagen staining

The total collagen in myocardial tissue specimens was stained with Picro-sirius Red F3BA (Polysciences, Northampton, UK) as described earlier [22,23]. Tissue sections of 5 μm thickness, were treated with 0.2% aqueous phosphomolybdic acid and incubated in 0.1% Picro-sirius Red. Before dehydration, the slides were treated with 0.01 N HCl and mounted. Slides were visualised under the light microscope and eventually collagen contents were quantified using video image analysis system.

Immunohistochemical localisation of fibronectin

For fibronectin staining, 5 μm thickness sections on slides were pre-treated for antigen retrieval in a microwave in pre-warmed citrate buffer and boiled for 20 minutes. Non-specific binding sites were blocked by 10% normal goat serum in phosphate buffered saline containing 5% bovine serum albumin. Specific primary antibodies against human fibronectin (Clone Ab-3, Neomarkers, Fremont, CA, USA) in 1 : 150 dilution were applied to the sections and incubated overnight at 4°C. Positive control was performed by using an anti-human mouse monoclonal alpha-smooth muscle actin (α-SMA) antibody (clone 1A4; BioGenex, San Ramon, CA, USA) in a dilution of 1 : 1000. Negative control was prepared by the omission of the primary antibody. After washing in 0.5% tween-20 in PBS solution, the sections were incubated with mouse biotinylated anti-rabbit IgG for 30 min and subsequently, with peroxidase conjugated streptavidin. Red color for fibronectin detection was developed during 30 minutes using a mixture, of Naphtol AS-MX phosphate (N5000), new fuchsine, sodium nitrite, Tris (pH 8.0) and levamisol. Sections were counter stained with haematoxylin, mounted and visualised under light microscope.

Quantitative video image analysis

Expression of fibronectin as well as collagens was quantitatively analysed using a video image analysis system. After staining, the sections were mounted and visualised under light microscope (Leica DM RBE, Leica GmbH, Wetzlar, Germany). From each section, series of 12 digital colour images from a representative area of the myocardium were taken and analysed for positive staining using Leica Qwin standard (Y2.2b) image analysis software package (Leica Imaging Systems Ltd., Cambrige, England). After optimisation of the staining detection levels for hue, saturation and intensity, all images derived from a single batch of staining were analysed. Interstitial expression was represented as staining per total tissue area, excluding vascular areas, whereas peri-vascular localisation was depicted as staining per peri-vascular area. Since the peri-vascular collagen area (PVCA) and vessel luminal area (VA) are positively correlated, the stained PVCA was normalised to the VA and represented as PVCA/VA ratio [15]. In the same way the peri-vascular fibronectin area (PVFA) was normalised for the VA and represented as PVFA/VA ratio. Myocyte cell size was measured with the same set-up and software. From each section 3–4 digital images were stored saved as "tif" file after visualising and photographing with a 20× (adult) or 40× (young) lens. The myocyte membrane, of at least 20 transversely cut myocytes containing a nucleus, per section were drawn manually and the myocyte surface area was calculated as μm^2.

Isolation of total cellular RNA and RT-PCR

Right ventricular tissue biopsies (50–100 mg) were homogenised in guanidinium isothiocyanate buffer and processed for the extraction of total cellular RNA according to the methods described elsewhere [38]. The RNA concentration was measured spectrophotometrically and RNA quality was tested on a denatured formaldehyde agarose gel. First strand cDNA was synthesised from 2 μg of total cellular RNA of each patient using Promega's Universal RiboClone cDNA Synthesis System (Promega, BNL, Leiden) with Molony murine Leukemia virus reverse transcriptase (M-MLV RT) and random hexamer primers (Promega, BNL, Leiden) in a final volume of 25 μl. For each PCR-reaction 2 μl cDNA, 0.5 μM specific forward and reverse primer were added to a PCR-reaction mixture containing 0.5 units of AmpliTaq Gold DNA polymerase (Perkin Elmer, Roche Molecular Systems Inc., New Jersey, USA) in a final volume of 20 μl. The PCR amplification profile involved an initial denaturation step at 94°C for 10 minutes, followed by 35 cycles of denaturation at 94°C for 1 minute, primer annealing at 55°C for 30 seconds, and extension at 72°C for 1 minute and 30 seconds, followed by a final extension step at 72°C for 10 minutes in a thermal cycler model PTC-100 (MJ Research, Inc., Watertown, USA). Appropriate oligonucleotide primers for the PCR reaction were designed from the published human specific sequences employing computer software, DNA-man (Version 3.2) (Lynnon, BioSoft.). Specific primers were designed for Collagen Iα [39]; (forward: 5′-GATGCCAATGTGGTTCGTGA-3′, reverse: 5′-GCTGTAGGTGAAGCGGCTGT-3′, collagen III [40] forward: 5′-CAGTGGAC CTCCTGGCAAAG-3′, reverse: 5′-TGTCCACCAGTGTTTCCGTG-3′ and for fibronectin [41] (forward: 5′-CACCATCCAACCTGCGTTTC-3′, reverse: 5′-TGTCCTACATTCGGCGGGT-3′) and purchased from Sigma-Genosys Ltd. (Sigma-Genosys Ltd., Cambridge, UK). Oligonucleotide primers for β-actin [42] (forward: 5′-TGACGGGGTCACCCACACTGTGCCCATCTA-3′, reverse: 5′-ACTCGTCATACTCCTGCTTGCTGATCCA-3′ were purchased from Gibco BRL Custom Primers (Life Technologies BV, Breda).

Quantitative analysis of PCR products

The PCR amplified products for collagen Iα, III and fibronectin were analysed on a 1.5% agarose gel and compared with the β-actin bands. The gels were digitally photographed with an alpha-Imager 950 (Version 3.24) documentation system (Biozym, Landgraaf, The Netherlands). Quantification was done by measuring the intensity of the bands with a molecular analyst (Version 1.5) image analysis program (Biorad Laboratories, Hercules, CA) after correcting for the background. The intensity values of bands for individual molecule were divided with β-actin band of each respective patient and fold induction of collagens or fibronectin was assessed. The specific primer set originally designed for a 531 bp fibronectin product, also amplified a splice variant of the 456 bp. The two products appeared to be the result of alternative splicing of a common precursor. When the quantitative PCR analysis was done, both the bands were taken for optical density measurements.

Statistical analysis

The video-image analysis and mRNA expression quantitative data were calculated from different groups and the results were expressed as mean ± SEM. Statistical probability was assessed by (non-parametric) Kruskal-Wallis one way analysis of variance as well as by student's "t" test. Results were accepted as statistically significant with $p \leq 0.05$.

RESULTS

In this study, we examined the level of cell hypertrophy and degree of fibrosis at different stages of the developing heart in patients with ToF. To assess the level of (cell) hypertrophy, we measured the surface area of transversely cut nucleated myocytes in right ventricular biopsies. We have also examined the magnitude of cardiac fibrosis by quantitatively investigating the total collagen and fibronectin expression both at protein and mRNA level in patients with ToF.

Assessment of myocardial cell hypertrophy

To determine the level of myocyte hypertrophy the myocyte (membrane) reticuline fibers were stained and the myocyte surface area was assessed by video image analysis. The myocyte surface area showed no significant increase in ToF-1a group as compared to age matched controls ($270 \pm 24\,\mu m^2$ vs. $203 \pm 70\,\mu m^2$), whereas in ToF-1b group, surface area was enhanced 1.7 times as compared to C-2 ($866.6 \pm 210\,\mu m^2$ vs. $498 \pm 50\,\mu m^2$, $p > 0.05$). However, the cell surface area in case of ToF-2 was found to be significantly increased as compared to age matched control C-2 ($1653 \pm 182\,\mu m^2$ vs. $498 \pm 50\,\mu m^2$, $p < 0.01$), indicating for clear myocardial hypertrophy.

Myocardial expression of collagen and fibronectin

Picro-sirius Red staining for total collagens depicted myocardial collagen localisation pattern in the interstitium as well as in peri-vascular areas in all patients. The extracellular matrix and myocyte distribution in ToF patients showed differences in the cellular organisation and myocyte shape compared to age matched controls [43]. Controls showed nice pattern of grouped uniform shaped myocytes in long muscle bundles surrounded by tight collagen bundles, which form a supportive network to the myocytes (Fig. 1). In the adult control group mean part of the collagen is localised in those thick long fibber bundles which serve as a border between myocyte bundles. The ToF-patients however, showed disarrayed, less uniform in shape and uncoordinated myocytes. At the sub-endocardial side collagen content has increased a lot as compared to the controls and tight collagen bundles were invading from the endocardium into the mid myocardium. In ToF-1a collagen fibres were randomly localised in the interstitium, in dots and smaller bundles (Fig. 1). The collagen layer around the myocytes in ToF-2 was increased as compared to control and especially near the sub-endocardium where some individual myocytes were surrounded by a tight collagen layer. The ToF-2 myocytes were disarrayed or they were arranged in smaller myocyte groups and could not form muscle bundles (data not shown). Video image analysis of interstitial collagen expression data is depicted in Fig. 2. The results showed significantly enhanced levels in ToF-2 as compared to ToF-1a ($p < 0.01$) and C-2 compared to C-1 ($p < 0.05$). In the normalised peri-vascular collagen area significant differences in the PVCA/VA ratio were found in ToF-1a as compared to C-1, C-2 and ToF-2 (all $p < 0.01$) and no differences were observed among C-1, C-2, ToF-2 and ToF1b. Interstitial collagen levels in PA/VSD patients remained unchanged as compared to controls (Fig. 2 panel A). However, for the normalised peri-vascular collagen area the PVCA/VA ratio was significantly lower in these patients as compared to controls ($p < 0.01$) (Fig. 2C).

Myocardial localisation of fibronectin in ToF-patients showed that the expression was confined to the interstitial and peri-vascular region, as well as to the cytoplasm of some cardio-myocytes. The staining pattern for fibronectin fibres was quite similar as for total collagen's, but less dense. Fibronectin fibres were localised more in dots, short fibres bundles and around the myocytes in ToF-patients as compared to respective controls. In control patients fibronectin fibres bundles support and co-ordinate the myocyte bundles and tissue, whereas in the ToF patients there was a disarray of myocytes. Furthermore, fibronectin fibres around the myocytes were more abundant and more randomly distributed in ToF-1 as compared to C-1 [44]. In ToF-2 the fibronectin layer around the myocytes was missing but at the sub endocardial side the fibronectin was abundantly available. Video image analysis of interstitial expression of fibronectin in ToF patients showed unaltered expression of this extracellular matrix protein as compared to the respective controls except in case of PA/VSD group where the fibronectin levels decreased as compared to the age matched control ($p < 0.05$). The normalised peri-vascular fibronectin area, the PVFA/VA ratio was significantly higher in the ToF-2 group as compared to the age matched control (7.1 ± 1.2 vs. 3.7 ± 0.5, $p < 0.03$). Fibronectin levels were also higher in ToF-2 when compared to ToF-1a (5.8 ± 0.6) and ToF-1b (4.2 ± 1.3). Interestingly, in ToF-1a the fibronectin levels remained unchanged when compared with the age matched C-1 (3.5 ± 1.1). The normalised peri-vascular fibronectin stained area, the PVFA/VA ratio showed a significantly decreased level in the PA/VSD group as compared to controls ($p = 0.02$).

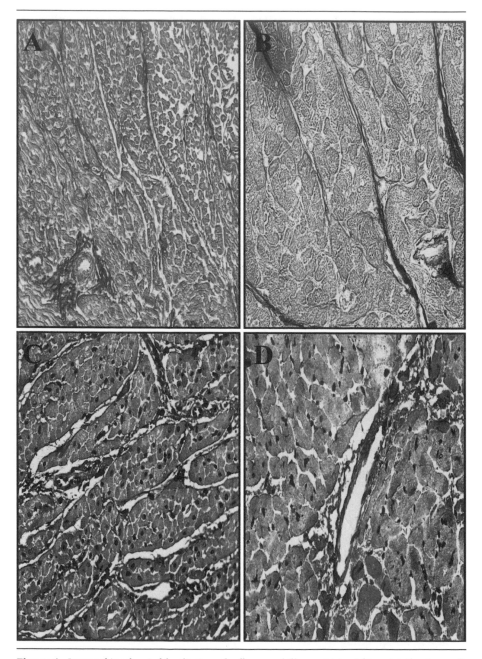

Figure 1. Immunohistochemical localisation of collagen and fibronectin in right ventricular tissue of patients with PA/VSD and age matched controls. Micro-photographs (200× magnification) showing human right ventricular tissue stained with picro-sirius red for collagen (A and B) and with human specific antibodies for fibronectin (C and D) (as described in Materials and methods). Panel A and C depict control donors whereas, panel B and D represent the patients from PA/VSD group. The staining represents collagen and fibronectin fibres localised in peri-vascular as well as in interstitial tissue area.

Tissue Specific Expression of Fibrosis Markers

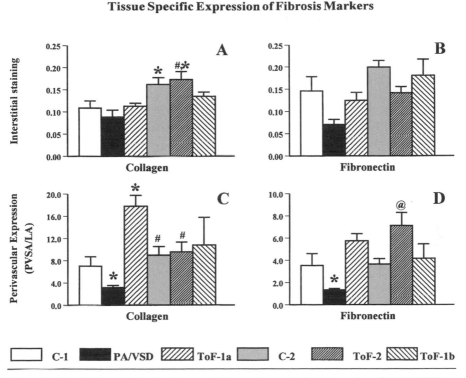

| C-1 | PA/VSD | ToF-1a | C-2 | ToF-2 | ToF-1b |

Figure 2. Quantitative analysis of collagen and fibronectin protein levels in patients with PA/VSD and tetralogy of Fallot. The protein levels of collagen and fibronectin in PA/VSD and ToF-patients were quantified using video image analysis for interstitial (panel A and B) and peri-vascular (panel C and D) areas. The results were presented as the ratio between interstitial red stained area and total tissue area (panel A and B) and peri-vascular fibronectin stained area (PVSA) corrected for the vessel luminal area (LA) (panel B and C). Values are shown as mean ± SEM. The significance differences (p < 0.05) were marked as compared; * with C-1; # with ToF-1 and @ with C-2.

Analysis of fibronectin and collagen mRNAs by RT-PCR

RT-PCR was performed to assess the mRNA expression levels of collagen and fibronectin in PA/VSD patients and control donors in a semi-quantitative way. We determined collagen Iα, collagen III and fibronectin mRNA expression in 9 patients who underwent surgery for PA/VSD and compared the levels with 3 age matched controls. Optical densitometric analysis of the amplified products showed that collagen III gene expression levels were significantly higher (p = 0.03) in patients with PA/VSD as compared to controls. Whereas, collagen Iα and fibronectin mRNA levels in patients with PA/VSD did not alter as compared to the respective controls.

DISCUSSION

In this study we have shown that right ventricular hypertrophy in patients who underwent secondary surgery for ToF is verified at the level of cardiomyocytes as

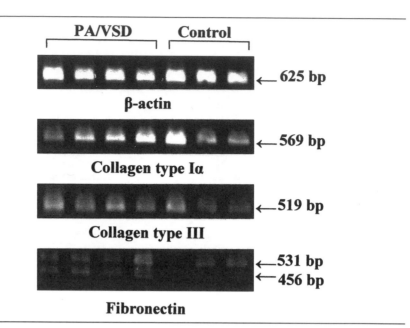

Figure 3. RT-PCR analysis of fibronectin, collagen Iα and collagen III expression. Using specific oligonucleotide primers, fibronectin, collagen Iα and collagen III and the internal standard β-actin mRNAs were amplified by RT-PCR and analysed on an agarose gel by ethidium bromide staining. The RT-PCR products for fibronectin (531 and 456 bp—two splice variants), collagen Iα (569 bp) and collagen III (519 bp) in PA/VSD patients and controls were quantitatively compared with the internal standard β-actin (625 bp).

being the surface area of these cells highly enlarged. Our data further elaborate on the histopathological findings from the right ventricular myocardium in preoperative ToF that show interstitial fibrosis, myofibrillar disorganisation, disarray and degenerative changes in addition to myocardial cell hypertrophy. These finding on myocardial fibrosis are in agreement and an elaboration on previous studies done on a fewer number of patients with ToF [45,6].

The amount of fibrosis in young ToF-1a patients was not much altered as compared to age matched controls which is in accordance with earlier findings of Schwartz and colleagues [6]. In our study the adult patients, ToF-1b have lower fibrotic levels, most probably because those patients got primary correction at adult age due to the complications earlier in life where less severe. Although, ToF-1a patients showed no or less increase in fibrotic levels and myocyte surface size their myocardium has already responded to the stress factors which are expressed in the clear difference in myocardial localisation of collagen and fibronectin fibres and disarray of myocytes as described in the results. Other morphometrical studies also report that increased myocardial fibrosis in ToF is associated with increased myocyte diameter and myocardial disarray [45]. Furthermore post mortem analysis of ToF myocardium showed normal degree of fibrosis levels in the left ventricle and abnormal increased levels in the right ventricle of patients older then 1 year with an increase in outflow tract and sub-endocardium [6]. Taken together, our data on myocardial fibrosis supports the policy for primary repair at a young age to diminish the myocardial damage.

Our findings on the peri-vascular collagen and fibronectin expression indicate that the levels are already high in patients with ToF at a very young age (ToF-1a) and remains elevated later in life (ToF-2). This might indicate that surgical correction at young age could be an adequate treatment to regulate peri-vascular fibrosis. The early increase of (peri-vascular) collagen deposition in the right ventricle as found in our study at early primary correction may occur because the original myocardial extracellular matrix has been expanded and weakened due to the hemodynamic overload. The myocardium perhaps would attempt to compensate until enough new collagen has been produced to restore tensile strength and to resist the distending forces. Our findings in the ToF-1a and ToF-2 group fit into this concept as the ToF-2 showed a more prominent increase in the amount of collagen as compared to ToF-1a. Corrective surgery limits the myocardial overload and may therefore limit the amount of damage to the myocardial collagen matrix [31].

When we compare the expression levels of the fibrosis markers in patients with PA/VSD and ToF-1a, we found unchanged patterns for interstitial collagen as well as fibronectin, whereas the peri-vascular collagen area corrected for lumen area were higher in ToF-1a and lower in patients with PA/VSD as compared to their age matched controls. These results suggest a poor accumulation of collagen and fibronectin matrix around the vessels in PA/VSD patients and point to a less well developed extracellular matrix support for their coronary blood vessels. An altered biosynthesis of the collagen and fibronectin net work may be responsible for abnormal cardiac performance in these patients. As fibronectin binds to collagen and modulates the collagen fibrillogenesis, resulting in higher collagen subtype Iα and a lower collagen type III expression [34]. Decreased levels of fibronectin would consequently result in less fibrillogenesis resulting in lower collagen type Iα and higher collagen type III levels, as we found in our study. As collagen type I accounts for 80% of the total collagen content in the cardiac tissue, a down regulation of this gene would result in decreased levels of fibrosis. Enhanced levels for collagen III could also be attributed to the altered myocardial architecture towards hypoxic as well as hypertrophic state in patients with PA/VSD. Furthermore, the enhanced levels of collagen III mRNA in PA/VSD group may also arise due to the decreased degradation of the mRNA for collagen III. Interestingly, enhanced levels of collagen III mRNA could not lead to the elevated levels of total collagen protein as we observed unchanged values for total collagen in two groups studied indicating for its enhanced mRNA stability. Other studies have shown that cardiac collagen from normal and hypertrophied myocardium differs qualitatively [46]. In this study also we observed qualitative differences in the collagen localisation in patients with ToF as compared to controls. The decreased absolute cardiac contents for collagens in PA/VSD patients in their hypertrophied myocardium could be attributed to the relative low extractability of these collagens, due to decreased intramolecular cross-linking [46].

The changes as found in our study for collagen and fibronectin expression may be attributed to an altered structure or function of the myocardium. We believe that changes in gene expression accompanying cardiac hypertrophy are the result of a multifactorial process and the observed changes may therefore be concomitant phenomena. The changes in the right ventricular collagen expression in ToF patients could be a result of increased hemodynamic load with a parallel increase in ventricular mass [6,14]. Although in our study myocardial staining for collagens seems to be intense, it has been reported earlier that the myocardium near the right ventricular outflow tract contains higher collagen levels [6] compared to areas around the septum or apex. Furthermore the myocyte cell size has increased in the hypertrophied heart which might influence our data on the myocardial fibrosis. We expressed our staining data as a ratio between the area of staining and total tissue area but it should bear in mind that the enlarged cells will increase the total tissue area per digital image and consequently decrease the staining ratio. Consequently, an increased myocardial fibrosis in a hypertrophied heart may not be noted.

SUMMARY AND CONCLUSIONS

In conclusion, from the data presented in this chapter, it becomes evident that the patients with ToF have abnormal myocardial architecture as the expression pattern of two major fibrosis markers, collagen and fibronectin were altered both at mRNA and protein levels. The study provides further evidence for the increased amount of myocardial extracellular matrix deposition in the interstitium as well as around the vessels in the right ventricular tissue of ToF-patients. Beside the enhanced fibrotic levels, increased myocyte surface area and myocytes disarray was observed in patients who underwent surgery for ToF, which is a clear sign for a cellular hypertrophic state of the myocardium. Interestingly, in patients with extreme form of ToF, the PA/VSD patients interstitial collagen and fibronectin contents remained unchanged which could be due to a fact of a poor quality of collagen and fibronectin fibres giving rise to low values under video image analysis. Furthermore in these patients, peri-vascular collagen as well as fibronectin levels even decreased indicating for a poorly developed extracellular matrix support for their coronary vessels. The disorganisation and disarray of myocardial extracellular matrix in patients with ToF and PA/VSD could play an important functional role in the development of arrhythmias as observed prior to the primary and secondary surgery in these patients. Our data support the notion for the early surgical intervention in patients with ToF and could assist in contemporary patient management and care. Our findings might also help in further improvement of clinical treatment of patients with ToF and PA/VSD, especially in the timing for surgery, and possibly predict for long term postoperative prognosis.

ACKNOWLEDGEMENTS

Financial support from the Netherlands Heart Foundation (NHS 96.082) is gratefully acknowledged. We thank the Heart Valve Bank, Rotterdam for providing us with control biopsies.

REFERENCES

1. Bogers AJ, van der Laarse A, Vliegen HW, Quaegebeur JM, Hollaar L, Egas JM, Cornelisse CJ, Rohmer J, Huysmans HA. 1988. Assessment of hypertrophy in myocardial biopsies taken during correction of congenital heart disease. Thorac Cardiovasc Surgeon 36:137–140.
2. Pozzi M, Trivedi DB, Kitchiner D, Arnold RA. 2000. Tetralogy of Fallot: what operation, at which age. Eur J Cardiothorac Surg 17:631–636.
3. Starnes VA, Luciani GB, Latter DA, Griffin ML. 1994. Current surgical management of tetralogy of Fallot. Ann Thorac Surg 58:211–215.
4. Warner KG, Anderson JE, Fulton DR, Payne DD, Geggel RL, Marx GR. 1993. Restoration of the pulmonary valve reduces right ventricular volume overload after previous repair of tetralogy of Fallot. Circulation 88:II189–197.
5. Murphy JG, Gersh BJ, Mair DD, Fuster V, McGoon MD, Ilstrup DM, McGoon DC, Kirklin JW, Danielson GK. 1993. Long-term outcome in patients undergoing surgical repair of tetralogy of Fallot. N Engl J Med 329:593–599.
6. Schwartz SM, Gordon D, Mosca RS, Bove EL, Heidelberger KP, Kulik TJ. 1996. Collagen content in normal, pressure, and pressure-volume overloaded developing human hearts. Am J Cardiol 77:734–738.
7. Arai M, Matsui H, Periasamy M. 1994. Sarcoplasmic reticulum gene expression in cardiac hypertrophy and heart failure. Circ Res 74:555–564.
8. Mitsuno M, Nakano S, Shimazaki Y, Taniguchi K, Kawamoto T, Kobayashi J, Matsuda H, Kawashima Y. 1993. Fate of right ventricular hypertrophy in tetralogy of Fallot after corrective surgery. Am J Cardiol 72:694–698.
9. Seliem MA, Wu YT, Glenwright K. 1995. Relation between age at surgery and regression of right ventricular hypertrophy in tetralogy of Fallot. Pediatr Cardiol 16:53–55.
10. Bishop SP. 1984. Structural alterations in the hypertrophied and failing myocardium. In: Functional aspects of the normal hypertrophied and failing heart. Eds. FL Abel and WH Hewman, 278–300. The Hague: Martinus Nijhoff Publishing.
11. Boheler KR, Dillmann WH. 1988. Cardiac response to pressure overload in the rat: the selective alteration of in vitro directed RNA translation products. Circulation Res 63:448–456.
12. Brand T, Sharma HS, Schaper W. 1993. Expression of nuclear proto-oncogenes in isoproterenol-induced cardiac hypertrophy. J Mol Cell Cardiol 25:1325–1337.
13. Tomanek RJ, Torry RJ. 1994. Growth of the coronary vasculature in hypertrophy: mechanisms and model dependence. Cell Mol Biol Res 40:129–136.
14. Vikstrom KL, Bohlmeyer T, Factor SM, Leinwand LA. 1998. Hypertrophy, pathology, and molecular markers of cardiac pathogenesis. Circ Res 82:773–778.
15. Brilla CG, Janicki JS, Weber KT. 1991. Impaired diastolic function and coronary reserve in genetic hypertension. Role of interstitial fibrosis and medial thickening of intramyocardial coronary arteries. Circ Res 69:107–115.
16. Brilla CG, Janicki JS, Weber KT. 1991. Cardioreparative effects of lisinopril in rats with genetic hypertension and left ventricular hypertrophy. Circulation 83(5):1771–1779.
17. Weber KT, Brilla CG. 1991. Pathological hypertrophy and cardiac interstitium. Fibrosis and renin-angiotensin-aldosterone system. Circulation 83(6):1849–1865.
18. Schwartz K, Carrier L, Mercadier JJ, Lompre AM. 1993. Molecular phenotype of the hypertrofied and failing myocardium. Circulation 87:VII5–10.
19. Pelouch V, Dixon IM, Golfman L, Beamish RE, Dhalla NS. 1994. Role of extracellular matrix proteins in heart function. Mol Cell Biochem 129:101–120.
20. Ignotz RA, Massague J. 1986. Transforming growth factor-beta stimulates the expression of fibronectin and collagen and their incorporation into the extracellular matrix. J Biol Chem 261(9):4337–4345.
21. Chapman D, Weber KT, Eghbali M. 1990. Regulation of fibrillar collagen types I and III and basement membrane type IV collagen gene expression in pressure overloaded rat myocardium. Circ Res 67.787–794.
22. Volders PG, Willems IE, Cleutjens JP, Arends JW, Havenith MG, Daemen MJ. 1993. Interstitial collagen is increased in the non-infarcted human myocardium after myocardial infarction. J Mol Cell Cardiol 25:1317–1323.
23. Bishop JE, Rhodes S, Laurent GJ, Low RB, Stirewalt WS. 1994. Increased collagen synthesis and decreased collagen degradation in right ventricular hypertrophy induced by pressure overload. Cardiovasc Res 28:1581–1585.

24. Weber KT, Sun Y, Tyagi SC, Cleutjens JP. 1994. Collagen network of the myocardium: function, structural remodeling and regulatory mechanisms. J Mol Cell Cardiol 26:279–292.
25. Caspari PG, Gibson K, Harris P. 1976. Changes in myocardial collagen in normal development and after β-blockade. Rec Adv Card Struct Metab 7:99–104.
26. van Bilsen M, Chien KR. 1993. Growth and hypertrophy of the heart: towards an understanding of cardiac specific and inducable gene expression. Cardiovasc Res 27:1140–1149.
27. Zak R. 1973. Cell proliferation during cardiac growth. Am J Cardiol 31:211–219.
28. Farhadian F, Contard F, Corbier A, Barrieux A, Rappaport L, Samuel JL. 1995. Fibronectin expression during physiological and pathological cardiac growth. J Mol Cell Cardiol 27:981–990.
29. Borg TK, Caulfield JB. 1981. The collagen matrix of the heart. Fed Proc 20:2037–2041.
30. Factor SM, Robinson TF, Dominitz R, Cho S. 1986. Alterations of the myocardial skeletal framework in acute myocardial infarction with and without ventricular rupture. Am J Cardiovasc Pathol 1:91–97.
31. Whittaker P. 1997. Collagen and ventricular remodeling after acute myocardial infarction: concepts and hypotheses. Basic Res Cardiol 92:79–81.
32. Samuel JL, Barrieux A, Dufour S, Dubus I, Contard F, Koteliansky V, Farhadian F, Marotte F, Thiery JP, Rappaport L. 1991. Accumulation of fetal fibronectin mRNAs during the development of rat cardiac hypertrophy induced by pressure overload. J Clin Invest 88:1737–1746.
33. McLenachan JM, Dargie HJ. 1990. Ventricular arrhythmias in hypertensive left ventricular hypertrophy. Relationship to coronary artery disease, left ventricular dysfunction, and myocardial fibrosis. Am J Hypertens 3:735–740.
34. Speranza ML, Valentini G, Calligaro A. 1987. Influence of fibronectin on the fibrillogenesis of type I and type III collagen. Coll Relat Res 7:115–123.
35. Bogers AJJC, Roofthooft M, Pisters H, Spitaels SEC, Bos E. 1994. Longterm follow-up of gamma irradiated transannular homograft patch in surgical treatment of tetralogy of Fallot. Thorac Cardiovasc Surgeon 42:337–339.
36. Hokken RB, Bogers AJJC, Spitaels SEC, Hess J, Bos E. 1995. Pulmonary homograft insertion after repair of pulmonary stenosis. J Heart Valve Dis 4:182–186.
37. Bancroft JD, Cook HC. 1994. Manual of Histological Techniques and Their Diagnostic Aplication, Eds. JD Bancroff and HC Cook, 53. London: Churchil livingstone.
38. Sharma HS, van Heugten HA, Goedbloed MA, Verdouw PD, Lamers JM. 1994. Angiotensin II induced expression of transcription factors precedes increase in Transforming Growth Factor-β1 mRNA in neonatal cardiac fibroblasts. Biochem Biophys Res Comm 205:105–112.
39. Bernard MP, Chu ML, Myers JC, Ramirez F, Eikenberry EF, Prockop DJ. 1983. Nucleotide sequence of complementary deoxyribonucleic acids for the pro alpha 1 chain of human type 1 procollagen. Statistical evaluation of structures that are conserved during evolution. Biochem 22:5213–5223.
40. Ala-Kokko L, Kontusaari S, Baldwin CT, Kuivaniemi H, Prockop DJ. 1989. Structure of cDNA clones coding for the entire prepro alpha 1 chain of human type III procollagen. Differences in protein structure from type I procollagen and conservation of codon preferences. Biochem J 260:509–516.
41. Kornblihtt AR, Vibe-Petersen K, Baralle FE. 1983. Isolation and characterization of cDNA clones for human and bovine fibronectins. Proc Natl Acad Sci USA 80(11):3218–3222.
42. Yamaguchi T, Iwano M, Kubo A, Hirayama T, Akai Y, Horii Y, Fujimoto T, Hamaguchi T, Kurumatani N, Motomiya Y, Dohi K. 1996. IL-6 mRNA synthesis by peripheral blood mononuclear cells (PBMC) in patients with chronic renal failure. Clin Exp Immunol 103:279–328.
43. Peters TH, Sharma HS, Yilmaz E, Bogers AJ. 1999. Quantitative analysis of collagens and fibronectin expression in human right ventricular hypertrophy. Ann N Y Acad Sci 874:278–285.
44. Sharma HS, Peters THF, Bogers AJJC. 2000. Angiogenesis and fibrosis during right ventricular hypertrophy in human tetralogy of Fallot. In: The hypertrophied heart, Eds. N Takeda, M Nagano and NS Dhalla, 227–241. Boston, USA: Kluwer Academic Publishers.
45. Kawai S, Okada R, Kitamura K, Suzuki A, Saito S. 1984. A morphometrical study of myocardial disarray associated with right ventricular outflow tract obstruction. Jpn Circ J 48:445–456.
46. Limoto DS, Covell JW, Harper E. 1988. Increase in crosslinking of type I and type III collagens associated with volume–overloaded hypertrophy. Circ Res 63:399–408.

B. Ostadal, M. Nagano and N.S. Dhalla (eds.).
CARDIAC DEVELOPMENT. Copyright © 2002.
Kluwer Academic Publishers. Boston.
All rights reserved.

HUMAN HIBERNATING MYOCARDIUM-DEVELOPMENT TO DEGENERATION

ALBRECHT ELSÄSSER, SAWA KOSTIN,[1] and JUTTA SCHAPER[1]

Department of Cardiology, University of Freiburg/Brsg, Germany
[1] *Department of Experimental Cardiology, Max-Planck-Institute, Bad Nauheim, Germany*

Summary. The term hibernating myocardium applies to regional left ventricular dysfunction caused by chronic ischemia. It has been postulated that this phenomenon represents a functional adaptation to the chronic lack of oxygen but our own morphological-clinical studies are in contrast to this hypothesis. Recently, we described in human hibernating myocardium a self-perpetuating continuous vicious circle of cellular degeneration, which leads to progressive tissue damage. Here, we put forward the assumption that this vicious circle of structural deterioration is initiated by a disturbed steady state between myocardial oxygen supply and demand followed by intracellular degenerative processes and extracellular repair mechanisms. Structural alterations of cardiomyocytes characterized by a reduced rate of protein synthesis and predominating degradation induce sequestration of cellular particles into the interstitial space accompanied by atrophy of cardiomyocytes. Consecutively, repair mechanisms in the extracellular matrix are initiated. During the inflammatory and fibrogenic phases of this reaction, replacement fibrosis is synthesized leading to a reduction of cell-cell-contacts and of intra- and extracellular coupling followed by derangement of mechanical and signal transduction. Due to the increasing degree of replacement fibrosis, microvascular density is reduced while the oxygen diffusion distance is increased until the oxygen supply to the cardiomyocytes becomes critical resulting in a further progression of intracellular degeneration. For this reason, we propose that this vicious circle is a self-perpetuating process of tissue injury leading to further reduction of regional left ventricular function. This circle can only be interrupted by restoration of an adequate myocardial perfusion.

Corresponding author: Albrecht Elsässer, M.D., Dept. Of Cardiology, University of Freiburg, Hugstetter Str. 3, D-79106 Freiburg/Br., Germany. Voice: ++49 (0) 761 270-3618; Fax: ++ (0) 761 270-3775;
e-mail: elsässer@med1.ukl.uni-freiburg.de

Key words: hibernating myocardium, degeneration, replacement fibrosis

INTRODUCTION

Rahimtoola defined human hibernating myocardium as persistently impaired left ventricular function at rest due to chronically reduced blood flow that can be partially or completely restored to normal after revascularisation. A new equilibrium between reduced oxygen supply and myocardial demand should be established, that preserves the structural integrity of the tissue [1,2].

This definition is based on retrospective observations of the clinical time course of patients with coronary artery disease and chronic left ventricular dysfunction that improved upon revascularization. Therefore, the term hibernating myocardium describes solely a clinical situation and not a pathophysiological or pathological entity.

The central theme of the clinical and experimental studies concerning hibernating myocardium is the altered supply/demand ratio and its physiological, biochemical and structural consequences. However, a comparison of the results reveals a limited validity of the animal data obtained so far and therefore, there is no experimental model available yet to represent the condition of human hibernating myocardium [3,4].

Initially, the intent of the clinical studies was to evaluate the reliability of different diagnostic methods. The data showed that positron emission tomography (PET), thallium scintigraphy with reinjection and stress echocardiography are suitable, comparable, and accurate methods to detect hibernating myocardium. They also are reliable predictors of the functional improvement after revascularization [5–12]. The diagnostic efficacy can be improved by combining two methods [12].

Based on the clinical results, numerous concepts of pathomechanisms were postulated. It was proposed that left ventricular dysfunction might thus result from a disturbed myocardial perfusion ranging from a permanent reduction of blood flow at rest to repetitive stunning due to limited coronary reserve [13–15].

The aim of the this review was to summarize our published data on ultrastructural changes, gene expression and synthesis rate of different intracellular and extracellular proteins and their reciprocal involvement including the role of cytokines and of angiotensin converting enzyme (ACE). Finally, consequences on the functional capacity of hibernating myocardium will be discussed [12,16–18]. On the basis of the data presented here, a hypothesis concerning the pathomechanism of hibernating myocardium will be presented.

Alterations in human hibernating myocardium

Cardiomyocytes

In light and electron microscopy revealed myocytes varying in size between hypertrophy, normal size and atrophy. A disorganization of contractile apparatus caused by a loss of contractile material and by disorganization of the cytoskeleton was evident (Fig. 1). An accumulation of numerous small or giant mitochondria presenting as

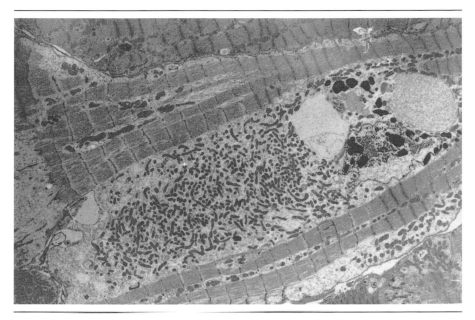

Figure 1. Electron micrograph of human hibernating myocardium. Note the loss of contractile material in the center of the large cardiomyocyte. Bar = 2.5 μm.

intracellular clusters was observed. In addition, areas containing nonspecific cytoplasm, membrane limited vacuoles, myelin figures, and lipid droplets were observed. Glycogen storage was a prominent feature in human hibernating myocardium.

The nuclei were varying in size and shape and chromatin clumping was documented.

More detailed information about different cell compartments was gained using immunohistochemistry and confocal microscopy. The contractile proteins actin and myosin as well as the sarcomeric skeleton protein titin were reduced. The cytoskeletal proteins desmin and alpha-actinin were focally accumulated and disorganized.

The mRNA content of the proteins described above was documented by in situ hybridization which showed a decrease and an inhomogeneous distribution of mRNA labeling.

The cellular organization of the myocardium was disturbed and a loss of gap junctions was observed by connexin-43 labeling (Fig. 2). This results in a reduction of cell–cell contacts and isolation of cardiomyocytes surrounded by large amounts of fibrotic tissue [16–18].

Interstitial cells and extracellular matrix

The ultrastructural changes were an augmentation of ground substance, collagen fibrils and elastic fibers as well as an increased number of fibroblasts and

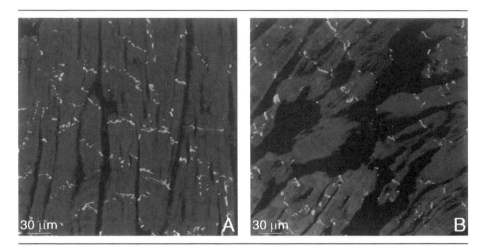

Figure 2. Confocal microscopy of connexin-43 labeling in slightly altered (A) and severely altered human hibernating myocardium. Note the irregular characterization of intercalated discs by the antibody which is more pronounced in B that shows a higher degree of fibrosis (black unlabeled area in the center) than in A.

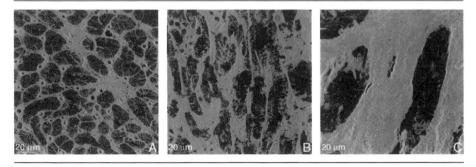

Figure 3. Confocal microscopy of labeling with fibronectin of human hibernating myocardium. A shows a slight degree of fibrosis and B a more severe degree. In C two cardiomyocytes are visible that are isolated by large amounts of fibrotic tissue. Fibrosis is white and cardiomyocytes are black. Fine "pseudo-intracellular" labeling caused by staining of the inner lining of invaginating T-tubules is evident in all pictures.

macrophages. In the widened extracellular space cellular debris originating from cardiomyocytes was abundant.

By immunohistochemistry a significant increase of extracellular matrix proteins was detected. The structural proteins collagen I, III and VI as well as the adhesive protein fibronectin were accumulated. As components of the basallamina laminin and collagen IV were augmented and thick layers of these proteins were surrounding the myocytes (Fig. 3).

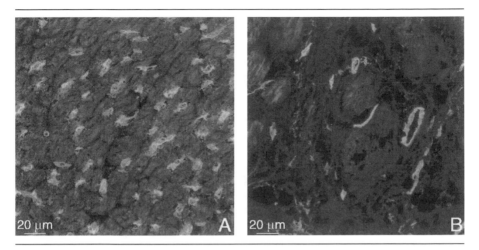

Figure 4. Confocal microscopy of PECAM labeling shows that the number of capillaries (white) in human hibernating myocardium is significantly reduced (B) as compared to normal human myocardium.

The number of fibroblasts, macrophages and lymphocytes was elevated, whereas capillary and arteriolar density was reduced (Fig. 4).

The mRNA levels of collagen I and fibronectin were increased and were distributed over the cells of the connective tissue.

An obvious finding was the increase of gene expression and protein content of TGF-β1 and ACE as compared to human control myocardium (Fig. 5) [16–18].

Changed interactions between the intracellular and extracellular compartments and between myocytes

The changes observed and described here were interpreted as degenerative changes in human hibernating myocardium resulting from permanent or temporary and repetitive imbalance between a reduced oxygen supply and the myocardial demand. The intracellular degeneration characterized by diminished synthesis rate and predominating degradation of proteins will lead to a continuous structural deterioration resulting in cellular atrophy by sequestration of cell particles into the extracellular space and initiation of repair mechanisms with increased synthesis of extracellular proteins summarized as a replacement fibrosis. It is interesting to note that, in contrast to the cardiomyocytes, the cellular components of the extracellular matrix showed a normal or increased synthetic function despite the situation of a reduced oxygen supply [16–18].

The extracellular repair mechanisms initiated in human hibernating myocardium consist of an inflammatory reaction and fibrogenic processes. Immigration of lymphocytes and phagocytotic activity of macrophages characterize the inflammatory reaction. Summarized as the fibrogenic phase, an increased numbers of fibroblasts

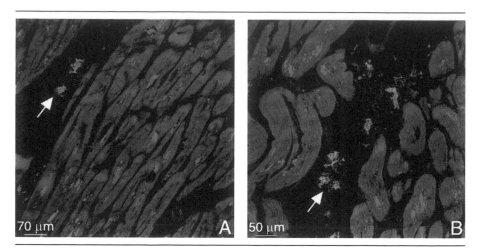

Figure 5. TGF-β1 is present in small amounts in fibroblasts (arrow) in normal myocardium. In human hibernating myocardium, the number of positive structures (arrow) is greatly increased.

produce the different proteins of the extracellular matrix [19]. The dimeric fibronectin is an adhesive extracellular protein that connects via integrins myocytes with components of the extracellular matrix such as heparin, collagen, factor VIII, growth factors and others [20,21]. It plays an important role in wound healing and scar formation [22]. Accordingly, in hibernating myocardium the amount of fibronectin was increased.

Fibronectin and laminin are the major components of the basal laminia of myocytes which was thickened in hibernating myocardium [23].

Collagen I and III are fibrillar proteins, whereas collagen VI is a globular molecule. Collagen III forms a network connecting the cross-striated, thick fibrils of collagen I and VI, which insert into the cardiomyocytes and endothelial cells and are coupled with the domains of fibronectin [24,25]. In human hibernating myocardium the different types of collagen are increased in the same degree as fibronectin.

The increase in the rate of synthesis of the extracellular proteins as a consequence of an increased transcriptional activity leads to a synthesis of scar tissue. This replacement fibrosis produces a disintegration of the structural organization of the myocardium with disturbances of the intra- and extracellular connections as well as a separation of cell groups and reduction of the cell-cell coupling points by loss of gap junctions [18,19,25].

Important factors of the degenerative processes

Both inflammatory as well as fibrogenic phases appear simultaneously in human hibernating myocardium suggesting these processes are active and in continuous progression. Factors involved in extracellular repair mechanisms are TGF-β1 and ACE, whose mRNA and proteins are overexpressed [18].

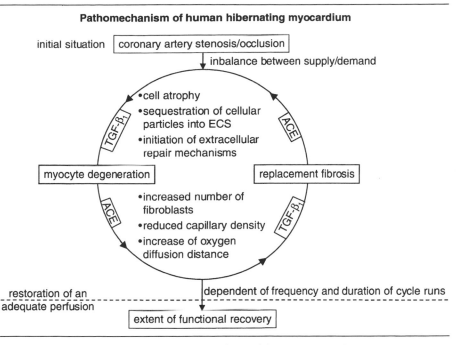

Figure 6. Vicious circle of tissue deterioration in human hibernating myocardium.

TGF-β1 is synthesized by macrophages, fibroblasts and myofibroblasts [25,26]. As detected by a minor increase in lymphocytes and macrophages in human hibernating myocardium, TGF-β1 suppresses the inflammatory cell response and it acts as a strong chemotactic stimulus for further immigration of fibroblasts, which were found in great numbers in the extracellular space. Furthermore, TGF-β1 stimulates the transformation of fibroblasts to myofibroblasts and promotes collagen turnover and wound contraction [20,27–29].

Fibroblasts, myofibroblasts and endothelial cells produce ACE, which contributes to local healing as well as matrix remodeling and leads to vasoconstriction through inhibition of bradykinin. Resulting increased concentrations of angiotensin II promote cell migration and synthesis of collagen as well as vascular hyperplasia [25,30–32].

In addition, the number of vessels is reduced in human hibernating myocardium. As consequences of the diminished vessel density and of altered morphology of the vascular wall a further reduction of the blood supply to the myocytes occur.

Hypothesis on the pathomechanism of human hibernating myocardium

Summarizing the results, we propose that a vicious circle of structural deterioration is established in hibernating myocardium (Fig. 6). This leads to progression of tissue damage with consecutive functional deterioration in the following way [17,18]:

At the beginning of myocardial underperfusion the reduced contractile function may be interpreted as an adaptation to a reduced oxygen supply preserving the myocardial integrity through a reduced metabolic rate. The steady state between oxygen supply and demand is delicate and can be disturbed easily and immediately by a further reduction of the oxygen supply caused by a progression of the coronary artery disease or by an increased cellular oxygen demand. A imbalance leads to intracellular degeneration, which involves all cell compartments. Since the mRNA of the contractile and cytoskeletal proteins was reduced, cellular degradation may be predominant over synthesis leading to a loss of structural components. The resulting cell atrophy is caused by a sequestration of cell particles into the extracellular space, which initiates an extracellular response with inflammatory and fibrogenic phases. This replacement fibrosis is responsible for the disarrangement and isolation of cell groups and an encapsulation of the myocytes by thickening of the basal lamina. The consequence is a reduction of cell-cell-contacts and of intra- and extracellular coupling. The myocardial syncytium that is the basis for differentiation, organization, proliferation and contractile function is annihilated [24,33,34].

In human hibernating myocardium, the capillary density is reduced and the oxygen diffusion distance is increased until the supply to the myocytes becomes critical. With this, intracellular degeneration is in progression and a new circle is started.

The end point of repetitive runs of vicious circles is a severe loss of intracellular structures, especially the contractile and cytoskeletal proteins, and a marked fibrosis, which therefore represent the limiting steps for functional recovery. We propose that in human hibernating myocardium a continuous remodeling takes place caused by a self-perpetuating vicious circle, which can only be stopped by restoration of an adequate perfusion.

Functional consequences

The correlation between clinical data and the myocardial structural alterations shows that the extent of functional recovery of the hibernating area after restoration of an adequate perfusion is dependent of the severity of the intracellular degeneration and the degree of extracellular changes. These include the development of replacement fibrosis, a reduction of vessel density and an increase in intercapillary diffusion distance [16–18].

Two types of fibrosis are differentiated which are identified as reactive and replacement fibrosis. Reactive fibrosis is observed in chronic volume and/or pressure overloading of the myocardium. The tissue is characterized by hypertrophy of the myocytes and by small isolated perivascular areas of fibrosis. In contrast, replacement fibrosis is initiated by a loss or atrophy of myocytes and fills up the resulting gap. Therefore there is a direct correlation between the reduction of the numbers or volume of myocytes and the degree of fibrosis. Whereas the synthesis of replacement fibrosis is an irreversible process, reactive fibrosis can disappear after removal of the triggering agents [19,25,35].

A reduction of vessel density causes an increase in intercapillary distance as a result of which the oxygen diffusion way is extended.

On the basis of the present results a quantification was performed using morphometry and the values were correlated to clinical data of the study population. An extent of fibrosis >32% of total tissue, a capillary density of <660/mm^2 and an intercapillary distance of >39 μm represent the limitations of capacity of the tissue to resume structural integrity. Only a partial functional recovery after restoration of an adequate perfusion will occur in this situation. Therefore, the extracellular alterations seem to determine the functional improvement of the revascularized hibernating area and are suitable markers to predict the extent of functional improvement [18].

To interrupt a progressive tissue damage with irreversible degeneration caused by the self-perpetuating vicious circle, human hibernating myocardium should be revascularized as soon as possible after establishment of the clinical diagnosis.

REFERENCES

1. Rahimtoola SH. 1989. The hibernating myocardium. Am Heart J 117:211–221.
2. Rahimtoola SH. 1993. The hibernating myocardium in ischaemia and congestive heart failure. Eur Heart J 212–220.
3. Heusch G. 1998. Hibernating myocardium. Physiol Rev 78:1055–1085.
4. Schulz R, Rose J, Martin C, Brodde OE, Heusch G. 1993. Development of short-term myocardial hibernation. Its limitation by the severity of ischemia and inotropic stimulation. Circulation 88:684–695.
5. Schelbert HR. 1991. Positron emission tomography for the assessment of myocardial viability. Circulation 84:122–131.
6. Brunken R, Schwaiger M, Grover-McKay M, Phelps ME, Tillisch J, Schelbert HR. 1987. Positron emission tomography detects tissue metabolic activity in myocardial segments with persistent thallium perfusion defects. J Am Coll Cardiol 10:557–567.
7. Dilsizian V, Bonow RO. 1993. Current diagnostic techniques of assessing myocardial viability in patients with hibernating and stunned myocardium [published erratum appears in Circulation 1993 Jun; 87(6):2070]. Circulation 87:1–20.
8. Altehoefer C, vom Dahl J, Buell U, Uebis R, Kleinhans E, Hanrath P. 1994. Comparison of thallium-201 single-photon emission tomography after rest injection and fluorodeoxyglucose positron emission tomography for assessment of myocardial viability in patients with chronic coronary artery disease. Eur J Nucl Med 21:37–45.
9. Bonow RO, Dilsizian V, Cuocolo A, Bacharach SL. 1991. Identification of viable myocardium in patients with chronic coronary artery disease and left ventricular dysfunction: comparison of thallium scintigraphy with reinjection and PET imaging with 18-fluorodeoxygluose. Circulation 83:26–37.
10. Baer F, Voth E, Deutsch HJ, Schneider CA, Schicha H, Sechtem U. 1994. Assessment of viable myocardium by dobutamine transoesophageal echocardiography and comparison with fluorine-18-fluorodeoxyglucose positron emission tomography. J Am Coll Cardiol 24:343–353.
11. Barilla F, Gheorghiade M. 1991. Low-dose dobutamine in patients with acute myocardial infarction identifies viable but not contractile myocardium and predicts the magnitude of improvement in wall motion abnormalities in response to coronary revascularization. Am Heart J 122:1522–1531.
12. Elsässer A, Müller KD, Vogt A, Strasser R, Gagel C, Schlepper M, Klövekorn WP. 1998. Assessment of myocardial viability: dobutamine echocardiography and thallium-201 single-photon emission computed tomographic imaging predict the postoperative improvement of left ventricular function after bypass surgery. Am Heart J 136:463–475.
13. Wijns WW, Vatner SF, Camici PG. 1998. Hibernating myocardium. N Engl J Med 339:173–181.

14. Gamici PG, Wijns W, Borgers M, De Silva R, Ferrari R, Knuuti J, Lammertsma AA, Liedtke AJ, Paternostro G, Vatner SF. 1997. Pathophysiological mechanisms of chronic reversible left ventricular dysfunction due to coronary artery desease. Circulation 96:3205–3214.
15. Vanoverschelde JL, Wijns W, Borgers M, Hendrickx G, Depre C, Flameng W, Melin JA. 1997. Chronic myocardial hibernation in humans. Circulation 95:1961–1971.
16. Elsässer A, Schlepper M, Klövekorn WP, Cai WJ, Zimmermann R, Müller KD, Strasser R, Kostin S, Gagel C, Münkel B, Schaper W, Schaper J. 1997. Hibernating myocardium—an incomplete adaptation to ischemia. Circulation 96:2920–2931.
17. Elsässer A, Schlepper M, Zimmermann R, Klövekorn WP, Schaper J. 1998. The extracellular matrix in hibernating myocardium—a significant factor causing structural defects and cardiac dysfunction. Mol Cell Biochem 186:147–158.
18. Elsässer A, Decker E, Kostin S, Hein S, Skwara W, Müller KD, Greiber S, Schaper W, Klövekorn WP, Schaper J. 2000. A self-perpetuating vicious cycle of tissue damage in human hibernating myocardium. Mol Cell Biochem 213:17–28.
19. Weber KT, Brilla CG, Janicki JS. 1993. Myocardial fibrosis: functional significance and regulatory factors. Cardiovasc Res 27:341–348.
20. Farhadain F, Contrad F, Corbier A, Barrieux A, Rappaport L, Samuel J. 1995. Fibronectin expression during phsiological and pathological cardiac growth. J Moll Cell Cardiol 27:981–990.
21. Knowlton AA, Connelly CM, Romo GM, Mamuya A, Apstein CS, Brecher P. 1992. Rapid expression of fibronectin in the rabbit heart after myocardial infarction with and without reperfusion. J Clin Invest 89:1060–1068.
22. Hynes RO. 1990. Fibronectins. Springer, New York 1–545.
23. Engel J, Odermatt E, Engel A, Madri J, Furthmayr H, Rohde H, Timpl R. 1981. Shapes, domain organizations and flexibility of laminin and fibronectin. J Mol Biol 150:97–120.
24. Weber K, Sun Y, Tyagi C, Cleutjens PM. 1994. Collagen network of the myocardium: function, structural remodeling and regulatory mechanims. J Moll Cell Cardiol 26:279–292.
25. Weber KT. 1997. Extracellular matrix remodeling in heart failure. Circulation 96:4065–4082.
26. Brand T, Schneider MD. 1995. The TGFβ superfamily in myocardium: ligands, receptors, transduction, and function. J Moll Cell Cardiol 27:5–18.
27. Brilla CG, Maisch B, Zhou G, Weber KT. 1995. Hormonal regulation of cardiac fibroblast function. Eur Heart J 16:45–50.
28. Sappino AP, Schürch W, Gabbiani G. 1990. Differentiation repertoire of fibroblastics cells: expression of cytoskeletal proteins as marker of phenotypic modulations. Lab Invest 63:144–161.
29. Willems I, Havenith MG, De Mey JGR, Daemen MJ. 1994. The alpha-smooth muscle actin positive cells in healing human myocardial scars. Am J Path 145:868–875.
30. Sun Y, Clentjens JPM, Diaz-Arias AA, Weber KT. 1994. Cardiac angiotensin converting enzyme and myocardial fibrosis in the rat. Cardiovasc Res 28:1423–1432.
31. Sun Y, Weber KT. 1996. Angiotensin converting enzyme and myofibroblasts during tissue repair in the rat heart. J Moll Cell Cardiol 28:851–858.
32. Nokimoto S, Yasue H, Fujimoto K, Sakata R, Miyamoto E. 1995. Increased angiotensin converting enzyme activity in left ventricular aneurysm of patients after myocardial infarction. Cardiovasc Res 29:664–669.
33. Adams JC, Watt FM. 1993. Regulation of development and differentiation by the extracellular matrix. Development 117:1183–1198.
34. Perlouch V, Dixon ICM, Golfman L, Beamish RE, Dhalla RS. 1993. Role of extracellular matrix proteins in heart function. Mol Cell Biochem 129:101–120.
35. Weber KT, Sun Y, Katwa LC, Cleutjens JPM. 1995. Connective tissue: a metabolic entity? J Moll Cell Cardiol 27:107–120.

B. Ostadal, M. Nagano and N.S. Dhalla
CARDIAC DEVELOPMENT. Copyrig
Kluwer Academic Publishers. Boston.
All rights reserved.

PROTECTION OF THE DEVELOPING HEART AGAINST OXYGEN DEPRIVATION

B. OŠŤA'DAL, I. OŠŤA'DALOVA', L. ŠKÁRKA, and F. KOLÁŘ

Institute of Physiology, Academy of Sciences of the Czech Republic and Center for Experimental Cardiovascular Research, Prague, Czech Republic

Summary. Cardiac tolerance to oxygen deprivation changes significantly during ontogenetic development: immature heart appears to be more resistant to ischemic/hypoxic injury as compared with the adult myocardium. The mechanisms of the higher resistance of the developing heart to oxygen deprivation have not yet been satisfactorily clarified. Adaptation to chronic hypoxia results in similarly enhanced cardiac resistance in animals exposed to hypoxia either immediately after birth or in adulthood. Preconditioning failed to improve ischemic tolerance just after birth but it developed during the early postnatal period, thus counteracting the decreasing tolerance to ischemia. It is, however, too early to reach a definitive conclusion on whether (i) the mechanism(s) involved in the protection of the immature heart differ or are identical with those of the adult myocardium and (ii) cardioprotection by adaptation to chronic hypoxia and preconditioning utilize the same or different pathways. Basic knowledge of the mechanisms which increase tolerance of the immature heart to oxygen deprivation may contribute to the design of therapeutic strategies for both pediatric cardiology and cardiac surgery.

Key words: cardiac development, cardiac protection, chronic hypoxia, ischemic preconditioning

INTRODUCTION

The most frequent (and hence most widely studied) diseases of modern times undoubtedly include hypoxic states of the cardiopulmonary system. In recent years,

Corresponding author: Bohuslav Ošťádal, Institute of Physiology, Vídeňská 1083, 142 20 Prague 4. Phone: +4202-4752553; Fax: +4202-4752125; e-mail: ostadal@biomed.cas.cz

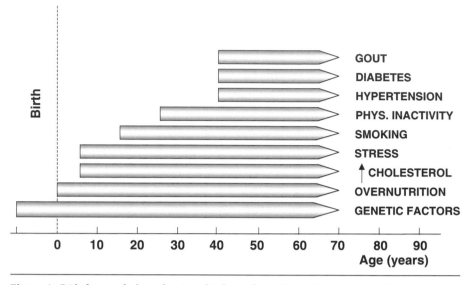

Figure 1. Risk factors of atherosclerosis and ischemic heart disease during ontogenetic development in humans. [Data from Fejfar (1).]

cardiological research has concentrated on the theoretical basis of rational prevention and therapy of the most serious cardiovascular problems, such as myocardial ischemia. Clinical-epidemiological studies have shown that the risk factors of atherosclerosis and ischemic heart disease are present during the early phases of ontogenetic development [1]. Some of these, including excessive food intake and increased levels of cholesterol, operate after birth, whereas genetic factors are present before birth (Fig. 1). Atherosclerosis and ischemic heart disease are thus no more the diseases of the fifth and higher decades of life, but their origin and consequences may be essentially influenced by risk factors acting already during early development. Furthermore, hypoxemia is a characteristic feature of many pediatric patients with cyanotic congenital heart defects; in addition, the immature heart of children who have undergone open-heart surgery is subjected to ischemic arrest. It follows, therefore, that experimental studies of the pathogenetic mechanisms of cardiac ischemia/hypoxia must shift to the early ontogenetic periods. Accordingly, the increased interest of theoretical and clinical cardiologists in the developmental approach is not surprising.

The degree of hypoxic injury depends, however, not only on the intensity and duration of the hypoxic stimulus but also on the level of cardiac tolerance to oxygen deprivation. This variable is determined by the relationship between myocardial oxygen supply and demand, i.e., myocardial blood flow and oxygen-carrying capacity of blood on the one hand, and the functional state of cardiac muscle (level of contractile function, systolic wall tension, heart rate, and external work) and basal metabolism, on the other [2]. Because most of these determinants change significantly during development, it is understandable that significant ontogenetic changes also underlie their common consequence, cardiac tolerance to oxygen deprivation [3].

ONTOGENETIC DIFFERENCES IN CARDIAC TOLERANCE TO OXYGEN DEPRIVATION

Over the past years, many experimental studies have compared the tolerance of the mature and immature heart to hypoxia and ischemia (for review see 3). However, they do not represent equivalent insults. Whereas coronary flow is reduced in ischemia, hypoxia involves the exposure of the myocardium to a perfusate with low P_{O2}. The latter condition provides a continuous supply of substrate, whereas removal of lactate prevents the intracellular acidosis that occurs with ischemia. Thus, by anaerobic glycolysis, the energy stores and ionic gradients can be maintained in the hypoxic heart for a considerable period of time [4].

Early evidence for an age-dependent decrease in resistance to hypoxia is found in studies on the survival time of the rat, cat, dog, guinea pig, and rabbit in anoxic environment [5]. It was found that in each species the survival time was inversely related to age and maturity of the newborn. The concept of greater tolerance of the neonatal heart has been supported by Su and Friedman [6] and Jarmakani and co-workers [7,8] in rabbits and dogs, by using isolated myocardium perfused for 30 min with 95% N_2 and 5% CO_2. The increase in lactate production during hypoxia was significantly greater in the newborn than in adults, indicating that the newborns are capable of maintaining adult levels of myocardial ATP. Several other studies have shown a greater posthypoxic preservation of variables, such as calcium handling [9] and mitochondrial function in the newborn heart [10]. The ontogenetic development of cardiac resistance to acute anoxia in vitro in rats showed a biphasic pattern [3]; the relatively high cardiac resistance at birth even increased up to the end of the weaning period in both male and female hearts. During further development this value decreased in males but remained unchanged in females; the adult female heart was thus significantly more resistant to hypoxia [11]. It may be concluded that cardiac sensitivity to hypoxia or anoxia changes significantly during ontogenetic development but the time-course may be different in males and females.

As with hypoxia, the immature myocardium also appears to be relatively resistant to ischemia. Riva and Hearse [12] and Awad et al. [13] have observed that the age-dependent changes in resistance to global ischemia in isolated male rat hearts (expressed as postischemic recovery of developed pressure) showed a biphasic pattern, with increasing tolerance from the end of the first postnatal week up to the weaning period, followed by a decline to adulthood. This time course is similar to that of cardiac resistance to hypoxia (see above). Detailed analysis of the tolerance of isolated rat hearts to global ischemia during the first week of life [14] has revealed a significant decrease from day 1 to 7 (Fig. 2), followed by an increase on day 10, suggesting a possible triphasic pattern of the ontogenetic development of cardiac sensitivity to ischemia, at least in rats. The sensitivity of the neonatal

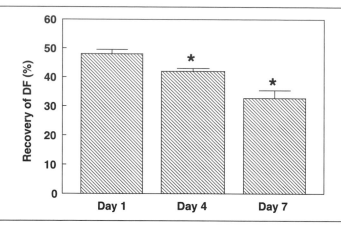

Figure 2. Tolerance of isolated perfused rat heart to global ischemia during first week of life expressed as recovery of developed force (DF) after ischemia (percentage of baseline values); *-p < 0.01. [Data from Ostadalova et al. [14].]

myocardium may be species–dependent: the neonatal pig heart is more susceptible to ischemia than the neonatal rabbit heart [15].

The mechanisms of the higher resistance of the immature heart to oxygen deprivation have not yet been satisfactorily clarified. It may be speculated that an explanation lies in the lower energy demand, greater anaerobic glycolytic capacity, and higher glycogen reserves of the neonatal heart [10,16,17]. The tolerance of the immature heart to ischemia may also be related to amino acid utilization by transamination [18]. Moreover, the ATP catabolic pathways change during development: ATP depletion occurs more rapidly in the mature heart [19]. In addition, AMP accumulates in the immature heart during ischemia which allows a rapid replenishment of ATP on reperfusion; on the other hand, de novo synthesis of ATP is required in the mature heart. These observations suggest that the immature heart is better equipped for ATP synthesis, a situation that may be advantageous in conditions of low substrate availability. The immature heart thus suffers less ischemic injury than the mature heart after the same ischemic insult. The role of mitochondria in the ontogenetic differences in cardiac tolerance to oxygen deprivation is not yet clear. We have observed [20] that mitochondrial membrane potential in the rat heart—one of the most important parameters of the mitochondrial energy state—changes significantly during ontogenetic development. Whether this change is related to the decreasing tolerance of the myocardium to hypoxia needs further analysis.

To the increased tolerance of the immature heart may contribute also the age–dependent changes in Ca^{2+} transport [21]. Calcium homeostasis is closely related to cell metabolism and is an accepted determinant of tissue injury during both oxygen deprivation and repletion [22]. Ca^{2+} transport in the neonate is different from that in the adult. The contraction of mammalian myocardium is known to depend on both transsarcolemmal Ca^{2+} influx and Ca^{2+} release from the sarcoplasmic reticulum. However, the relative contribution of the two mechanisms varies significantly during development. The contraction of neonatal myocardium where the sarcoplasmic reticulum is not fully developed depends to a large extent on the flux of Ca^{2+} across the sarcolemma via the Ca^{2+} channels. During further development, the ability of the sarcoplasmic reticulum to accumulate Ca^{2+} increases and there is a progressive maturation of Ca^{2+} release from the sarcoplasmic reticulum. Similarly, the Ca^{2+} sensitivity of cardiac myofilaments increases, reaching adult values in rats after two weeks of postnatal life [23]. Significant ontogenetic differences have been described in the subcellular localization of L-type Ca^{2+} channels which during maturation concentrate in junctional domains of the developing T-tubules associated with the sarcoplasmic reticulum [24]. This process together with the increasing functional role of Ca^{2+} release from the sarcoplasmic reticulum, may explain the decreasing sensitivity to the negative inotropic effect of calcium antagonists during development [25,26]. The role of acidosis may also be important: the negative inotropic effect of low pH was strikingly smaller in the neonatal rabbits which, according to Solaro et al. [27], can be accounted for by a lower myofibrillar Ca^{2+} sensitivity to low pH in this age group.

Another determinants of tissue injury are oxygen free radicals. According to Southworth et al. [28] the immature myocardium exposed to an ischemic insult suffers less injury than the mature heart and, as a consequence, produces fewer free radicals on reperfusion. The largest difference was in the guinea-pig heart observed after 20 min ischemia when the mature heart produced four times more free radicals than the immature heart. None of these observation can, however, fully explain the day-by-day changes in cardiac tolerance to ischemia that occur in rats during the first week of life [14].

PROTECTION OF THE IMMATURE HEART

As has been stated above, the degree of ischemic injury depends not only on the intensity and duration of the ischemic stimulus but also on the level of cardiac tolerance to oxygen deprivation. It is, therefore, not surprising that the interest of many experimental and clinical cardiologists during the past 40 years has been focused on the question of how cardiac tolerance to oxygen deprivation might be increased. The relatively short history of this endeavor represents a good example of the mutual inspiration and collaboration between experimental and clinical cardiologists.

Already in the late 1950s, the first observations appeared [29], showing that the incidence of myocardial infarction is lower in people living at high altitude. These epidemiological observations were confirmed in experimental studies [30,31] using simulated hypoxia. In the early 1970s the interest was concentrated on the possibilities of pharmacological limitations of infarct size (e.g. 32). This effort was, however, not successful, since it became more and more obvious that clinical observations did not correspond with the optimism of experimental results. After a period of skepticism, the discovery of the short-lasting adaptation of the myocardium, so

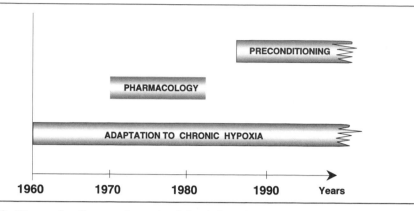

Figure 3. History of cardiac protection against ischemia/hypoxia.

called "preconditioning" by Murry et al. [33], opened the door to a new era of cardiac protection. As ischemic preconditioning represents now the most efficient form of temporal protection, it has attracted a great deal of attention and, in fact, considerable progress has been made in understanding this phenomenon over the past years (Fig. 3).

Whereas a substantial amount of data is available concerning protection of the adult myocardium, much less is known about this phenomenon in the developing heart. The data in the literature are scarce and often contradictory [3]. This short survey summarizes the results and hypotheses dealing with the ontogenetic differences in cardioprotection induced by adaptation to chronic hypoxia and ischemic preconditioning.

ADAPTATION OF THE IMMATURE HEART TO CHRONIC HYPOXIA

Chronic hypoxia is the main pathophysiological factor in severe disturbances of the cardiovascular system, represented by pulmonary, ischemic, and congenital heart disease and in cardiopulmonary changes induced by exposure to a high altitude environment. Adaptation to chronic hypoxia is characterized by a variety of functional changes to maintain homeostasis with a minimum expenditure of energy [34], which may protect the functionally overloaded heart from undue increased metabolic demands. It is interesting to note that the history of cardioprotection mediated by chronic hypoxia is quite different from that of preconditioning. Whereas the latter phenomenon was discovered in the laboratory, experimental investigation of the protective effects of adaptation to high altitude was stimulated by the above mentioned clinical epidemiological findings [29]. As far as the clinical relevance of the cardioprotective effect of adaptation to chronic hypoxia is concerned, in addition to populations living at high altitude, increased cardiac resistance to acute anoxia was described in children, operated for cyanotic congenital heart disease. Unfortunately, epidemiological data on the incidence of myocardial infarction in

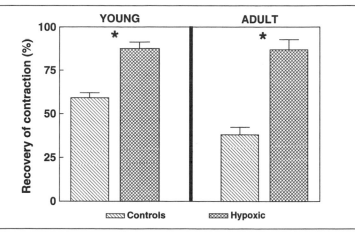

Figure 4. Effect of adaptation to simulated intermittent high-altitude hypoxia (barochamber, 7,000 m, 8 h/day, 5 days a week, a total of 24 exposures) on cardiac resistance to acute hypoxia (expressed as recovery of isotonic contraction of isolated papillary muscle, percentage of baseline values) in young (exposed from the 4th day of postnatal life) and adult (exposed from the 12th week) rats; *P < 0.01. [Data from Ostadal et al. [39].]

populations suffering from chronic obstructive lung disease or other clinical manifestations of chronic hypoxia are not available.

Under laboratory conditions, adaptation to chronic hypoxia protects the heart not only against acute ischemia, but also against acute anoxia *in vitro* and the necrogenic effect of beta-mimetic catecholamines [31]. Adaptation also reduces the severity and incidence of reperfusion arrhythmias [35] as well as the development of systemic hypertension and left ventricular hypertrophy in spontaneously hypertensive rats [36,37]. In contrast to the protective effect, adaptation to chronic hypoxia may, however, also exert an adverse influence on the cardiopulmonary system, including pulmonary hypertension and right ventricular hypertrophy, which may result in congestive heart failure [38].

As has been discussed above, the healthy immature myocardium is more tolerant to ischemia than that of adults. However, only a few authors have compared the tolerance to oxygen deprivation in chronically hypoxic versus normoxic immature hearts. We have observed [39] that chronic hypoxia, simulated in a barochamber, results in similarly enhanced cardiac resistance (expressed as the recovery of contractile function of the isolated right ventricle after acute anoxia *in vitro*) in rats exposed to chronic hypoxia either from the 4th day of postnatal life or in adulthood (Fig. 4). Adaptation to chronic hypoxia increased the tolerance in both sexes but the sex difference (i.e. increased tolerance in females) was maintained [11]. Similarly, Baker et al. [15] demonstrated that adaptation to chronic hypoxia increased the tolerance of the developing rabbit heart (days 7 to 28 of postnatal life). Postischemic recovery of aortic flow at these stages was better in chronically hypoxic hearts compared with age-matched controls. Our recent experiments have shown [40] that the protective effect of adaptation to chronic hypoxia is absent in newborn rats; this phenomenon develops only during the first week of life.

Unfortunately, despite the fact that the first experimental study on the cardio-protective effect of chronic hypoxia was published more than 40 years ago, no satisfactory explanation of this important phenomenon has yet been found. The possible protective mechanisms are summarized elsewhere [41,42]; they include alterations of e.g. oxygen carrying capacity of blood, capillarization, energy metabolism, heat shock proteins, prostaglandins and adenosine. Recently, it has been shown that long-term adaptation to chronic hypoxia results in enhanced activation of mitochondrial ATP-sensitive potassium channels (K_{ATP}) in the heart of adult rats [35] as well as in the myocardium of immature rabbits [43]. K_{ATP} channel opener diazoxide (which in micromolar range is selective for mitochondrial K_{ATP} channels) increased cardiac protection in normoxic hearts but its effect in hypoxic group was not significant. Conversely, K_{ATP} channel blocker 5-hydroxydecanoate (which selectively blocks mitochondrial K_{ATP} channels) attenuated the cardioprotective effect of chronic hypoxia but had no effect on postischemic recovery in normoxic hearts. This may suggest that adaptation to chronic hypoxia leads to activation of mitochondrial K_{ATP} channels which are then insensitive to their opener—diazoxide.

Mechanisms that may lead to activation of mitochondrial K_{ATP} channels in chronic hypoxia-induced cardioprotection are still unknown. Although several possibilities can be found in the literature, direct evidence is missing. Function of mitochondrial K_{ATP} channels can be regulated, for example, by protein kinase C [44] which is permanently activated in chronic hypoxia [45]. Baker et al. [46] and Shi et al. [47] have found that exposure of immature rabbit hearts to chronic hypoxia increased mRNA levels for eNOS, as well as release of nitrite, nitrate, and tissue cGMP content. Moreover, the NO donor GSNO increased the recovery of postischemic function in normoxic hearts but not in hearts chronically hypoxic from birth. Conversely, NOS inhibitors abolished the cardioprotective effect of hypoxia. A similar effect of NOS inhibitor was observed in neonatal rat hearts, adapted to high altitude hypoxia [40]. Baker et al. [46] proposed that increased production of NO in chronically hypoxic animals leads to activation of sarcolemmal and mitochondrial K_{ATP} channels via soluble guanylyl cyclase, causing accumulation of cGMP and activation of cGMP-dependent protein kinase. Thus, increased NO production in the immature hypoxic hearts may be an adaptive response as other proposed mechanisms like polycythemia and increased hemoglobin level [42].

It is, however, unclear at present how the opening of mitochondrial K_{ATP} channels results in cardiac protection. It has been suggested that the main function of these channels is to control mitochondrial matrix volume which, in turn, is thought to regulate electron transport and bioenergetics [48]. This hypothesis is in good agreement with the observation of Eells et al. [43] that the rate of ATP synthesis in immature hearts adapted to chronic hypoxia was significantly greater than that in normoxic hearts. Mitochondrial K_{ATP} channel activation may therefore be an essential component of signal transduction pathway calling for increased ATP production to support increased work of the heart or possibly to compensate for decreased oxygen availability. The reduction in the rate of ATP synthesis observed in mitochondria from hypoxic hearts treated with K_{ATP} channel blockers is consistent with this interpretation. These data support a role for mitochondrial K_{ATP} channel activation and its impact on mitochondrial bioenergetics as an important factor in the cardioprotective effect of adaptation to chronic hypoxia in both immature and adult hearts.

ISCHEMIC PRECONDITIONING

It is now 16 years since the phenomenon termed "ischemic preconditioning" has been formally recognized. In their seminal study, Murry et al. [33] reported that infarct size produced by sustained coronary occlusion could be markedly reduced if they first "preconditioned" the heart with episodes of brief ischemia. The observed phenomenon known as "classic" or "early" ischemic preconditioning has now been documented in all species tested as well as in human isolated cardiomyocytes and atrial muscle [49]. The window of protection is quite short; reports vary but the protection wears off in about one hour. Interestingly, a "second window of protection" (i.e. delayed preconditioning) appears 24 h after the initial stimulus and may persist for as long as 2 to 3 days. The classical stimulus for preconditioning is a critical reduction of myocardial blood flow, but other more unconventional strategies have also proved to be effective. Preconditioning can be induced by a reduction of regional or total coronary flow in isolated heart preparations, by hypoxic perfusion of isolated hearts, by hypoxia in non-perfused cardiac preparations, by rapid pacing and even in isolated cardiomyocytes, subjected to hypoxia. Moreover, there are several classes of pharmacological agents that may be able to mimic the protection conferred by ischemic preconditioning [50,51]. Preconditioning reduces not only infarct size but also the severity of ischemic and reperfusion arrhythmias and improves the postischemic contractile function.

Whereas extensive data are available on ischemic preconditioning in the adult myocardium, information on whether this protective phenomenon also occurs in immature heart is inadequate [3]. It has been shown [14] that classical ischemic preconditioning, at least in rats, is not present at birth and that the enhanced postischemic recovery of contractile function only develops during the first postnatal week (Fig. 5). Increased duration of the preconditioning cycle as well as the shortening of ischemic duration did not lead to the appearance of the protective effect [13]. However, on the basis of these results it cannot be excluded that ischemic preconditioning using an other indexes of injury (e.g. infarct size, incidence of arrhythmias), or in a different animal species, might have a different developmental pattern. Liu et al. [52] and Baker et al. [53] observed that preconditioning can be induced in isolated perfused immature rabbits hearts; data on the newborns are, however, lacking.

Some information on the neonatal hearts has also been obtained in cultured cells. Webster et al. [54] demonstrated that neonatal rat cardiac myocytes preconditioned by a 25 min exposure to hypoxia followed by reoxygenation were protected against

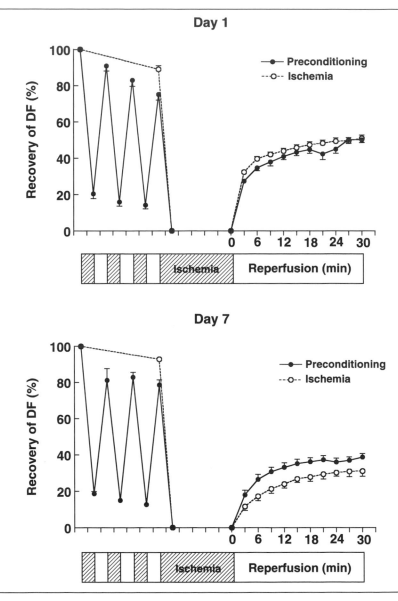

Figure 5. Time-course of post-ischemic recovery of developed force (DF, expressed as percentage of baseline values) in 1- and 7-day-old isolated perfused rat hearts. Controls-dotted line, preconditioned—continuos line. [Data from Ostadalova et al. [14].]

membrane damage for up to 6h of prolonged severe hypoxia, as determined by arachidonic acid release and contractile recovery. In contrast, non-preconditioned myocytes exhibited significant hypoxic damage after only 2–4h. It is obvious that contractile failure of myocytes in tissue culture occurs much more slowly in response to hypoxia than in working hearts, perhaps because of differences in the balance of energy supply and demand between the two situations. Similarly, Ovelgønne et al. [55] have shown that preconditioning can be induced in cultured neonatal myocytes after a 60-min exposure to hypoxia but not by heat shock proteins. However, because of the specific developmental features of this experimental model, information thus obtained is difficult to compare with the whole-heart studies.

The precise mechanisms of preconditioning in the adult myocardium are still unclear and the same is also valid for the immature heart (for review see 42). They almost certainly involve the initial release of "endogenous myocardial protective substances" [50] which probably include adenosine, bradykinin, prostacyclin, nitric oxide, the translocation of protein kinase C (PKC) to sarcolemmal and nuclear membranes and probably the effect on mitochondrial K_{ATP} channels. However, the possible age-dependent differences in triggers, signaling pathways and end effectors have to be taken into consideration. For example, PKC isoforms change during ontogenetic development: we have observed [14] that the levels of PKC isoforms α and δ in the rat heart changed significantly already during the first week of life. On the other hand, no sign of translocation of any PKC isoforms was observed on day 7, i.e. on the first day of postnatal life when ischemic preconditioning appeared. However, on the basis of this observation the role of PKC in the mechanism of preconditioning cannot be excluded; a study of further postnatal development of this protective phenomenon would be decisive in this respect.

Among the list of possible mediators of preconditioning, NO has been suggested to play an important role. It has been shown, that the early and late phases of this phenomenon can be blocked by the NO pathway inhibitors [56]. The precise mechanism is not known but the finding that NO can potentiate the K_{ATP} channels [57] raises the distinct possibility that NO could modulate the possible end-effector of ischemic preconditioning. Since all three sources of nitric oxide in the myocardium, i.e. endothelium of coronary vasculature, endocardial endothelium and cardiomyocytes undergo significant changes during ontogenetic development, age-related variations in the role of NO cannot be excluded.

Recently, increasing evidence has accumulated in support of mitochondrial K_{ATP} channels as a trigger and effector of cardioprotection [58]. Baines et al. [59] using infarct size as the end-point have observed, that diazoxide mimicked preconditioning in the adult rabbit heart and that 5-hydroxydecanoate blocked the protective effect of this phenomenon. Similarly, Baker et al. [53] have shown that 5-hydroxydecanoate completely abolished the protective effect of preconditioning in the immature rabbit heart. It seems therefore, that mitochondrial K_{ATP} channels are involved in the mechanism of preconditioning both in immature and adult hearts. In this connection it is necessary to mention the hypothesis of Downey and Cohen [60] that mitochondrial K_{ATP} channels act as triggers rather then mediators of protection: action of these channels involves mitochondrial generation of free radicals which then can stimulate downstream kinases. Whether the same would be valid also for the immature heart remains to be clarified.

It may be concluded that ischemic preconditioning as a potent cardioprotective mechanism is, at least in rats, not a genotypic phenomenon but that it develops very early during postnatal life. This fact might be of importance for potential clinical application of ischemic preconditioning before cardiac surgery in children with congenital heart disease. It is, however, too soon to reach a definitive conclusion as to whether the mechanisms involved in the preconditioning of the immature heart differ from that in the adult myocardium.

COMBINATION OF ADAPTATION TO CHRONIC HYPOXIA AND ISCHEMIC PRECONDITIONING

As compared with the temporal character of preconditioning, cardiac protection by adaptation to chronic hypoxia may persist long after the regression of other hypoxia-induced adaptive changes, such as polycythemia, pulmonary hypertension and right ventricular hypertrophy [38]. In this connection the question arises whether the cardioprotective mechanism of chronic hypoxia and ischemic preconditioning may share similar pathways, at least in part. Tajima et al. [61] addressed this problem and demonstrated that the protective effect of preconditioning against subsequent postischemic contractile dysfunction is additive to that afforded by adaptation to chronic hypoxia. This may suggest that the two phenomena are independent and utilize different mechanisms. In contrary, our recent experiments examining infarct size as the end-point of injury demonstrated that effects of chronic hypoxia and preconditioning are not additive [62]. Furthermore, Asemu et al. [35] using ischemic arrhythmias as the end-point, have shown that protection by a combination of chronic hypoxia and preconditioning was significantly more efficient than preconditioning alone in normoxic adult rats but the difference between the two preconditioned groups was rather small. Therefore, these results are not sufficiently conclusive as to whether the antiarrhythmic effect of the two phenomena are additive and may thus utilize different protective pathways. However, our experiments [35] revealed that adaptation to chronic hypoxia increased the antiarrhythmic threshold of ischemic preconditioning in adult animals: the stronger ischemic stimulus was needed to activate the signaling cascade leading to further short-term cardiac protection.

On the other hand, Baker et al. [53] have observed that whereas the isolated immature rabbit heart normoxic from birth, could be preconditioned (with recovery of contractile function as the end-point), isolated immature heart, chronically hypoxic from birth, could not be preconditioned even when the number of occlusion periods was increased. They have concluded that chronically hypoxic immature hearts are already protected and that additional cardioprotection by ischemic preconditioning is not possible. Our preliminary study suggests [40] that this is not valid for the neonatal rat heart, where the degree of ischemic tolerance can be significantly increased by a combination of the two protective phenomena.

Additional studies are therefore needed to define the relationship between adaptation to hypoxia, and ischemic preconditioning as well as their mechanisms in immature hearts. Nevertheless, it seems that in the immature heart both phenomena share a common final effector (or trigger?), mitochondrial K_{ATP} channels, even if the signal transduction pathway in the immature heart that results in increased activation of these channels is unknown [53].

REFERENCES

1. Fejfar Z. 1975. Prevention against ischemic heart disease: a critical review. In: Modern Trends in Cardiology. Ed. MF Oliver, 465–499. London and Boston: Butterworths.
2. Ardehali A, Ports TA. 1990. Myocardial oxygen supply and demand. Chest 98:699.
3. Ošt'ádal B, Ošt'ádalová I, Dhalla NS. 1999. Development of cardiac sensitivity to oxygen deficiency: comparative and ontogenetic aspects. Phys Rev 79:635–659.
4. Pridjan AK, Levitsky S, Krukenkamp I, Silverman NA, Feinberg H. 1988. Developmental changes in reperfusion injury. J Thorac Cardiovasc Surg 96:577–581.
5. Fazekas JF, Alexander FAD, Himwich HE. 1941. Tolerance of the newborn to anoxia. Am J Physiol 134:281–285.
6. Su JY, Friedman WF. 1973. Comparison of the responses of fetal and adult cardiac muscle to hypoxia. Am J Physiol 224:1249–1253.
7. Jarmakani JM, Nagamoto T, Nakazawa M, Langer GA. 1978. Effect of hypoxia on myocardial high-energy phosphates in the neonatal mammalian heart. Am J Physiol 235:H475–H481.
8. Jarmakani JM, Nakanishi T, George BL, Bers D. 1982. Effect of extracellular calcium on myocardial mechanical function in the neonatal rabbit. Dev Pharmacol Ther 5:1–13.
9. Nakanishi T, Nishioka K, Jarmakani JM. 1982. Mechanism of tissue Ca^{2+} gain during reoxygenation after hypoxia in rabbit myocardium. Am J Physiol 242:H437–H449.
10. Young HH, Shimizu T, Nishioka K, Nakanishi T, Jarmakani JM. 1983. Effect of hypoxia and reoxygenation on mitochondrial function in neonatal myocardium. Am J Physiol 245: H998–1006.
11. Ošt'ádal B, Procházka J, Pelouch V, Urbanová D, Widimský J. 1984. Comparison of cardiopulmonary responses of male and female rats to intermittent high altitude hypoxia. Physiol Bohemoslov 33:129–138.
12. Riva E, Hearse DJ. 1993. Age-dependent changes in myocardial susceptibility to ischemic injury. Cardiosci 4:85–92.
13. Awad WI, Shattock MJ, Chambers DJ. 1998. Ischemic preconditioning in immature myocardium. Circulation 98:II-206–II-213.
14. Ošt'ádalová I, Ošt'ádal B, Kolář F, Parratt JR, Wilson S. 1998. Tolerance to ischaemia and ischaemic preconditioning in neonatal rat heart. J Mol Cell Cardiol 30:857–865.
15. Baker EJ, Boerboom LE, Olinger GN, Baker JE. 1995. Tolerance of the developing heart to ischemia: impact of hypoxemia from birth. Am J Physiol 268:H1165–H1173.
16. Hoerter J. 1976. Change in the sensitivity to hypoxia and glucose deprivation in the isolated perfused rabbit heart during perinatal development. Pflügers Arch 363:1–6.
17. Bass A, Stejskalová M, Stieglerová A, Ošt'ádal B, Šamánek M. 2001. Ontogenetic development of energy-supplying enzymes in rat and guinea-pig heart. Physiol Res 50:237–245.
18. Julia P, Young HH, Buckberg GD, Kofsky ER, Bugyi HI. 1990. Studies of myocardial protection in the immature heart. II. Evidence for importance of amino acid metabolism in tolerance to ischemia. J Thorac Cardiovasc Surg 100:888–895.
19. Hohl CM. 1997. Effect of respiratory inhibition and ischemia on nucleotide metabolism in newborn swine cardiac myocytes. In: The Developing Heart. Ed. B Ostadal, M Nagano, N Takeda, NS Dhalla, 393–405. Philadelphia: Lippincott.
20. Škárka L, Baumruk F, Kopecký J, Jarkovská D, Ošt'ádal B. 2000. Ontogenetic development of mitochondrial membrane potencial in the rat heart. Exp Clin Cardiol 5:48.
21. Nijjar MS, Dhalla NS. 1997. Biochemical basis of calcium handling in developing myocardium. In: The Developing Heart. Ed. B Ostadal, M Nagano, N Takeda, NS Dhalla, 189–217. Philadelphia: Lippincott.
22. Rizutto R, Bernardi P, Pozzan T. 2000. Mitochondria as all-round players of the calcium game. J Physiol 529:37–47.
23. Vornanen M. 1997. Postnatal changes in cardiac calcium regulation. In: The Developing Heart. Ed. B Ostadal, M Nagano, N Takeda, NS Dhalla, 219–229. Philadelphia: Lippincott.
24. Wibo M, Bravo G, Godfraind T. 1991. Postnatal maturation of excitation-contraction coupling in rat ventricle in relation to the subcellular localization and surface density of 1,4-dihydropyridine and ryanodine receptors. Circ Res 68:662–673.
25. Škovránek J, Ošt'ádal B, Pelouch V, Procházka J. 1986. Ontogenetic differences in cardiac sensitivity to verapamil in rats. Pediatr Cardiol 7:25–29.
26. Kolář F, Ošt'ádal B, Papoušek F. 1990. Effect of verapamil on contractile function of the isolated perfused heart. Basic Res Cardiol 85:429–434.

27. Solaro RJ, Lee JA, Kentish JC, Allen DG. 1988. Effect of acidosis on ventricular muscle from adult and neonatal rats. Circ Res 63:779–787.
28. Southworth R, Shattock MJ, Kelly FJ. 1997. Age-related differences in the cardiac response to ischemia and free radical production on reperfusion. In: The Developing Heart. Ed. B Ostadal, M Nagano, N Takeda, NS Dhalla, 427–441. Philadelphia: Lippincott.
29. Hurtado A. 1960. Some clinical aspects of life at high altitudes. Ann Int Med 53:247–258.
30. Kopecky M, Daum S. 1958. Tissue adaptation to anoxia in rat myocardium (in Czech). Cs Fyziol 7:518–521.
31. Poupa O, Krofta K, Procházka J, Turek Z. 1966. Acclimatization to simulated high altitude and acute cardiac necrosis. Fed Proc 25:1243–1246.
32. Maroko PR, Deboer LWV. 1972. Infarct size reduction: a critical review. Adv Cardiol 27:282–316.
33. Murry CE, Jennings RB, Reimer KA. 1986. Preconditioning with ischemia: a delay of lethal cell injury in ischemic myocardium. Circulation 74:1124–1136.
34. Durand J. 1982. Physiologic adaptation to altitude and hyperexis. In: High Altitude Physiology and Medicine. Ed. W Brendel and RA Zink RA, 209–211. New York: Springer-Verlag.
35. Asemu G, Papoušek F, Ošt'ádal B, Kolář F. 1999. Adaptation to high altitude hypoxia protects the rat heart against ischemia-induced arrhythmias. Involvement of mitochondrial K_{ATP} channel. J Mol Cell Cardiol 31:1821–1831.
36. Meerson FZ, Ustinova EE, Manukhina EB. 1989. Prevention of cardiac arrhythmias by adaptation: regulatory mechanisms and cardiotropic effect. Biomed Biochim Acta 48:583–588.
37. Henley WN, Belush LL, Notestine MA. 1992. Reemergence of spontaneous hypertension in hypoxia-protected rats returned to normoxia as adults. Brain Res 579:211–218.
38. Ošt'ádal B, Ošt'ádalová I, Kolář F, Pelouch V, Dhalla NS. 1998. Cardiac adaptation to chronic hypoxia. Adv Organ Biol 6:43–60.
39. Ošt'ádal B, Kolář F, Pelouch V, Widimský J. 1995. Ontogenetic differences in cardiopulmonary adaptation to chronic hypoxia. Physiol Res 44:45–51.
40. Ošt'ádalová I, Ošt'ádal B, Kolář F. 2000. Adaptation to chronic hypoxia and ischaemic preconditioning in neonatal rat heart. Exr Clin Cardiol 5:43.
41. Kolář F. 1996. Cardioprotective effects of chronic hypoxia: relation to preconditioning. In: Myocardial Preconditioning. Ed. Wainwright CL, Parratt JR, 261–275. Berlin: Springer Verlag.
42. Ošt'ádal B, Kolář F. 1999. Cardiac Ischemia: From Injury to Protection. 173pp. Boston, Dordrecht, London: Kluwer Academic Publishers.
43. Eells JT, Henry MH, Gross GJ, Baker JE. 2000. Increased mitochondrial K_{ATP} channel activity during chronic myocardial hypoxia. Is cardioprotection mediated by improved bioenergetics? Circ Res 87:915–921.
44. Sato T, O'Rourke B, Marban E. 1998. Modulation of mitochondrial ATP-dependent K^+ channels by protein kinase C. Circ Res 83:110–114.
45. Sahai A, Mei C, Zavosh A, Tannen RL. 1997. Chronic hypoxia induces LL-PK 1 cell proliferation and dedifferentiation by the activation of protein kinase C. Am J Physiol 272: F809–F815.
46. Baker JE, Boerboom LE, Olinger GN. 1998. Age related changes in the ability of hypothermia and cardioplegia to protect ischemic rabbit myocardium. J Thorac Cardiovasc Surg 96:717–724.
47. Shi Y, Pritchard KA, Holman P, Rafiee P, Griffith OW, Kalyanaraman B, Baker JE. 2000. Chronic myocardial hypoxia increases nitric oxide synthase and decreases caveolin-3. Free Radical Biol Med 29:695–703.
48. Garlid KD. 1996. Cation transport in mitochondria—the potassium cycle. Biochim Biophys Acta 1275:123–126.
49. Downey JM, Cohen MV. 1997. Preconditioning: what it is and how it works. Dialogues Cardiovasc Med 2:179–196.
50. Parratt JR. 1995. Possibilities for the pharmacological exploitation of ischaemic preconditioning. J Mol Cell Cardiol 27:991–1000.
51. Yellon DM, Baxter GF, Garcia-Dorado D, Heusch D, Sumeray MS. 1998. Ischaemic preconditioning: present position and future directions. Cardiovasc Res 37:21–33.
52. Liu H, Cala PM, Anderson SE. 1998. Ischemic preconditioning: effects on pH, Na and Ca in newborn rabbit hearts during ischemic/reperfusion. J Mol Cell Cardiol 30:685–697.
53. Baker JE, Holman P, Gross GJ. 1999. Preconditioning in immature rabbit hearts. Role of K_{ATP} channels. Circulation 99:1249–1254.
54. Webster KA, Discher DJ, Bishopric NH. 1995. Cardioprotection in an in vitro model of hypoxic preconditioning. J Mol Cell Cardiol 27:453–458.

55. Ovelgønne JH, Van Wijk R, Verkleij AJ, Post JA. 1996. Cultured neonatal rat heart cells can be preconditioned by ischemia, but not by heat shock. The role of stress proteins. J Mol Cell Cardiol 28: 1617–1629.
56. Vegh A, Komori S, Szekeres L, Parratt JR. 1992. Antiarhythmic effects of preconditioning in anaesthetized dogs and rats. Cardiovasc Res 26:487–495.
57. Shinbo A, Ijima T. 1997. Potentiation by nitric oxide of the ATP-sensitive K^+ current induced by K^+ channel openers in guinea-pig ventricular cells. Br J Pharmacol 120:1568–1574.
58. O'Rourke B. 2000. Pathophysiological and protective roles of mitochondrial ion channels. J Physiol 529:23–30.
59. Baines CP, Wang L, Cohen MV, Downey JM. 1999. Myocardial protection by insulin is dependent on phosphatidylinositol 3-kinase but not protein kinase C or K_{ATP} channels in the isolated rabbit hearts.
60. Downey JM, Cohen MV. 2000. Do mitochondrial K_{ATP} channels serve as triggers rather than end-effectors of ischemic preconditioning's protection? Basic Res Cardiol 95:272–274.
61. Kolář F, Asemu G, Neckář J, Papoušek F, Ošt'ádal B. 1999. Cardioprotection following chronic hypoxia. Physiol Res 48:S7
62. Tajima M, Katayose D, Bessho M, Isoyama S. 1994. Acute ischaemic preconditioning and chronic hypoxia independently increase myocardial tolerance to ischaemia. Cardiovasc Res 28:312–319.

B. Ostadal, M. Nagano and N.S. Dhalla (eds.).
CARDIAC DEVELOPMENT. Copyright © 2002.
Kluwer Academic Publishers. Boston.

MOLECULAR AND PHARMACOLOGICAL ASPECTS OF THE DEVELOPING HEART

SATYAJEET S. RATHI, PRAVEEN BHUGRA,
and NARANJAN S. DHALLA

Institute of Cardiovascular Sciences, St. Boniface General Hospital Research Centre, and Department of Physiology, Faculty of Medicine, University of Manitoba, Winnipeg, Canada

Summary. From the evidence presented in this article, it is quite clear that fetal and newborn hearts are functionally less developed as compared to adult hearts. In immature hearts, different pharmacological responses differ from the adult hearts but these are species dependent. Regulation of the sympathetic system and β-adrenoceptor blocking agents which modulate the sympathetic activity affect the myocardium differently at various stages of development from fetus, neonates and adulthood. The role of the renin-angiotensin system is crucial in development as angiotensin II receptors are increased during fetal development and morphogenesis but these decline after birth. Ca^{2+}-handling in neonates is not the same as in adult hearts as the intracellular Ca^{2+} in newborns is mainly regulated by mechanisms such as Ca^{2+}-influx via L type Ca^{2+}-channels and Na^+-Ca^{2+} exchange in sarcolemma. Furthermore, Ca^{2+}-uptake, storage and release by sarcoplasmic reticulum in neonatal hearts are less developed and thus the effects of various Ca^{2+}-antagonists and other such agents are mediated through the Ca^{2+}-channels and Na^+-Ca^{2+} exchange. Responses to cardiac glycosides that modulate Na^+-K^+ ATPase and Na^+-Ca^{2+} exchange activities are also determined by developmental changes in the heart. Since phosphodiesterases, which hydrolyze cAMP, undergo developmental changes, the responses of the heart to phosphodiesterase inhibitors vary markedly during the development. Although our understanding of the developmental aspects of the heart has increased significantly, the complexity of the developing heart and the mechanisms of action of different pharmacological agents in the immature heart still remain to be examined carefully.

Address for correspondence: Dr. Naranjan S. Dhalla, Institute of Cardiovascular Sciences, St. Boniface General Hospital Research Centre, 351 Tache Avenue, Winnipeg, MB, R2H 2A6, Canada. Tel: (204) 235-3417; Fax: (204) 233-6723; e-mail: cvso@sbrc.ca

INTRODUCTION

Acquisition of different functions of the cardiovascular system at various stages of development from fetus to adulthood takes place by cell division, cell differentiation and cell growth. It is now well known that the fetal and newborn hearts have less functionality and are therefore immature in comparison to the adult heart. This view is based on experimental evidence which demonstrated that the developed tension per unit cross-sectional area of the isolated cardiac muscle in young animals was less than that generated by the adult hearts [1–3]. There are also numerous studies describing differences in functional responses elicited by various pharmacological agents in neonatal and adult hearts from different species and experimental animals. Although our understanding of the developmental aspects of cardiovascular function and differences in drug responses has improved considerably over the past 50 years, the information regarding the mechanisms of drug responses in the developing heart as well as changes which take place after the action of drugs is still lacking. The purpose of this article is to present an overview regarding the pharmacological responses and the molecular mechanisms of developmental variations in the cardiovascular function. It is proposed to discuss this topic in the following categories: (a) sympathetic system and β-adrenoceptors, (b) renin-angiotensin system, (c) calcium channel activity, (d) sodium-calcium exchange and (e) cyclic nucleotide phosphodiesterase system.

SYMPATHETIC SYSTEM AND β-ADRENOCEPTORS

Cardiac function is controlled by the autonomic nervous system (i.e. sympathetic system and parasympathetic system), which elicits actions through the participation of adrenoceptors and muscarinic-cholinergic receptors, respectively. At least nine adrenoceptor and five muscarinic receptor subtypes have been shown to exist in the myocardium. The adrenoceptors are classified into two types (Fig. 1) which are further categorized by the pharmacological and molecular cloning into nine subtypes [4]. It has been demonstrated that the sympathetic innervation of the ventricles remains incomplete for several days after birth [2,5,6]; this is associated with the immaturity of myocardium, disorganization of myofibrils and different mechanism for the excitation-contraction coupling [7–10]. In early neonatal stages, β-adrenergic receptors are abundant on the cell membrane of cardiomyocytes [11–13] and therefore there occurs an increase in contractile force development by the β-agonists. The density of β-adrenoceptors is maximum at birth and declines slowly thereafter. It has been demonstrated that the density of receptors and the sympathetic innervation may vary with the species. For example, in rabbit and dog, the sympathetic innervation of the heart is incomplete during the developing phase [14,15]. In cultured isolated rat myocytes, the sympathetic innervation improves the cardiac contractility [16,17] indicating that the amount of sympathetic innervation plays a vital role in inotropic response of myocardium to β-adrenoceptor agonists during the developmental phases.

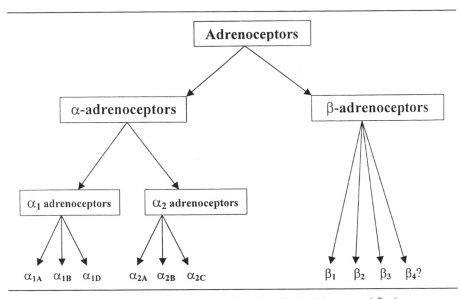

Figure 1. The classification of adrenoceptors which are broadly divided in α- and β-adrenoceptors. These are further subtypes as shown above.

In adult human heart, β_1- and β_2-adrenoceptors are coupled to G_s-proteins for the activation of adenylyl cyclase leading to an increase in the intracellular level of cAMP. The second messenger results in the activation of protein kinase A (PKA) which phosphorylates several proteins including L-type Ca^{2+}-channels in the sarcolemmal (SL) membrane and phospholamban in the sarcoplasmic reticulum (SR) [18,19]. Phosphorylation of the L-type Ca^{2+}-channels promotes Ca^{2+}-influx and thus leads to enhanced contraction. It is also suggested that phosphorylation of phospholamban may be involved in enhanced diastolic relaxation by increasing Ca^{2+}-uptake into the SR tubules. G_s-proteins have also been shown to activate L-type Ca^{2+}-channels directly in mammalian cardiomyocytes [20,21]. Xiao and colleagues [22–24] have proposed that the β_2-adrenoceptors can also couple to G_i-proteins in adult rat ventricular cardiomyocytes. Han et al. (1989) have reported that postnatal rat heart consisted of pertussis toxin-sensitive G-protein and that both G_i- and G_o-subtypes of G-proteins are substrate for ADP ribosylation [25]. Moreover, Luetje et al. [26] have observed that $G_{i\alpha}$-protein contents in neonates rat ventricle were 3.3-fold higher as compared to the adult heart. The rat ventricular tissues from different age groups (1, 7 and 30 day old rats) showed an increase in the efficiency of β-adrenergic signal transduction due to reduction of the G_i-proteins and dominance of the $G_{s\alpha}$-linked pathway in the postnatal rat heart [27]. Although developmental regulation of α-subunit of G-proteins has been shown to occur, the factors influencing their impact upon contractile responses are unclear. Furthermore, very little information is available regarding developmental changes in G_s-proteins in the heart.

It is now well established that the binding of an appropriate agonist to β-adrenoceptors results in a change in the receptor conformation, activation of G_s-proteins, stimulation of adenylyl cyclase and generation of cAMP. Therefore it is thought that the positive inotropic response of the heart to β-adrenergic receptor agonist during cardiac maturation requires an intact adenylyl cyclase system. Although adenylyl cyclase activity in developing mammalian myocardium is responsive to activation by GTP and GTP analogues, this effect is thought to be mediated by $G_{s\alpha}$-proteins. Tanaka and Shigenobu [28], demonstrated the adrenergic binding site density and stimulation of adenylyl cyclase activity by isoprenaline in ventricular preparations obtained from 15 day fetal, one day old and seven day old rats. It has been suggested that the β-receptors and adenylyl cyclase system are well developed independently in late fetal and early newborn animals but the functional coupling of β-receptors to adenylyl cyclase in these hearts may be weaker in comparison to the adult heart. This suggestion is supported by the observation that the maximal inotropic response in papillary muscles from newborn rabbits to forskolin, a direct activator of G_s-proteins, is substantially greater than that elicited by isoprenaline [29]. However, the ability of isoprenaline in the presence of GTP to stimulate adenylyl cyclase activity is diminished in late fetal and early newborn preparation. In myocardium from 14 to 16 day old rabbits, the maximal effect of isoprenaline and forskolin were quantitatively similar suggesting that the functional coupling of β-adrenoceptors to adenylyl cyclase is completed by two weeks of age in the rabbit [28,30,31]. It has also been demonstrated that the SR phospholamban content in fetal sheep is reduced [32] and troponin isoforms change during perinatal maturation in the rat [33] and rabbit [34].

Increase in Ca^{2+}-current was noticed upon stimulation of α_1-adrenoceptors by phenylephrine after pretreatment with propranolol, a β-adrenoceptor blocker. Prazosin blocked the stimulatory effect of α_1-adrenoceptor activation in neonatal cardiomyocytes; however, this effect was not observed in young rat myocytes. Thus it was proposed that the coupling of the α_1-adrenoceptor to Ca^{2+}-channels may switch during development [35]. Inayatulla et al. [36] studied the positive inotropic response of sympathetic agents in relation to the myocardial adrenoceptors in rat and concluded that the positive inotropic response of the heart to sympathomimetic amines declines with age and this change in response is more marked in the case of α_1-adrenoceptor mediated effects. Accordingly, it was suggested that these alterations in response may not be due to a decrease in the number or affinity of α_1- and β_1-adrenoceptors [36].

It has been observed that the maximum developed tension in response to isoproterenol in the isolated left ventricular papillary muscle from 21 day old rabbit was 3- to 4-fold higher as compared to the adult rabbit. These differences in responses may be due to higher sensitivity of isoproterenol in the developing heart. The number of specific [³H] dihydralprenolol binding sites in the young heart is 3- to 21-fold higher in comparison to the adult rats [28]. Thus it was concluded that the increase in cardiac contractility by catecholamines during development is directly proportional to the increase in density of beta adrenoreceptors. On the other hand, no change in the activation of adenylyl cyclase by forskolin during the same period of development was observed whereas there was a significant reduction in isoproterenol-induced activation of adenylyl cyclase with the further development leading to decrease in chronotropic and inotropic sensitivity to β-adrenoceptor agonists in the adult heart. This change could be partly due to reduction in density of β-adrenoceptors or may be due to a weaker coupling of receptors of adenylyl cyclase with G_s-proteins [28,37]. It was interesting to observe that treatment of animals with terbutalin (a $β_2$-adrenoceptor agonist) and dexamethasone in late gestation produced an increase in the adenylyl cyclase activity and β-receptor binding in cardiac membrane leading to delayed peak of adenylyl cyclase activity immediately after birth [38]. Thus it was concluded that β-adrenergic stimulation serves as a tropic factor controlling the ontogenic rise of the adenylyl cyclase activity; this regulation appears to involve the enzyme itself rather than changes in receptor binding capabilities or receptor specific linkage.

The sympathetic nervous system by releasing noradrenaline and activating β-adrenergic activation regulates Ca^{2+}-entry into cardiomyocytes [39,40]. Release of ATP has also been shown to occur upon stimulation of the sympathetic nervous system and produce an increase in Ca^{2+}-influx [41–43]. ATP responses in myocardium are thought to be independent of cAMP but may be mediated by specific receptors on the SL membrane [44,45]. At the cell surface, ATP interacts with its purinergic receptors causing an increase in the intracellular concentration of Ca^{2+} and thus increasing the contractile force; the increase in contraction induced with ATP may be mediated by enhanced turnover of inositol containing lipids [46,47]. Thus it is possible that ATP linked mechanisms in addition to β-adrenoceptors may also be involved in the determination of changes in sympathetic responses of the heart during development.

Driscoll and colleagues [48] have reported that the positive inotropic effects of adrenoceptor agonists, dopamine (which has pharmacological action on the dopamine receptor and β-adrenoceptor as well as in very high concentration on α-adrenoceptor) and isoprenaline (which has pharmacological action on the β-adrenoceptors) are less in newborn puppies as compared to adult dogs. The response of isoprenaline in rabbit ventricular papillary muscles isolated from one day old rabbit was comparatively less than that from seven day old or four month old rabbits; however, the EC_{50} values were higher in one day old rabbits as compared to the adult [49]. It has also been demonstrated that the effect of isoprenaline were similar in both age groups with the maximum inotropic effect greater in newborn than in the adult [29,50]. Due to these conflicting data, it is concluded that differences in isoprenaline or dopamine responses due to developmental stages of the heart are species-dependent.

RENIN-ANGIOTENSIN SYSTEM

Angiotensin II (Ang II), an important component of the renin-angiotensin system (Fig. 2), is known to be a potent vasoconstrictor and thereby leads to an increase in blood pressure. The vasoconstrictor effect of Ang II influences renal tubules to retain sodium and water as well as to stimulate aldosterone release from the adrenal

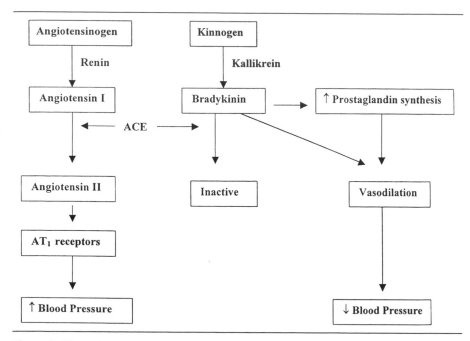

Figure 2. The renin–angiotensin system and kinnogen pathway. Angiotensinogen in the presence of renin is converted to angiotensin I. Angiotensin itself is inactive and is converted by the angiotensin converting enzyme (ACE) to angiotensin II which acts on the angiotensin receptors (AT₁) leading to vasoconstriction and salt/water retention. The ACE is also known as kinase II and it inactivates the bradykinin and thus inhibits the vasodilatory effect of bradykinin.

gland [51]. The action of angiotensin II is mediated mainly by two subtypes of receptors, namely AT_1 and AT_2 receptors; existence of these receptors was first documented by using pharmacological approach through various Ang II receptor antagonists [52]. AT_1 receptor was first cloned independently by Murphy et al. and Sasaki et al. in 1991 [53,54]. Studies on the structure and function analysis in rats and mice suggest that AT_1 receptors are present in two subtypes ($AT_{1\alpha}$ and $AT_{1\beta}$ receptors) which have 94% homology with regards to amino acid sequence and show similar pharmacological nature and distribution in tissues. AT_1 receptors mediate most of the pharmacological effects of Ang II such as elevation of blood pressure, vasoconstriction, increase in cardiac contractility, aldosterone release and catecholamine release from nerve ending as well as renal sodium and water absorption.

The selective AT_2 receptor ligands available are PD123177, PD123319, CGP42112, L162,686, L162,638, EXP801 and CGP42112A. Cloning of AT_2 receptors in human, rat and mouse tissues showed that these receptors are expressed all over in developing fetal tissues. Therefore it has been suggested that AT_2 receptors may play a role during fetal development and morphogenesis. The expression of AT_2 receptor rapidly decreases after birth and these become restricted only to uterus,

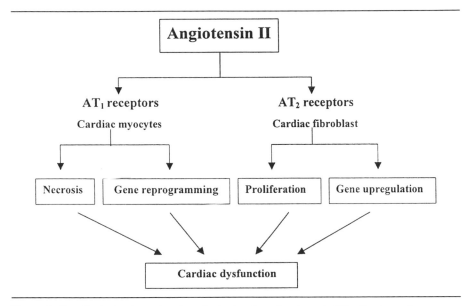

Figure 3. Broadly depict the various hypothesized action of angiotensin II leading to cardiac dysfunction (for details refer to renin-angiotensin system in the review).

ovary, certain brain nuclei, heart and adrenal medulla in adults. There is no evidence for the subtypes of AT_2 receptors available in the literature; however, recent research data provide evidence that AT_2 receptors are coupled with the G_i-proteins [55,56]. AT_2 receptors activate protein tyrosine kinase, inhibit cell growth [57] and induce apoptosis [58] in various cell lines. Both AT_1 and AT_2 are expressed in cardiomyocytes but it has been demonstrated that the response of Ang II leading to cardiac dysfunction is mostly medicated through AT_1 receptors [59–61] (Fig. 3).

It has also been demonstrated that Ang II induces hypertrophy in neonatal cardiomyocytes [60,62,63] and adult cardiomyocytes [64–66]. Ang II can directly induce expression of the fetal gene phenotype such as β-myosin heavy chain (β-MHC), skeletal α-actin and atrial natriuretic factor (ANF) in neonatal rat cardiomyocytes suggesting the involvement of AT_1 receptor in cardiac gene reprogramming in vitro [63]. The immediate early genes (including c-fos, c-jun, jun-b, Egr-1 and c-myc) are also stimulated by Ang II [63]. However, the role of Ang II in the induction of early gene and their role in hypertrophy of cardiomyocyte reprogramming requires more studies to understand the exact mechanism. In cardiomyocytes, AT_1 receptors are coupled to hetrotrimeric G_q-proteins. Ang II stimulates phosphatidylinositol-specific phospholipase C (PLC)-β isoform through G-proteins, causing an increase in the concentrations of inositol triphosphate (IP_3) and diacylglycerol (DAG); IP_3 releases Ca^{2+} from SR whereas DAG leads to the activation of protein kinase C (PKC). Apart from the above mentioned basic signal transduction pathway via G_q-proteins, various reports have suggested that Ang II in neonatal rat cardiomyocytes activates tyrosine kinases [67] through extracellular signal regulated kinases (ERKs) and c-Jun amino-terminal kinases (JNKs) [68]. Ang II also activates 70 kDa ribosomal S6 kinase (p70RSK) [69] and 90 kDa ribosomal S6 kinase (p90RSK) [67]; activation of phospholipase A_2 and phospholipase D increase the concentrations of phosphatidic acid and arachidonic acid [60]. In neonatal rat cardiac myocytes it was observed that AT_1 receptor has no intrinsic tyrosine kinase activity but it induces rapid phosphorylation of Jauus kinase2 as well as of a signal transducer and activator of transcription (STAT); $STAT_1$ and $STAT_2$ are phosphorylated within 30 min whereas $STAT_3$ is phosphorylated within 120 min [70]. While the significance of these findings is not known, the activation of RhoA by Ang II is responsible for the Ang II–induced sarcomeric actin organization and ANF expression [71].

Hypertrophic mechanism by Ang II in neonatal cardiomyocytes is poorly understood at present. It has been observed that Ang II activates p70S6K in myocytes whereas rapamycin, an immunosuppressant, abolished the Ang II–induced protein synthesis without antagonizing the ERK activation or c-fos mRNA induction, suggesting the role of p70S6K in Ang II–induced hypertrophy [69]. At present, no information regarding the involvement of ERK activation in cardiac hypertrophy or gene expression induced by Ang II is available. It has been suggested that ERK activation may be involved in myocyte hypertrophy with other hypertrophic stimuli such as phenylephrine [61,72,73]. Since Ang II is known to generate reactive oxygen intermediates in neonatal rat heart and since butylated hydroxyanisole, an antioxidant, inhibited the Ang II–induced ^{3}H-leucine incorporation in cardiomyocytes, it appears that reactive oxygen intermediates may play an important role in Ang II–induced hypertrophy [74].

Most of the work with Ang II has been done in cultured neonatal rat cardiomyocytes because these cells in the presence of serum have the ability to divide whereas adult cardiomyocytes are terminally differentiated and have no ability to divide suggesting a significant level of difference in phenotype between neonatal and adult cardiomyocytes. Stretching of neonatal rat cardiomyocyte is the most popular research tool for investigating the effect of load on cardiomyocytes (in vitro model), leading to cardiac hypertrophy and gene reprogramming [60]. Ito et al. [75] suggested that Ang II stimulates endothelin-1 production in neonatal rat myocytes by activating PKC, which may be involved in Ang II–induced myocyte hypertrophy via an autocrine mechanism. Sadoshima et al. [76] suggested that myocyte secretes Ang II which acts as a central component for stretch induced hypertrophy. Some studies on the isolated perfused adult rat heart or the isolated perfused adult feline heart were conducted to demonstrate that an increase in protein synthesis or c-fos and c-myc mRNA due to systolic pressure overload was not abolished by AT_1 receptor antagonist [77,78]. This observation regarding the pressure-induced growth response in adult heart appears to be inconsistent with the molecular mechanism of Ang II–induced hypertrophic response in neonatal cardiomyocytes. Therefore, it is concluded that there are many unresolved questions regarding the mechanism of Ang II–mediated cardiovascular response.

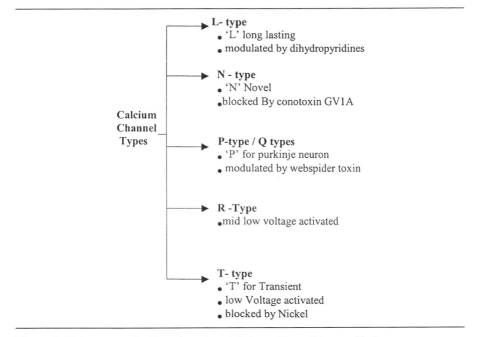

Figure 4. Various types of calcium channels and their specific modulator or blocker.

CALCIUM CHANNEL ACTIVITY AND PHARMACOLOGICAL AGENTS

Calcium serves two vital biological roles (a) it regulates membrane electrical potential and cation transport; and (b) it serves as a cellular messenger and controls several important processes such as contraction, cell architecture and enzyme activation. In fact, the Ca^{2+}-mediated processes are vital to the health and welfare of the cell. Calcium enters muscle cells through the voltage-gated channels, receptor-operated channels, sodium–calcium exchange mechanism and to a small degree, according to its own gradient [79,80]. The Ca^{2+}-channels through which Ca^{2+} enters the cell are broadly divided into five subtypes (Fig. 4). It has now become increasingly evident that the voltage dependent Ca^{2+}-channels are subject to regulatory influences. These influences may be physiological, pathological or pharmacological in nature [81].

Voltage-gated Ca^{2+}-channels are physiologically and pharmacologically important in many excitable cells, including the heart, where these contribute not only to impulse generation and conduction but also serve as a major route for Ca^{2+} entry. Ca^{2+} modulates regulatory protein kinases, activation of contractile proteins and gene expression [82,83]. It is established that Ca^{2+} entry through L-type channels is regulated by the β-adrenergic signaling pathway. The binding of agonist to β-adrenoceptor is coupled to an intracellular signal transduction by the stimulatory G_s-protein. Agonist occupancy activates adenylyl cyclase to increase the intracellular concentration of cAMP, which in turn activates cAMP-dependent protein kinase

(PKA) by dissociating the inactive holoenzyme into regulatory and catalytic sub-units. In adult cardiomyocytes, this sequence increases L-type channel activity, in part through changes in gating caused by phosphorylation of the channel by a closely associated protein, PKA [84–88], or through direct membrane G-protein interactions with the channel protein [89]. The L-type Ca^{2+} channel is a multisub-unit complex consisting of primary pore forming α_1-subunit along with additional accessory α_2, δ, γ and β_2 subunit [90]. It has been reported that L-type channel modulation by PKA is enhanced by co-expression of α_1- and β_2-subunits in het-erologous expression system [91,92]; α_1-subunit alone can also be the target of PKA [93].

During development, modulatory response to catecholamine is affected by changes in the relative expression levels of β-adrenergic signaling transduction com-ponents and/or the type and architecture of L-type channel subunits. There is also evidence to suggest that alternative splicing of the cardiac L-type channel α_1-subunit may take place during development [94]. In addition, there is evidence regarding changes in the cAMP signaling pathway during early stages of development of hearts from several species [95]. It has also been observed that the physiological (i.e. pos-itive inotropic and chronotropic) response to β-adrenergic stimulation of the devel-oping heart lag behind the expression of β-adrenoceptor and adenylyl cyclase in most of the species and the mouse in particular [96–98]. Furthermore, total PKA activity in the murine embryonic heart increases most markedly during the 6 days before birth, a period in which the physiological response to β-adrenergic stimula-tion also becomes apparent [99]. Similarly, there is improved coupling between β-adrenoceptors and physiological responses in the fetal rat heart during the late embryonic stages [100]. In chronic heart failure, there occurs a reduced responsive-ness to β-adrenoceptor agonists which may contribute to a reduction in contrac-tile activity due in part to the downregulation and sequestration of receptors [101]. The uncoupling of receptors from downstream steps in signaling transduction are partly mediated by β-adrenoceptor kinases and β-arrestin [102–106]. In addition, dilated cardiac hypertrophy, a hallmark of heart failure, is accompanied by the reac-tivation of genes which are expressed during the heart development [107,108]. Accordingly, it has been suggested that understanding of the fetal programming of β-adrenergic signal transduction pathway and its interactions with L-type Ca^{2+}-channel is likely to provide valuable insight into the processes contributing to cardiac dysfunction due to heart disease. Recent advances in genetically modified mice have revealed some steps in the β-adrenoceptor system are specifically targeted in the heart [109,110].

Since the SR tubules are not well developed in immature hearts, it has been pro-posed that the entry of Ca^{2+} through the SL membrane not only participates in release of Ca^{2+} from the intracellular stores of Ca^{2+} but it also provides Ca^{2+} directly to the contractile proteins during the development. Therefore, it has been postu-lated that SL has a greater role in regulating the intracellular Ca^{2+} concentration at the contractile proteins in developing heart [111–118]. Various reports available in the literature regarding underdeveloped SR at the time of birth in a number of mammalian species [32,111,112,115] suggest that the extracellular requirement of Ca^{2+} to maintain normal contraction is more in immature heart than in the developed heart [119,120]. It has also been suggested that if the newborn heart is relatively more dependent for calcium entry via the SL membrane to initiate contraction then the sensitivity to Ca^{2+}-channel blockers may also be more in the immature heart. Later Klitzner and colleagues [117,118] supported the concept that cardiac contraction in neonatal rabbit is relatively more dependent on transarcolemmal Ca^{2+}-influx than in adults. However, Wetzel et al. [119] studied the transsarcolemmal Ca^{2+}-current in rabbit myocytes isolated from neonates (1–5 days) versus adult myocytes and suggested that neonatal rabbit cardiac myocytes exhibit lower current density of L-type calcium channels and prevalence of T-type channels compared with adult cardiomyocytes.

To investigate the role of Ca^{2+} and its channels in developing heart, different investigators used various Ca^{2+}-channel blockers which are also known as Ca^{2+}-antagonists. The Ca^{2+}-antagonists are a structurally diverse group of compounds and have different pharmacological actions such as negative inotropic, chronotropic and dormotropic effects on the heart and vasodilator action in the vascular smooth muscle [122]. Ostadal et al. [123] studied ontogenic differences in cardiac sensitivity to calcium antagonists in chick embryo and postnatal immature rat hearts. They observed that verapamil exhibits no protective effect on isoprenaline-induced changes of the chick embryonic heart but instead it increased the mortality of experimental embryos. It was also observed that the mortality in verapamil treated rats due to isoprenaline was age dependent as it was increased with decreasing the age of animal. Similarly, the intensity of negative inotropic response of the isolated right ventricular myocardium and isolated perfused rat heart to verapamil was significantly greater in the youngest age groups suggesting possible negative consequences of the clinical use of Ca^{2+}-antagonists during the early phases of ontogeny. Klitzener and colleagues [124] studied the effect of diltiazem in myocytes obtained from the right ventricular papillary muscle of rabbit (>7 days old) using standard voltage clamp method to measure the inward Ca^{2+}-current. They demonstrated that diltiazem blocked the inward Ca^{2+}-current and reduced the twitch tension in the isolated papillary muscle and concluded that in neonatal rabbit myocytes Ca^{2+}-influx through the diltiazem-sensitive calcium channels is not the only source of extracellular calcium for excitation contraction coupling.

Interaction of various agonists (hormones, neurotransmitters and drugs) on the outer membrane of the cell activates Ca^{2+}-channels and because of this interaction, it is thought that a series of effects may lead to increase in Ca^{2+}-influx, increase in intracellular Ca^{2+} and muscle contraction [37,98]. Dodd and Boucek [125] evaluated the effect of Bay K8644 in right ventricular papillary muscle isolated from 12 to 20 day old and adult rabbits and reported that there was no difference in the magnitude of the increase contractility between different age groups. Ventricular papillary muscles from 12 to 20 day old rabbits showed a positive lusitropic effect at higher concentrations of Bay K8644 versus the adult muscle which failed to exert this response. It was suggested that this positive inotropic effect of Bay K8644 or similar agents could be more in less mature preparation due to greater dependence on transarcolemmal Ca^{2+}-influx [125].

Na$^+$ AND Ca^{2+} EXCHANGER

By virtue of their ability to regulate Ca^{2+} movements directly or indirectly, both Na^+-K^+ ATPase and Na^+-Ca^{2+} exchange system are important in excitation-contraction coupling in the heart [126,127]. The physiological and pharmacological role of the Na^+-Ca^{2+} exchanger have been extensively studied in mature myocardium [128–130]; however, the level of information in developing heart as compared to adult heart is relatively sparse. As a consequence of immature SR in the developing heart, the role of Na^+-Ca^{2+} exchange in the SL membrane assumes relatively greater importance in modulating Ca^{2+} fluxes [126,131]. It should be pointed out that cardiac glycosides (i.e. digitalis and its derivatives and similar agents) increase myocardial contractility by inhibiting the membrane Na^+-K^+ ATPase pump leading to a rise in the intracellular Na^+ gradient and subsequent increase in the intracellular Ca^{2+} through Na^+-Ca^{2+} exchange mechanism [132]. Thus it has been hypothesized that the activity of Na^+-Ca^{2+} exchanger should be considered in determining the sensitivity of digitalis because the exchanger is ultimately responsible for Na^+-related alteration in the intracellular Ca^{2+} [133–135]. Chen et al. [136] have shown that the Na^+-Ca^{2+} exchanger protein was predominantly located in the peripheral SL membrane before and during the development of T tubules in rabbit myocytes. This was based upon performing indirect immunofluorescent studies in isolated myocytes from immature (5, 11, 17 and 30 days) and adult rabbits for localization of the Na^+-Ca^{2+} exchange system. Carafoli [137] demonstrated that varying degrees of Ca^{2+}-uptake by Na^+-loaded SL vesicles isolated from the fetal (28 days gestation), neonatal (24–48 hours), immature (14–16 days) and adult rabbit was stimulated by valinomycin and inhibited by amiloride suggesting the developmental regulation of Na^+-Ca^{2+} exchange.

Nankanshi and colleagues [112,138] studied the effect of acetyl stropanthandin and ouabain on isolated arterially perfused ventricular septal preparation in fetal (28 days gestation), newborn (3–7 days) and adult rabbits. They demonstrated that the relative magnitude of the positive inotropic effect was more in fetus and newborn as compared to adult hearts [112,138]. Apart from the differences in the magnitude of positive inotropic effect, it was highlighted that the cardiotoxicity of cardiac glycosides was high in fetal and adult but was nearly absent in newborn hearts. However, by employing the right ventricular papillary muscles from different age groups, i.e. immature (1–2 week, 1 month and 2 months of age) and adult rabbit, it was reported that muscles from immature rabbit were less sensitive to ouabain (higher EC_{50}) in comparison to adults [139]. In canine myocardium from neonatal (7 days old) and adult rabbit, the sensitivity and maximum response to ouabain were reported to be similar among these groups [140]. It has also been demonstrated that ouabain produced a positive inotropic effect at 3, 7 and 11 days reaching the maximum on the 14th day and then slowly declined to a typical mild negative inotropic effect in adult rat myocardium [141]. These results make us conclude that the response of myocardium to ouabain may be highly dependent on species and age. Furthermore, the variation in response to ouabain may be related to the change occurring in Na^+-Ca^{2+} exchange system during the development phase.

It has been suggested that the role of Na^+-Ca^{2+} exchange may be greater in one week old rabbit than in adults [138]. This view was further strengthened by an independent work in rabbit myocardium based upon detailed myocellular morphometry and contractile response to changes in the extracellular Na^+ during development of cardiac tissue [111]. Thus on the basis of the above results and additional morphological data, it is evident that Na^+-Ca^{2+} exchange is relatively important in regulating relaxation in immature rabbit hearts [111,142]. In chick hearts, Na^+-Ca^{2+} exchange activity in the SL membrane was reported to be higher in fetus (embryonic day 4 to newborn 10th day) [143] whereas in rabbit it has been demonstrated that the Na^+-Ca^{2+} exchange activity was comparable in two week old and adult rabbits [144]. It has also been proposed that alternative mechanism may be involved in controlling the trans-sarcolemmal Ca^{2+} movements and regulating tension in newborn rabbit myocardium [121,124]. It is thus concluded that there are many unanswered questions regarding the pharmacological aspect of the developmental heart due to the lack of inhibitors and agonists of the Na^+-Ca^{2+} exchanger. The drugs mostly used as experimental tools such as cardiac glycosides are pharmacologically known to have a narrow margin of safety and their long-term efficacy is also doubtful.

CYCLIC NUCLEOTIDE PHOSPHODIESTERASE INHIBITORS

In contrast to the stimulation of β-adrenoceptor mechanism, Artman [131] suggested an alternative approach of increasing the intracellular concentration of cAMP. This was based on inhibiting the hydrolysis cAMP which would lead to accumulation of cAMP, causing activation of cAMP-dependent protein kinase and ultimately an increase in contractility. Since a family of cyclic nucleotide phosphodiesterase is known to catalyse the hydrolysis of cAMP, cAMP-specific phosphodiesterase distribution and their activity are thought to be important factors during myocardial development. It should be noted that phosphodiesterases are classified into five types (Fig. 5). The positive inotropic effect by cAMP phosphodiesterase inhibitors requires (a) increase in basal level of cAMP from adenylyl cyclase, (b) activatable cAMP dependent protein kinase and phosphorylation of appropriate regulatory proteins. Amrinone and milrinone (phosphodiesterase inhibitors) did not show response in myocardium of newborn dogs and rabbits [29,145,146], whereas in two week old rabbits the response to milrinone was more than that of the adult rabbit myocardium [29,147]. Such differences in data may be due to the changes taking place in phosphodiesterase activities during development.

Milrinone, a cardiotonic agent, causes positive inotropic effect in adult myocardium due to its selective inhibition of a high affinity cAMP phosphodiesterase activity in the SR [148,149]. Specific inhibitor of class type III has been

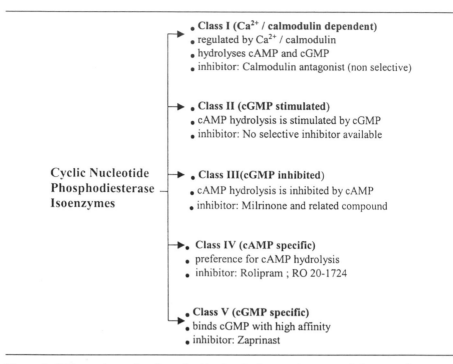

Cyclic Nucleotide Phosphodiesterase Isoenzymes

- **Class I (Ca²⁺ / calmodulin dependent)**
  - regulated by Ca²⁺ / calmodulin
  - hydrolyses cAMP and cGMP
  - inhibitor: Calmodulin antagonist (non selective)

- **Class II (cGMP stimulated)**
  - cAMP hydrolysis is stimulated by cGMP
  - inhibitor: No selective inhibitor available

- **Class III(cGMP inhibited)**
  - cAMP hydrolysis is inhibited by cAMP
  - inhibitor: Milrinone and related compound

- **Class IV (cAMP specific)**
  - preference for cAMP hydrolysis
  - inhibitor: Rolipram ; RO 20-1724

- **Class V (cGMP specific)**
  - binds cGMP with high affinity
  - inhibitor: Zaprinast

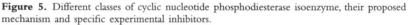

Figure 5. Different classes of cyclic nucleotide phosphodiesterase isoenzyme, their proposed mechanism and specific experimental inhibitors.

documented to be insensitive in newborn myocardium with respect to the SR associated with cAMP phosphodiesterase activity [148]. Cytosole has high affinity for cAMP phosphodiesterase in adult rabbit to milrinone; however, phosphodiesterase in cytosolic fractions in newborn myocardium belongs to Class IV cGMP-insensitive and milrinone-insensitive form [148]. Therefore Artman [131] concluded that Class III phosphodiesterase selective inhibitors are insensitive in newborn which may be due to the absence of phosphodiesterase activity. The Class IV phosphodiesterase inhibitors, R020-1724 and SQ65442, were evaluated for their contractile response and it was observed that these drugs failed to exert any positive inotropic effect in newborn as well as in adult rabbit myocardium. Thus it was indicated that the selective inhibitors of the two major forms of high affinity cAMP produce a positive inotropic effect in the myocardium of newborn rabbits [131].

Isobutylmethyl xanthine, a non-selective phosphodiesterase inhibitor evaluated in newborn rabbit myocardium exhibited approximately two-fold increase in tension development. Ogawa et al. [150] evaluated trequinsin on right ventricular papillary muscle from newborn rabbits and observed that it produced a 3.5-fold increase in contractility [150]. It was further suggested that the response was age-dependent and restricted to the newborns because the response decreased to minimal by two weeks and was more or less similar to the adult response. The difference in contractile response observed with trequinsin is not due to the difference in the ability of inhibition of hydrolysis of cAMP or cGMP in cytosolic fractions obtained from newborns, two week old and adult myocardium. It was suggested that complicity of the data obtained through experimental studies on fetal rabbit did not correspond to the pharmacological action of milrinone and therefore these may not be due to cAMP accumulation as there was increase in cAMP content but fetal myocardium did not show any inotropic effect of milrinone or isobutylmethyl xanthine [150,151].

ACKNOWLEDGEMENTS

This work was supported by a grant from the Canadian Institutes of Health Research (CIHR) Group in Experimental Cardiology. NSD holds the CIHR/Pharmaceutical Research & Development Chair in Cardiovascular Research. BP was a visiting scientist from Department of Pharmacology, Pramukswami Medical College, Karamsad, Gujurat, India.

REFERENCES

1. Downing SE, Talner NS, Gardner TH. 1965. Ventricular function in the newborn lamb. Am J Physiol 208:931–937.
2. Friedman WF. 1972. Intrinsic physiologic properties of the developing heart. Prog Cardiovasc Dis 15:87–111.
3. Hopkins SF, McCutcheon FP, Wekstein DR. 1973. Postnatal changes in rat ventricular function. Circ Res 32:685–691.
4. Alexender SPH, Peters JA. 1999. Trends in Pharmacological Sciences Receptors and Ion Channel Nomenclature Supplements, 10th ed., Elsevier Trend Journals, Cambridge.
5. Gauthier P, Nadeau RA, De Champlain J. 1975. The development of sympathetic innervation and functional state of the cardiovascular system in newborn dogs. Can J Physiol Pharmacol 53:763–776.
6. Lebowitz EA, Norick JS, Rudolph AM. 1972. Development of myocardial sympathetic innervation in the fetal lamb. Pediatr Res 6:887–893.
7. Langer GA, Brady AJ, Tan ST, Sarena SD. 1975. Correlation of the glycosides response, the force staircase and the action potential configuration in the neonatal rat heart. Circ Res 36:744–752.
8. Legato MJ. 1979. Cellular mechanisms of normal growth in the mammalian heart. I. Qualitative and quantitative features of ventricular architecture in the dog from birth to five months of age. Circ Res 44:250–262.
8a. Legato MJ. 1979. Cellular mechanisms of normal growth in the mammalian heart. II. A quantitative comparison between the right and left ventricular myocytes in the dog from birth to five months of age. Circ Res 44:263–280.
9. Page E, Earley J, Power B. 1974. Normal growth of ultrastructures in rat left ventricular myocardial cells. Circ Res 35:12–16.
10. Smith HE, Page E. 1977. Ultrastructural changes in rabbit heart mitochondria during the perinatal period: Neonatal transition to aerobic metabolism. Dev Biol 57:109–117.
11. Roeske WR, Wildenthal K. 1981. Responsiveness to drugs and hormones in the murine model of cardiac ontogenesis. Pharmacol Ther 14:55–66.
12. Cheng JB, Goldfin A, Cornett LE, Roberts JM. 1981. Identification of β-adrenergic receptors using [³H] dihydroalprenolol in fetal sheep heart: direct evidence of qualitative similarity to the receptors in adult sheep heart. Pediatr Res 15:1083–1087.
13. Feng ZP, Dryden WF, Gordon T. 1989. Postnatal development of adrenergic responsiveness in the rabbit heart. Can J Physiol Pharmacol 67:883–889.
14. Friedman WF, Pool PE, Jacobowitz D, Seagren SC, Braunwald E. 1968. Sympathetic innervation of the developing rabbit heart. Circ Res 23:25–32.

15. Ursell PC, Ren CL, Danillo P. 1990. Anatomic distribution of autonomic neural tissue in the developing dog heart. I. Sympathetic innervation. Anat Res 226:71–80.
16. Lloyd TR, Marvin WJ. 1989. Sympathetic innervation improves the contractile performance of neonatal cardiac myocytes in culture. J Mol Cell Cardiol 2:333–342.
17. Tucker DC, Gautier CH. 1990. Role of sympathetic innervation in cardiac development in oculo. Ann NY Acad Sci 588:120–129.
18. Walsh DA, Van Patten SM. 1994. Multiple pathway signal transduction by the cAMP dependent protein kinase. FASEB J 8:1227–1236.
19. Kaumann AJ, Molenaar P. 1997. Modulation of human cardiac function through 4 beta adrenoceptor populations. Naunyn-Schmiedeberg's Arch Pharmacol 355:667–681.
20. Clapham DE. 1994. Direct G protein activation of ion channel. Annu Rev Neurosci 17:441–464.
21. Schneider T, Igellmund P, Hescheler J. 1997. G protein interaction with K$^+$ and Ca^{2+} channels. Trends Pharmacol Sci 18:8–11.
22. Xiao R-P, Lakatta EG. 1993. β_1-adrenoceptors stimulation and β_2-stimulation differ in their effects on contraction, cytosolic Ca^{2+} current in single rat ventricular cells. Circ Res 73:286–300.
23. Xiao R-P, Hohl C, Altshuld R, Jones L, Livingston B, Ziman B, Tantini B, Lakatta EG. 1994. β_2-adrenergic receptor stimulated increase in cAMP in rat heart cells is not coupled to changes in Ca^{2+} dynamics, contractility or phospholamban phosphorylation. J Biol Chem 269:19151–19156.
24. Xiao R-P, Ji X, Lakatta EG. 1995. Functional coupling of the β_2-adrenoceptors to pertussis toxin-sensitive G protein in cardiac myocytes. Mol Pharmacol 47:322–329.
25. Han HM, Robinson RB, Bilezikian JP, Steinberg SF. 1989. Developmental changes in guanine nucleotide regulatory proteins in the rat myocardial α_1-adrenergic receptors complex. Circ Res 65:1763–1773.
26. Luetje CW, Tietje KM, Christian JL, Nathanson NM. 1988. Differential tissue expression and developmental regulation of guanine nucleotide binding regulatory proteins and their messenger RNAs in rat heart. J Biol Chem 263:13357–13365.
27. Bartel S, Karczewski P, Krause EG. 1996. G-proteins, adenylyl cyclase and related phosphoproteins in the developing rat heart. Mol Cell Biochem 163/164:31–38.
28. Tanaka H, Shigenobu K. 1990. Role of β-adrenoceptors-adenylate cyclase system in the development decrease in sensitivity to isoprenaline in fetal and neonatal rat heart. Br J Pharmacol 100:138–142.
29. Artman M, Kithas PA, Wike JS, Strada SJ. 1988. Inotropic responses change during postnatal maturation in rabbit. Am J Physiol 255:H335–H342.
30. Schumacher WA, Sheppard JR, Mirkin BL. 1982. Biological maturation and beta-adrenergic effectors: pre and postnatal development of the adenylate cyclase system in the rabbit heart. J Pharmacol Exp Ther 223:587–593.
31. Hatijis CG. 1986. Forskolin-stimulated adenylate cyclase activity in fetal and adult rabbit myocardial membranes. Am J Obstet Gynecol 155:1326–1331.
32. Mahony L, Jones LR. 1986. Developmental changes in cardiac sarcoplasmic reticulum in sheep. J Biol Chem 261:15257–15265.
33. L'Ecuyer TJ, Schulte D, Lin JJ-C. 1991. Thin filament changes during in vivo rat heart development. Pediatr Res 30:232–238.
34. McAuliffe JJ, Gao L, Solaro RJ. 1990. Changes in myofibrillar activation and troponin T isoform switching in developing rabbit heart. Circ Res 66:1204–1216.
35. Liu QY, Karpinski E, Pang PK. 1994. Changes in alpha-1-adrenoceptor coupling to Ca^{2+} channels during development in rat heart. FEBS Lett 338:234–238.
36. Inayatulla A, Li DY, Chemtob S, Verma DR. 1994. Ontogeny of positive inotropic responses to sympathomimetic agents and of myocardial adrenoceptors in rats. Can J Physiol Pharmacol 72: 361–367.
37. Kojima M, Ishima T, Taniguchi N, Kimura K, Sada H, Sperelakis N. 1990. Developmental changes in beta-adrenoceptors, muscarinic cholinoceptors and Ca^{2+} channels in rat ventricular muscles. Br J Pharmacol 99:334–339.
38. Navarro HA, Kudlacz EM, Slotkin TA. 1991. Control of adenylate cyclase activity in developing rat heart and liver: Effects of prenatal exposure to terbutaline or dexamethasone. Biol Neonate 60:127–136.
39. Reuter H. 1985. Calcium movements through cardiac cell membranes. Med Res Rev 5:427–440.
40. Tsien RW. 1983. Calcium channels in excitable cell membranes. Annu Rev Physiol 45:341–358.
41. Burnstock G. 1972. Purinergic nerves. Pharmacol Rev 24:509–581.

42. De Young MB, Scarpa A. 1987. Extracellular ATP induces Ca^{2+} transients in cardiac myocytes which are potentiated by norepinephrine. FEBS Lett 223:53–58.
43. Danziger RS, Raffaeli S, Moreno-Sanchez R, Sakai M, Capagrossi MC, Spurgeon HA, Hanford RG, Lakatta EG. 1988. Extracellular ATP has a potent effect to enhance cytosolic calcium and contractility in single ventricular myocytes. Cell Calcium 9:193–199.
44. Williams M. 1987. Purine receptors in mammalian tissues: Pharmacology and functional significance. Annu Rev Pharmacol Toxicol 27:315–345.
45. Zhao D, Dhalla NS. 1990. [^{35}S] ATP gamma S binding sites in purified heart sarcolemma membrane. Am J Physiol 258:C185–C188.
46. Scamps F, Maejoux E, Charlemagne D, Vassort G. 1990. Calcium current in single cells isolated from neonatal and hypertrophied rat heart. Effect of beta-adrenergic stimulation. Circ Res 67:1007–1016.
47. Legssyer A, Poggioli J, Renard D, Vassort G. 1988. ATP and other adenine compounds increase mechanical activity and inositol trisphosphate production in rat heart. J Physiol 401:185–199.
48. Driscoll DJ, Gillette PC, Ezrailson EG, Schwartz A. 1978. Inotropic response of the neonatal canine myocardium to dopamine. Pediatr Res 12:42–45.
49. Park MK, Sheridan PH, Morgan WW, Beck N. 1980. Comparative inotropic response of newborn and adult papillary muscle to isoproterenol and calcium. Dev Pharmacol Ther 1:70–82.
50. Nishioka K, Nakanashi T, George BL, Jamakarni JM. 1981. The effect of calcium on the inotropy of catecholamine and paired electrical stimulation in the newborn and adult myocardium. J Mol Cell Cardiol 13:511–520.
51. Timmermans PBMWM, Wong PC, Chiu AT, Herblin WF, Benfield P, Carini DJ, Lee RJ, Wexler R, Saye J, Smith R. 1993. Angiotensin II receptors and angiotensin II receptor antagonist. Pharmacol Rev 45:205–251.
52. Chiu AT, Herblin WF, McCall DE, Ardecky RJ, Carini DJ, Dunica JV, Pease LJ, Wong PC, Wexler RR, Johnson AL, Timmermans PBMWM. 1989. Identification of angiotensin II receptor subtypes. Biochem Biophys Res Commun 165:196–203.
53. Murphy TJ, Alexander RW, Griendling KK, Runge MS, Bernstein KE. 1991. Isolation of a cDNA encoding the vascular type-1 angiotensin II receptor. Nature (Lond) 351:233–236.
54. Sasaki K, Yamano Y, Bardhan S, Iwai N, Murray JJ, Hasagawa M, Matsuba Y, Inagami T. 1991. Cloning and expression of a complementary DNA encoding a bovine adrenal angiotensin II type 1 receptor. Nature (Lond) 351:230–233.
55. Hayashida W, Horiuchi M, Dzau VJ. 1996. Intracellular third loop domain of angiotensin type-2 receptor. Role in mediating signal transduction and cellular function. J Biol Chem 271:21985–21992.
56. Zhang J, Pratt RE. 1996. The AT_2 receptor selectively associates with G_i-alpha-2 and G_i-alpha 3 in the rat fetus. J Biol Chem 271:15026–15033.
57. Matsubara H. 1998. Pathophysiological role of angiotensin II type 2 receptor in cardiovascular and renal diseases. Circ Res 83:1182–1191.
58. Yamada T, Horiuchi M, Dzau VJ. 1996. Angiotensin II type 2 receptor mediates programmed cell death. Proc Natl Acad Sci USA 99:156–160.
59. Baker KM, Booz GW, Dostal DE. 1992. Cardiac actions of angiotensin II: Role of an intracardiac renin angiotensin system. Annu Rev Physiol 54:227–241.
60. Sadoshima J, Izumo S. 1997. The cellular and molecular response of cardiac myocytes to mechanical stress. Annu Rev Physiol 59:551–571.
61. Sugden PH, Clerk A. 1998. Cellular mechanism of cardiac hypertrophy. J Mol Med 76:725–746.
62. Baker KM, Aceto JF. 1990. Angiotensin II stimulation of protein synthesis and cell growth in chick heart cells. Am J Physiol 259:H610–H618.
63. Sadoshima J, Izumo S. 1993. Molecular characterization of angiotensin II induced hypertrophy of cardiac myocytes and hyperplasia of cardiac fibroblasts: Critical role of the AT_1 receptor subtype. Circ Res 73:413–423.
64. Wada H, Zile MR, Ivester CT, Cooper GT, McDermott PJ. 1996. Comparative effects of contraction and angiotensin II receptors on rat cardiac fibroblasts. Circulation 88:2849–2861.
65. Liu Y, Leri A, Li B, Wang X, Cheng W, Kajstura J, Anversa P. 1998. Angiotensin II stimulation in vitro induces hypertrophy of normal and postinfarcted ventricular myocytes. Circ Res 82:1145–1159.
66. Ritchie RH, Schiebinger RJ, LaPointe MC, Marsch JD. 1998. Angiotensin II induced hypertrophy of adult rat cardiomyocytes is blocked by nitric oxide. Am J Physiol 275:H1370–H1374.

67. Sadoshima J, Qiu Z, Morgan JP, Izumo S. 1995. Angiotensin II and other hypertrophic stimuli mediated by G protein-coupled receptors activate tyrosine kinase, mitogen-activated protein kinase, and 90-kD S6 kinase in cardiac myocytes. The critical role of Ca^{2+}-dependent signaling. Circ Res 76:1–15.

68. Kudoh S, Komuro I, Mizumo T, Yamazaki T, Zou Y, Shiojima I, Takekoshi N, Yazaki Y. 1997. Angiotensin II stimulates cJun NH_2 terminal kinase in cultured cardiac myocytes of neonatal rats. Circ Res 80:139–146.

69. Takano H, Kumuro I, Zou Y, Kudoh S, Yamazaki T, Yazaki Y. Activation of p70S6 protein kinase in necessary for angiotensin II-induced hypertrophy in neonatal rat cardiac myocytes. FEBS Lett 379:255–259.

70. Kodoma H, Fuduka K, Pan J, Makino S, Sano M, Takashi T, Hori S, Ogawa S. 1998. Biphasic activation of the JAK/STAT pathway by angiotensin II in rat cardiomyocytes. Circ Res 82:244–250.

71. Akoi H, Izumo S, Sadoshima J. 1998. Angiotensin II activates Rho A in cardiac myocytes: A critical role of RhoA in angiotensin induced premyofibrils formation. Circ Res 82:666–676.

72. Force T, Pombo CM, Avruch JA, Bonnventure JV, Kyriakis JM. 1996. Stress activated protein kinases in cardiovascular disease. Circ Res 44:322–329.

73. Glennon PE, Kaddoura S, Sale EM, Sale GJ, Fuller SJ, Sugden PH. 1996. Depletion of mitogen-activated protein kinase using an antisense oligodeoxynucleotide approach downregulates the phenylephrine-induced hypertrophic response in rat cardiac myocytes. Circ Res 78:954–961.

74. Nakamura K, Fushini K, Kouch H, Mihara K, Miayazaki M, Ohe T, Namba M. 1998. Inhibitory effects of antioxidants on neonatal rats cardiac myocytes hypertrophy induced by tumor necrosis factor-α and angiotensin II. Circulation 98:794–799.

75. Ito H, Hirata Y, Adachi S, Tanaka M, Tsujino M, Koike A, Nogami A, Murumo F, Hiroe M. 1993. Endothelin-1 is an autocrine/paracrine factor in the factor in the mechanism of angiotensin II-induced hypertrophy in cultured rat cardiomyocytes. J Clin Invest 92:398–403.

76. Sadoshima J, Xu Y, Slayer HS, Izumo S. 1993. Autocrine release of angiotensin II mediates stretch-induced hypertrophy of cardiac myocytes in vitro. Cell 75:977–984.

77. Thienelt CD, Weinberg EO, Bartunek J, Lorell BH. 1997. Load-induced growth response in isolated adult rat hearts: role of the AT_1 receptor. Circulation 95:2677–2683.

78. Kent RL, McDermot PJ. 1996. Passive load and angiotensin II evoke differential response of gene expression and protein synthesis in cardiac myocytes. Circ Res 78:829–838.

79. Rasmussen H. 1986. The calcium massager system (1). N Engl J Med 314:1094–1101.

80. Wood AJ. 1989. Calcium antagonist pharmacological differences and similarities. Circulation 80 (Suppl. IV):184–188.

81. Ferrante J, Triggle DJ. 1990. Drug and disease induced regulation of voltage-dependent calcium channel. Pharmacol Rev 42:29–44.

82. Kass RS. 1994. Ionic basis of electrical activity in the heart. In: Sperelakis N, ed. Physiology and Pathophysiology of the Heart. 3rd ed. Norwell, MA: Kluwer Academic Publishers, 77–90.

83. Tsien RW, Ellinor PT, Horne WA. 1991. Molecular diversity of voltage-dependent Ca channels. Trends Pharmacol Sci 12:349–354.

84. Kameyama M, Hescheler J, Hofmann F, Trautwein W. 1986. Modulation of Ca current during the phosphorylation cycle in guinea-pig heart. Pflugers Arch 407:123–128.

85. McDonald TF, Pelzer S, Trautwein W, Pelzer DJ. 1994. Regulation and modulation of calcium channels in cardiac, skeletal, and smooth muscle cells. Physiol Rev 74:365–507.

86. Herzig S, Patil P, Neumann J, Staschen CM, Yue DT. 1993. Mechanisms of β-adrenergic stimulation of cardiac Ca^{2+} channels revealed by discrete-time Markov analysis of slow gating. Biophys J 65:1599–1612.

87. Yue DT, Herzig S, Marban E. 1990. β-adrenergic stimulation of calcium channels occurs by potentiation of high-activity gating modes. Proc Natl Acad Sci USA 87:753–757.

88. Reuter H, Kokubun S, Prodhom B. 1986. Properties and modulation of cardiac calcium channels. J Exp Biol 124:191–201.

89. Brown AM. 1993. Membrane-delimited cell signaling complexes: direction channel regulation by G proteins. J Membr Biol 131:93–104.

90. Catterall WA. 1991. Functional subunit structure of voltage-gated calcium channels. Science 253: 1499–1500.

91. Klockner U, Itagaki K, Bodi I, Schwartz A. 1992. Beta subunit expression is required for cAMP-dependent increase of cloned cardiac and vascular calcium current. Pflugers Arch 420:413–415.

92. Haase H, Karczewski P, Beckert R, Krause EG. 1993. Phosphorylation of the L-type calcium channel beta subunit in involved in beta-adrenergic signal transduction in canine myocardium. FEBS Lett 335:217–222.
93. Sculptoreanu A, Rotman E, Takahashi M, Scheuer T, Catterall WA. 1993. Voltage-dependent potentiation of the activity of cardiac L-type calcium channel alpha 1 subunits due to phosphorylation by cAMP-dependent protein kinase. Proc Natl Acad Sci USA 90:10135–10139.
94. Diebold RJ, Koch WJ, Ellinor PT, Wang JJ, Muthuchamy M, Wieczorek DF, Schwartz A. 1992. Mutually exclusive axon splicing of the cardiac calcium channel alpha 1 subunit gene generates developmentally regulated isoforms in the rat heart. Proc Natl Acad Sci USA 89:1497–1501.
95. Sperelakis N, Haddad GE. 1995. Developmental changes in membrane electrical properties of the heart. In: Sperelakis N, ed. Physiology and Pathophysiology of the Heart. Norwell, MA: Kluwer Academic Publishers, 669–700.
96. Chen FM, Yamamura HI, Roeske WR. 1979. Ontogeny of mammalian myocardial beta-adrenergic receptors. Eur J Pharmacol 58:255–264.
97. Chen FC, Yamamura HI, Roeske WR. 1982. Adenylate cyclase and beta adrenergic receptor development in the mouse heart. J Pharmacol Exp Ther 222:7–13.
98. Kojima M, Sperelakis N, Sada H. 1990. Ontogenesis of transmembrane signaling systems of control of cardiac Ca^{2+} channels. J Dev Physiol 14:181–219.
99. Haddox MK, Roeske WR, Russell DH. 1979. Independent expression of cardiac type I and II cyclic AMP-dependent protein kinase during murine embryogenesis and postnatal development. Biochim Biophys Acta 585:527–534.
100. Slotkin TA, Lau C, Seidler FJ. 1994. Beta-adrenergic receptor overexpression in the fetal rat: distribution, receptor subtypes, and coupling to adenylate cyclase activity via G-proteins. Toxicol Appl Pharmacol 129:223–234.
101. Yu SS, Lefkowitz RJ, Hausdorff WP. 1993. Beta-adrenergic receptor sequestration: a potential mechanism of receptor resensitization. J Biol Chem 268:337–341.
102. Ungerer M, Böhm M, Elce JS, Erdmann E, Lohse MJ. 1993. Altered expression of β-adrenergic receptor kinase and β₁-adrenergic receptors in the failing human heart. Circulation 87:454–463.
103. Ungerer M, Parruti G, Böhm M, Puzicha M, DeBlasi A, Erdmann E, Lohse MJ. 1994. Expression of β-arrestins and β-adrenergic receptor kinases in the failing human heart. Circ Res 74:206–213.
104. Gilbert EM, Olsen SL, Renlund DG, Bristow MR. 1993. Beta-adrenergic receptor regulation and left ventricular function in idiopathic dilated cardiomyopathy. Am J Cardiol 71:23C–29C.
105. Bristow MR, Feldman AM. 1992. Changes in the receptor-G protein-adenylyl cyclase system in heart failure from various types of heart muscle disease. Basic Res Cardiol 87 (Suppl 1):15–35.
106. Dhalla NS, Dixon IM, Suzuki S, Kaneko M, Kobayashi A, Beamish RE. 1992. Changes in adrenergic receptors during the development of heart failure. Mol Cell Biochem 114:91–95.
107. Pennica D, King KL, Shaw KJ, Luis E, Rullamas J, Luoh SM, Darbonne WC, Knutzon DS, Yen R, Chien KR. 1995. Expression cloning of cardiotrophin 1, a cytokine that induces cardiac myocyte hypertrophy. Proc Natl Acad Sci USA 92:1142–1146.
108. Chien KR, Knowlton KU, Zhu H, Chien S. 1991. Regulation of cardiac gene expression during myocardial growth and hypertrophy: molecular studies of an adaptive physiologic response. FASEB J 5:3037–3046.
109. Koch WJ, Ellinor PT, Schwartz A. 1990. cDNA cloning of a dihydropyridine-sensitive calcium channel from rat aorta. J Biol Chem 265:17786–17791.
110. Gaudin C, Ishikawa Y, Wight DC, Madhavi V, Nadal-Ginard B, Wagne T, Vatner DE, Homcy CJ. 1995. Overexpression of Gₛ alpha protein in hearts of transgenic mice. J Clin Invest 95:1676–1683.
111. Hoerter J, Mazet F, Vassort G. 1981. Perinatal growth of the rabbit cardiac cell: possible implication for the mechanism of relaxation. J Mol Cell Cardiol 13:725–740.
112. Nakanishi T, Jarmakani JM. 1984. Development changes in myocardial mechanical function and subcellular organelles. Am J Physiol 246:H615–H625.
113. Boucek RJ, Shelton ME, Artman M, Landon E. 1985. Myocellular calcium regulation by the sarcolemmal membrane in the adult and immature rabbit heart. Basic Res Cardiol 80:316–325.
114. Artman M, Graham TP, Boucek RJ. 1985. Effects of postnatal maturation on myocardial contractile response to calcium antagonists and changes in contraction frequency. J Cardiovasc Pharmacol 7:850 855.
115. Seguchi M, Harding JA, Jarmakani JM. 1986. Developmental change in the function of sarcoplasmic reticulum. J Mol Cell Cardiol 18:189–195.

116. Seguchi M, Jarmakani JM, George BL, Harding JA. 1986. Effects of calcium antagonists on mechanical function in the neonatal heart. Pediatr Res 20:838–842.
117. Klitzner T, Friedman WF. 1988. Excitation-contraction coupling in developing mammalian myocardium: evidence from voltage clamp studies. Pediatr Res 23:428–432.
118. Chin TK, Friedman WF, Klitzner TS. 1989. Developmental changes in cardiac myocyte Ca^{2+} regulation. Circ Res 67:574–579.
119. Jarmakani JM, Nakanishi T, George BL, Bers D. 1982. Effect of extracellular calcium on myocardial mechanical function in neonatal rabbit. Dev Pharmacol Ther 5:1–13.
120. Boucek RJ, Citak M, Graham TP, Artman M. 1987. Effects of postnatal maturation on postrest potentiation in isolated rabbit atria. Pediatr Res 22:524–530.
121. Wetzel GT, Chen FH, Klitzner TS. 1991. L- and T- type calcium channels in acutely isolated neonatal and adult cardiac myocytes. Pediatr Res 30:80–89.
122. Fleckenstein A. 1993. Calcium Antagonism in Heart and Smooth Muscle. J Willey and Sons, New York.
123. Ostadal B, Skovranek J, Kolar F, Janatova T, Krause EG, Ostadalova I. 1987. Calcium antagonist and the developing heart. Biomed Biochem Acta 46:S522–S526
124. Klitzner TS, Chen F, Raven RR, Wetzel GT, Friedman WF. 1991. Calcium current and tension generation in immature mammalian myocardium: effects of diltiazem. J Mol Cell Cardiol 23:807–815.
125. Dodd DA, Boucek RJ Jr. 1989. Altered calcium channel agonist effects in newborn rabbits. Pediatr Res 25:23A.
126. Sperelakis N. 1972. (Na^+-K^+)-ATP activity of embryonic chick heart and skeletal muscles as a function of age. Biochem Biophys Acta 266:230–237.
127. Hanson GL, Schilling WP, Michael LH. 1993. Sodium-potassium pump and sodium and calcium exchange in adult and neonatal canine cardiac sarcolemma. Am J Physiol 264:H320–H326.
128. Barry WH, Bridge JH. 1993. Intracellular calcium homeostasis in cardiac myocytes. Circulation 87:1806–1815.
129. Katz AM. 1992. Physiology of the Heart. New York: Raven Press.
130. Philipson KD, Nicoll DA. 1993. Molecular and kinetic aspects of sodium-calcium exchange. Int Rev Cytol 137C:199–227.
131. Artman M. 1992. Developmental changes in myocardial contractile response to inotropic agents. Cardiovasc Res 26:3–13.
132. George BL, Nakanshi T, Jamakarni JM. 1979. The effect of developmental changes in membrane permeability to Ca^{2+} on cardiac function. Pediatr Res 13:344–347.
133. Khatter JC, Agbanyo M, Navaratnam S, Hoeschen RJ. 1989. Mechanisms of developmental increase in the sensitivity to ouabain. Dev Pharmacol Ther 12:128–136.
134. Khatter JC, Navaratnam S, Hoeschen RJ. 1988. Protective effect of verapamil upon ouabain-induced arrhythmias. Pharmacology 38:380–389.
135. Goshima K, Wakabayashi S. 1981. Involvement of a Na^+, Ca^{2+} exchange system in the genesis of ouabain-induced arrhythmias of cultured myocardial cells. J Moll Cell Cardiol 13:489–509.
136. Chen F, Molline G, Killner TS, Philipson KD, Frank JS. 1995. Distribution of Na^+/Ca^{2+} exchange protein in developing rabbit myocytes. Am J Physiol 268:C1126–C1132.
137. Carafoli E. 1987. Intracellular calcium homeostasis. Annu Rev Biochem 56:395–433.
138. Nakanshi T, Jaymakani JM. 1981. Effect of extracellular sodium on mechanical function in the newborn rabbit. Dev Pharmacol Ther 2:188–200.
139. Boerth RC. 1975. Decreased sensitivity of newborn myocardium to the positive inotropic effects of ouabain. In: Morselli PL, Garattini S, Serenit F, eds. Basic and New Therapeutic Aspects of Perinatal Pharmacology. New York: Raven Press 191–199.
140. Lathrop DA, Varro A, Gaum WE, Kaplan S. 1989. Age related changes in electromechanical properties of canine ventricular muscle: effect of ouabain. J Cardiovasc Pharmacol 14:681–687.
141. Vornanen M. 1987. Effects of caffeine on the mechanical properties of developing rat heart ventricles. Comp Biochem Physiol 78C:239–334.
142. Hoerter J, Vassort G. 1982. Participation of the sarcolemma in the control of relaxation of the mammalian heart during perinatal development. In: Chazov E, Smirnov V, Dhalla NS, eds. Advances in Myocardiology. New York: Plenum Medical, 373–380.
143. Vetter R, Will H. 1986. Sarcolemmal Na-Ca exchange and sarcoplasmic reticulum calcium uptake in developing chick heart. J Mol Cell Cardiol 18:1267–1275.
144. Meno H, Jarmakani JM, Philipson KD. 1988. Sarcolemmal calcium kinetics in the neonatal heart. J Mol Cell Cardiol 20:585–591.

145. Binah O, Leagato MJ, Danilo P, Rosen MR. 1983. Developmental changes in the cardiac effect of amrinone in the dog. Circ Res 52:747–752.
146. Klitzner TS, Shapir Y, Ravin R, Friedman WF. 1990. The biphasic effect of amrinone on tension development in newborn mammalian myocardium. Pediatr Res 27:144–147.
147. Artman M, Kithas PA, Wike JS, Crump DB, Sarda SJ. 1989. Inotropic response to cyclic nucleotide phosphodiesterase inhibitors in immature and adult rabbit myocardium. J Cardiovasc Pharmacol 13:146–154.
148. Kithas PA, Artman M, Thompson WJ, Strada SJ. 1989. Subcellular distribution of high-affinity type IV cyclic AMP phosphodiesterase activities in rabbit ventricular myocardium: relation to post-natal maturation. J Mol Cell Cardiol 21:507–517.
149. Kithas PA, Artman M, Thompson WJ, Strada SJ. 1988. Subcellular distribution of high-affinity type IV cyclic AMP phosphodiesterase activity in rabbit ventricular myocardium: relation to the effects of cardiotonic drugs. Circ Res 62:782–789.
150. Ogawa S, Nakanshi T, Kamata K, Takao A. 1987. Effect on milirone on myocardial mechanical and cyclic AMP content in fetal rabbit. Pediatr Res 22:282–285.
151. Okuda H, Nakanshi T, Nakazawa M, Takao A. 1987. Effect of isoproterenol on myocardial mechanical function and cyclic AMP content in the fetal rabbit. J Mol Cell Cardiol 19:151–157.

B. Ostadal, M. Nagano and N.S. Dhalla (eds.).
CARDIAC DEVELOPMENT. Copyright © 2002.
Kluwer Academic Publishers. Boston.

INCREASED CONSUMPTION OF VITAMIN A IN THE HEART UNDER OXIDATIVE STRESS

PAWAN K. SINGAL, VINCE P. PALACE, MICHAEL F. HILL,
NEELAM KHAPER DINENDER KUMAR, and IGOR DANELISEN

Institute of Cardiovascular Sciences, St. Boniface General Hospital Research Center and Department of Physiology, Faculty of Medicine, University of Manitoba, Winnipeg, Canada

Summary. Epidemiological and clinical studies examining the relationship between vitamin A and cardiovascular disease have traditionally used plasma concentrations as the sole indicator of vitamin A status with conflicting results. Using radiolabelled vitamin A, we show that under increased oxidative stress conditions in the heart failure subsequent to myocardial infarction, the heart increased its utilization of vitamin A. Steady state concentrations of vitamin A in these hearts or in the plasma were not affected. In the absence of a continuous supply of retinol through the plasma, vitamin A levels decreased significantly in an *ex vivo* oxidatively stressed isolated perfused heart. *In vivo* vitamin A levels in the heart failure may have been maintained by an increase in the mobilization of retinol from the liver through an increase in the activity of the bile salt dependent-retinol ester hydrolase enzyme. It is suggested that monitoring of the plasma concentrations of vitamin A may not be the best approach for assessing the utilization of vitamin A.

Key words: Retinol, Retinol Ester Hydrolase, Heart Failure

INTRODUCTION

During the last two decades, researchers have been able to establish that the development and progression of several forms of heart disease involve the production of

Address for Correspondence: Dr. Pawan K. Singal
Address for all Authors: Institute of Cardiovascular Sciences, St. Boniface General Hospital Research Center, 351 Tache Ave., Room 3022, Winnipeg, Manitoba, Canada. Tel: (204) 235-3485; Fax: (204) 233-6723; e-mail: psingal@sbrc.umanitoba.ca

free radicals and a resulting condition known as oxidative stress. Oxidative stress arises when oxygen, which is normally reduced by the simultaneous addition of four electrons during the final stages of aerobic cellular energy production, is only partially reduced by the sequential addition of one electron at a time. Partially reduced forms of oxygen, or free radicals, are extremely reactive because of unpaired electrons in their structures. These can react with and initiate damage to cellular components including membrane lipids, proteins and DNA [1]. Using a variety of techniques, it has been shown that free radicals and the damage that they can initiate are important factors in the development of congestive heart failure after a myocardial infarction [2–5], atherosclerosis and coronary artery disease [6–8], diabetes related heart disease [9,10] and cardiotoxicity associated with some of the drugs used for cancer chemotherapy [11–13].

As the evidence for the involvement of free radicals in heart disease has accumulated, so too has the interest in therapeutic interventions aimed at reducing oxidative stress in the heart during these disease conditions. Antioxidant vitamins are particularly attractive therapeutic agents because they are inexpensive, readily available, and non-toxic over a wide dose range and for long exposures [14,15]. Already, several epidemiological, clinical and experimental studies have shown that increased intake of vitamin E provides protection against cardiovascular disease [16–19]. However, there is still a great deal of confusion regarding the beneficial effects of other antioxidant vitamins in cardiovascular disease.

While experimental evidence for the protective effects of dietary vitamin A and provitamin A compounds like β–carotene against cardiovascular disease are strong, results from epidemiological and clinical studies can best be described as contradictory [20]. These discrepancies may arise from methodological oversights in some of the existing studies. More specifically, studies which report no relationship between vitamin A and cardiovascular disease have often used plasma concentrations as the sole indicator of vitamin A status. The plasma appears to be a logical choice since the delivery of vitamin A to tissues, including the myocardium, is achieved via the plasma. However, a series of experiments presented here confirm that while the myocardium does increase its metabolism of vitamin A after an oxidative stress-inducing cardiovascular event, this increased metabolic demand is not reflected in its altered concentrations in the plasma, but rather in losses of vitamin A from visceral storage organs.

Myocardial infarction, oxidative stress and vitamin A utilization

A rapid occlusion of the coronary artery due to thrombosis superimposed on atherosclerotic plaque results in acute ischemia. The myocardial cells downstream of this blockage undergo necrosis to produce a myocardial infarction (MI). In 15 to 25% of MI survivors, a condition called congestive heart failure (CHF) [21] develops. CHF is characterized by a loss of contractile function and has been shown to closely correlate with an increase in oxidative stress as well as a depletion of endogenous antioxidants in the myocardium [2–5]. It is also well established that reperfusion of a previously ischemic tissue results in the production of free radicals and oxidative stress within the tissue [22,23]. Thus, both MI and ischemia-reperfusion injury are thought to generate oxidative stress in the surviving myocardium.

Using an *in vivo* surgical model of MI in rats [2], we examined whether vitamin A is consumed during the evolution of CHF subsequent to MI. Animals in the MI group had depressed cardiac function as indicated by an increase (341%) in left ventricular end diastolic pressure and a decrease (20%) in left ventricular systolic pressure. The animals were considered to be at a stage of moderate heart failure [2]. Animals at this stage of heart failure showed significant decrease (53%) in redox ratio (GSH:GSSG) which is inversely correlated with oxidative stress [22]. However, myocardial and plasma content of vitamin A in rats that had been subjected to MI was not different from control rats. Earlier, it has been reported that both vitamin A and its long chain fatty acid storage forms are depleted in the liver and kidney of rats with MI compared with the controls [16].

Mechanism of the delivery of vitamin A to the heart

It should be noted that vitamin A storage organs and an intricate system of intra- and extra-cellular binding proteins are responsible for tightly regulating the concentration of vitamin A in the plasma [20]. Therefore, a lack of change in the vitamin A level of the heart or plasma coupled with a drop in the storage organ concentrations allowed us to speculate that vitamin A was being mobilized from the storage organs for delivery to the oxidatively stressed heart after MI. In order to test this hypothesis, we examined the metabolism of a specific pool of vitamin A under post-MI and control conditions. In order to achieve this, radiolabelled ^{3}H-vitamin A bound to its plasma carrier protein was injected into the tail vein of control and MI animals. Surgery for myocardial infarction and sham controls was performed as previously described [2]. Nine weeks after the surgery, rats were anesthetized and a heparin rinsed catheter was inserted into the tail vein. 50 μL of ^{3}H-retinol suspended in plasma, prepared as described [24], was injected into each rat followed by 200 μL of physiological saline. The total amount of retinol injected was 0.0334 μg with an activity of 5 μCi. Previous work has shown that this amount of retinol contributes <1% to the total plasma pool of retinol [16,25]. Four days after the injection, plasma, liver, kidney and myocardium were analyzed for the labelled vitamin A. HPLC purified vitamin A fractions were collected and counted by liquid scintillation [16].

Although the steady state myocardial content of vitamin A (i.e. labeled +unlabeled) was not different between the two groups, a greater proportion of the total was ^{3}H-vitamin A in the myocardium of rats with MI compared with the controls. This confirmed that the remaining viable myocardium in the MI group had an elevated metabolism of vitamin A compared with the controls. Furthermore, the radiolabelled vitamin A was carried in the plasma, where ^{3}H-vitamin A was also proportionally higher (44%) in MI animals compared with controls. Finally, we observed decrease in concentrations of ^{3}H-vitamin A in both the kidney and liver which is consistent with the notion that the elevated proportion of labeled vitamin

A in the myocardium and plasma were achieved at the expense of storage organ concentrations [16]. It should be noted that other tissues, including adipose [26] and bone marrow [27] can also store significant amounts of vitamin A compounds, but their ability to mobilize these stores after MI remains to be investigated.

Evidence for increased myocardial consumption of vitamin A

The question of whether or not sustained levels of vitamin A in these oxidatively stressed hearts are really due to its constant supply, was also addressed. Vitamin A content in isolated perfused rat hearts was compared under conditions of normal perfusion as well as under oxidative stress imposed by global ischemia-reperfusion. Isolated perfused hearts were subjected to global ischemia (45 min) and reperfusion (15 min). Control hearts were perfused for an equivalent time (60 min). The isolated heart perfusion system as well as buffer used were the same as previously described [28]. Vitamin A content was significantly lower (30%, $p < 0.05$) in the myocardium of the ischemic-reperfused hearts ($0.081 \pm 0.002 \mu g/g$) compared with the continually perfused hearts ($0.105 \pm 0.010 \mu g/g$). This indicated that metabolism of the antioxidant vitamin A increased within the myocardium under oxidative stress. Clearly, vitamin A in the *in vivo* oxidatively stressed hearts after MI was not depleted because the *in situ* conditions likely allowed the plasma to deliver vitamin A to the myocardium.

Basis of in situ vitamin A mobilization

For mobilization of vitamin A from the storage organs to the plasma, retinyl esters, which are long chain fatty acid storage forms of vitamin A, must first be hydrolyzed before retinol can be made available to apo-retinol binding protein for export to the plasma. This hydrolysis is performed by enzymes, collectively termed as retinol ester hydrolases (REH) [27,29]. REH activity in the liver is of two types: bile salt dependent and bile salt independent. The former is localized in the cytosol and the latter in the microsomal fraction. Enzyme assays of the livers of rats in this study [30,31] revealed that the bile salt dependent activity was approximately 3 fold higher in the MI animals than in sham controls and may account for the loss of stored vitamin A from this storage organ. Indeed, ^{3}H-retinyl esters in the liver were significantly lower (55%) in the MI group. The bile salt independent-REH activity in the microsomal fraction revealed no significant difference between MI and control animals. While additional studies are required to determine the precise mechanism of the increase in bile salt dependent REH activity after MI, recently it has been shown that oxidative metabolites can increase the bile salt dependent ester hydrolase activity in human aortic endothelial cells [32].

The results of the present study clarify some of the confusion regarding the relationship between vitamin A and cardiovascular disease. Specifically, the analysis of plasma concentrations of vitamin A to ascertain links to cardiac conditions may be inappropriate, at least during the early stages of the evolution of heart failure. Instead, other storage pools are more likely to be depleted as they maintain the plasma concentrations during oxidative stress of the myocardial tissue. Furthermore, the mobilization of vitamin A from the liver appears to be facilitated by an increase in the enzyme system that hydrolyzes vitamin A esters. While visceral concentrations of vitamin A would be useful indicators of increased metabolism of vitamin A in cardiovascular disease patients, it is not practical to obtain samples of these tissues. Fortunately, methods have recently been developed which allow the study of overall vitamin A status without biopsy samples [33,34]. Constant consumption of vitamin A in oxidatively stressed sites may ultimately deplete these backup vitamin A stores during the late stages of heart failure where monitoring of vitamin A in the plasma may provide more relevant information. Thus, therapeutic interventions to reduce myocardial vitamin A depletion may reduce oxidative damage and modulate the pathogenesis of heart failure.

ACKNOWLEDGMENTS

Supported by the Canadian Institutes for Health Research (CIHR) Group Grant in Experimental Cardiology (PKS). Drs. Palace and Hill were postdoctoral fellows of the Manitoba Health Research Council and CIHR respectively. Ms. Khaper was a student research fellow of the Canadian Heart and Stroke Foundation. Igor Danelisen is a student fellow of the MHRC.

REFERENCES

1. Singal PK, Petkau A, Gerrard JM, Hrushovctz S, Foerster J. 1988. Free radicals in health and disease. Mol Cell Biochem 84:121–122.
2. Hill M, Singal PK. 1997. Right and left myocardial antioxidant responses during heart failure subsequent to myocardial infarction. Circulation 96:2414–2420.
3. Keith M, Geranmayegan A, Sole MJ, Kurian R, Robinson A, Omran AS, Jeejeebhoy KN. 1998. Increased oxidative stress in patients with congestive heart failure. J Am Coll Cardiol 31:1352–1356.
4. Khaper N, Singal PK. 1997. Effects of afterload-reducing drugs on pathogenesis of antioxidant changes and congestive hear failure in rats. J Am Coll Cardiol 29:856–861.
5. Singh RB, Niaz MA, Rastogi SS, Rastogi S. 1996. Usefulness of antioxidant vitamins in suspected acute myocardial infarction (the Indian experiment of infarct survival-3). Am J Cardiol 77:232–236.
6. Chakravarti RN, Kirshenbaum LA, Singal PK. 1991. Atherosclerosis: Its pathophysiology with special reference to lipid peroxidation. J Applied Cardiol 6:91–112.
7. McMurray J, McLay J, Chopra M, Bridges A, Belch JJF. 1990. Evidence for enhanced free radical activity in chronic congestive heart failure secondary to coronary artery disease. Am J Cardiol 65: 1261–1262.
8. Prasad K, Kalra J. 1993. Oxygen free radicals and hypercholesterolemic atherosclerosis: effect of vitamin E Am Heart J 125:958–973.
9. Collier A, Wilson R, Bradley H, Thomson JA, Small M. 1990. Free radical activity in type 2 diabetes. Diabetic Medicine 7:27–30.
10. Kaul N, Siveski-Iliskovic N, Hill M, Khaper N, Seneviratne C, Singal PK. 1996. Probucol treatment reverses antioxidant and functional deficit in diabetic cardiomyopathy. Mol Cell Biochem 160/161:283–288.
11. Singal PK, Iliskovic N, Li T, Kumar D. 1997. Adriamycin cardiomyopathy: pathophysiology and prevention. FASEB J 11:931–936.
12. Singal PK, Iliskovic N. 1998. Doxorubicin-induced cardiomyopathy. New Engl J Med 24:339(13): 900–905.
13. Siveski-Iliskovic N, Kaul N, Singal PK. 1994. Probucol promotes endogenous antioxidants and provides protection against adriamycin-induced cardiomyopathy in rats. Circulation 89:2829–2835.
14. Bendich A, Machlin LJ. 1988. Safety of oral intake of vitamin E Am J Clin Nutr 48:612–619.

15. Diplock AT. 1995. Safety of antioxidant vitamins and beta-carotene. Am J Clin Nutr 62(suppl): 1510S–1516S.
16. Palace VP, Hill MF, Farahmand F, Singal PK. 1999. Mobilization of antioxidant vitamin pools and hemodynamic function after myocardial infarction. Circulation 99(1):121–126.
17. Dhalla, AK, Hill MF, Singal PK. 1996. Role of oxidative stress in transition of hypertrophy to heart failure. J Am Coll Cardiol 28:506–514.
18. Rimm EB, Stampfer MJ, Ascherio A, Giovannucci E, Colditz GA, Willett WC. 1993. Vitamin E consumption and the risk of coronary heart disease in men. New Engl J Med 328:1450–1456.
19. Stampfer MJ, Hennekens CH, Manson JE, Colditz GA, Rosner B, Willett WC. 1993. Vitamin E consumption and the risk of coronary disease in women. New Engl J Med 328:1444–1449.
20. Palace VP, Khaper N, Qin Q, Singal PK. 1999. Antioxidant potentials of vitamin A and carotenoids and their relevance to heart disease. Free Rad Biol Med 26:746–761.
21. Francis GS, McDonald KM, Cohn JN. 1993. Neurohumoral activation in preclinical heart failure. Remodeling and the potential for intervention. Circulation 87(supplIV):90–96.
22. Ferrari R, Alfieri O, Curello S, Ceconi C, Cargoni A, Marzallo P, Pardini A, Caradonna E, Visioli O. 1990. Occurrence of oxidative stress during reperfusion of the human heart. Circulation 81:201–211.
23. Bolli R, Jeroudi MO, Patel BS, Aruoma OI, Halliwell B, Lai EK, McCay PB. 1989. Marked reduction of free radical generation and contractile dysfunction by antioxidant therap begun at the time of reperfusion. Evidence that myocardial "stunning" is a manifestation of reperfusion injury. Circ Res 65:607–622.
24. Palace VP, Klaverkamp JF, Baron CL, Brown SB. 1994. Metabolism of ^{3}H-retinol by lake trout (salvenius namacycush) pre-exposed to 3,3′,4′,5-pentachlorobiphenyl (PCB 126). Aquat Toxicol 39:332.
25. Green MH, Green JB, Berg T, Norum KR, Blumhoff R. 1993. Vitamin A metabolism in rat liver: a kinetic model. Am J Physiol 264:G509–521.
26. Parker RS. 1989. Carotenoids in human blood and tissues. J Nutr 119:101–104.
27. Harrison EH. 1993. Enzymes catalyzing the hydrolysis of retinyl esters. Biochim Biophys Acta 1170:99–108.
28. Khaper N, Rigatto C, Seniviratne C, Li T, Singal PK. 1997. Chronic treatment with propranolol induces antioxidant changes and protects against ischemia-reperfusion injury. J Mol Cell Cardiol 29:3335–3344.
29. Mata NL, Mata JR, Tsin ATC. 1996. Comparison of retinyl ester hydrolase activities in bovine liver and retinal pigment epithelium. J Lipid Res 37:1947–1952.
30. Cooper DA. 1990. Assay of liver retinyl ester hydrolase. Meth Enzymol 189:490–494.
31. Harrison EH, Gad MZ. 1989. Hydrolysis of retinyl palmitate by enzymes of rat pancreas and liver. Differentiation of bile salt-dependent and bile salt-independent, neutral retinyl ester hydrolases in rat liver. J Biol Chem 29:17142–17147.
32. Li F, Hui DY. 1989. Synthesis and secretion of the pancreatic-type carboxyl ester lipase by human endothelial cells. Biochem J 329:675–679.
33. Hammell DC, Franklin ST, Nonnecke BJ. 1998. Use of the relative dose response assay to determine vitamin A status of calves. FASEB 12:A520.
34. Tanumihardjo SA, Olson JA. 1998. Synthesis of ^{13}C$_4$- retinyl acetate and its use in an isotope dilution assay to assess vitamin A status. FASEB 12:A519.

INDEX